ahca

American Health Care Association

HOW TO BE A

NURSE
ASSISTANT

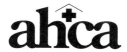

American Health Care Association

HOW TO BE A

NURSE ASSISTANT

*Career Training
in Long Term Care*

Margaret Casey, RN

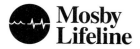
Mosby
Lifeline

St. Louis Baltimore Berlin Boston Carlsbad Chicago London Madrid
Naples New York Philadelphia Sydney Tokyo Toronto

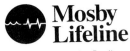
Mosby Lifeline

Dedicated to Publishing Excellence

Editor: Richard A. Weimer
Developmental Editor: Julie Scardiglia
Project Manager: Mark Spann
Production Editor: Amy Wastalu
Designer: David Zielinski
Manufacturing Supervisor: Betty Richmond

Printed in the United States of America.

Composition by Graphic World, Inc.
Color Separation by Color Dot, Inc.

Mosby-Year Book, Inc.
11830 Westline Industrial Drive
St. Louis, Missouri 63146

Library of Congress Cataloging-in-Publication Data

How to be a nurse assistant : career training in long term care /
    edited by Margaret Casey ; American Health Care Association,—1st
    ed.
        p.   cm.
      Includes bibliographical references and index.
      ISBN 0-8151-0133-3
      1. Long-term care of the sick. 2. Nursing. 3. Nurses' aides.
  I. Casey, Margaret. II. American Health Care Association.
    [DNLM: 1. Nurses' Aides—education. 2. Long-Term Care. WY 193
H847 1994]
RT120.L64H69 1994
610.73'06'98—dc20
DNLM/DLC   94-7574
for Library of Congress   CIP

95 96 97 98 99 / 9 8 7 6 5 4 3 2 1

"Well meant protectiveness gradually undermines any autonomy."
—Ellen Langer
Mindfulness

About the Author

Margaret Casey has been an enthusiastic and devoted educator of long term care professionals for more than 10 years. As a registered nurse and credentialed trainer, she has developed and implemented dozens of health care training programs for the American Red Cross. During the last 5 years, Ms. Casey's efforts have focused on training nurse assistants in long term care. Her work reflects her desire for quality long term care through the empowerment of nurse assistants. Ultimately, Ms. Casey's work has focused on care for residents with respect, dignity, and autonomy. The philosophy of *How to be a Nurse Assistant* balances nurse assistants' ability to provide the highest quality of care with the challenges of the environment.

CONTRIBUTING WRITERS

Many individuals contributed to the development of the written portion of this text. They are:

Kate Blumberg, PT
Physical Therapist
Contract Services
The Hillhaven Corporation
Lexington, Massachusetts
Chapters 8, 13, 20

Alyce Bosch, RN
Director of Nursing
Sunshine Terrace Foundation
Logan, Utah
Chapter 18

Carolyn Breeding, MS, RD, CN
Owner/Consultant
Dietary Consultants, Inc.
Richmond, Kentucky
Chapters 9, 16

Sherry Cruz, RN, MN, MBA
Rehabilitation Specialist
Intracorp
San Antonio, Texas
Chapters 2, 6, 21

Joan M. Dunbar, MBA, MSW
Coordinator of Commonwealth Restraint
   Minimization Project
Jewish Home and Hospital for the Aged
New York, New York
Chapter 19

Marguerite Jackson, RN, MS, CIC, FAAN
Administrative Director
Epidemiology Unit
University of California, San Diego
San Diego, California
Chapters 7, 23

Elizabeth H. Johnston, RN, BSN, C, MPA
Director of Nursing Service
Fir Lane Terrace Convalescent Center
Shelton, Washington
Chapter 12

Mary Lucero, BSH, NHA
President
Geriatric Resources, Inc.
Winter Park, Florida
Chapter 22

Kathleen M. Masucci, RN
Winthrop, Massachusetts
Chapters 14, 17

Raymond Miller, MSOSH
Director, Loss Prevention
Living Centers of America
Houston, Texas
Chapter 8

Patricia Montemerlo Siclari, RN, BA
Consultant
American Health Care Association
Pittsburgh, Pennsylvania
Chapter 5

Richard R. Neufeld, MD
Medical Director
Jewish Home and Hospital for the Aged
New York, New York
Chapter 19

PHOTOGRAPHER
Vincent Knaus
Springfield, Virginia

ILLUSTRATOR
Jack Pardue
Alexandria, Virginia

ACKNOWLEDGMENTS

The American Health Care Association would like to recognize the efforts of so many individuals dedicated to the quality of long-term care:

Margaret Casey for her tireless effort and creativity as author and codeveloper of this program and for her sensitivity and insight into the nurse assistant/resident relationship.

Patricia Montemerlo Siclari for her endless support and dedication as project manager and codeveloper. Also for her humor while keeping development on schedule, coordinating the writing staff, and managing the photography and illustration program.

Ellen Tishman of AHCA for bringing together the Casey-Siclari team and for her resourcefulness and availability.

Rob Watson and Deborah Ellsworth for their creativity and commitment to the project.

Linda Keegan of AHCA and Rick Weimer of Mosby for being progenitors of this project and visionary leaders.

Mosby Lifeline for lending its financial resources and for its commitment to long term health care education.

Julie Scardiglia of Mosby for her enthusiasm as coordinator of the editorial development and illustration program.

All contributing writers whose knowledge and experiences brought diversity and technical accuracy to this program.

Tom Lochhaas for his tireless editing and guidance and for being a team player.

Lisa Laing for her editing and word processing and for just being there.

Ruth Wiskind RN, MSN for her insight into instructing the psychosocial aspects of caregiving.

All reviewers whose comments further enhanced the quality and scope of this program.

Vincent Knaus for his ability to make the written word come alive through photography.

Jack Pardue for his creative illustrations.

Frank Siteman for his beautiful cover art.

A special thanks to the residents, staff and administration of the following nursing facilities for their willingness to open their doors, lend a caregiving hand and be the visual portion of this textbook.

Arcola Nursing and Rehabilitation Center
Wheaton, Maryland

Cardinal Sheehan Center Stella Maris
Towson, Maryland

Fernwood House
Bethesda, MD

Goodwin House
Alexandria, VA

Jefferson Hills Manor Inc.
Pleasant Hills, Pennsylvania

Lisner-Louise-Dickson-Hurt Home
Washington, D.C.

Mount Vernon Nursing Center
Alexandria, Virginia

Mt. Lebanon Manor Convalescent Center
Pittsburgh, Pennsylvania

Powhatan Nursing Home Inc.
Falls Church, Virginia

Woodbine Nursing Center
Alexandria, Virginia

South Hills Convalescent Center
Canonsburg, Pennsylvania

REVIEWERS

Dirk Anjewierden
Administrator
Alta Care Center
Salt Lake City, Utah

Sarah Greene Burger (Reviewer of Chapter 19)
Gerontological Nurse Consultant
National Citizens' Coalition for Nursing Home Reform
Washington, D.C.

Carla Carribino
Instructor
Christian City Convalescent Center
Union City, Georgia

Janet B. Chermak
Vice President of Professional Services
Hillhaven Corporation
Tacoma, Washington

Steven E. Chies
Administrator
North Cities Health Care
Coon Rapids, Minnesota

A.J. Dodson
Long-term Care Clinical Practice Specialist
American Health Care Association
Washington, D.C.

Judy Featherstone
Staff Development
North Cities Health Care
Coon Rapids, Minnesota

Marie Fisher
Director of Professional and Regulatory Services
Maine Health Care Association
Augusta, Maine

Janet George
Director of Quality Standards
Manor Healthcare Corporation
Silver Spring, Maryland

Tosia Hazlett
Manager, Clinical Training and Development
Manor Healthcare Corporation
Silver Spring, Maryland

Sandra Higgins
Owner/Administrator
Senior Citizen Nursing Home
Madisonville, Kentucky

Tammy Irwin
Consultant
Alta Care Center
Salt Lake City, Utah

Michael G. Maistros
Administrator
Bell Nursing Home
Belmont, Ohio

Cindy McClintock
Director of Nursing
North Cities Health Care
Coon Rapids, Minnesota

Linda McDaniels
Consultant
Senior Citizen Nursing Home
Madisonville, Kentucky

Mary Mitchell
Vice President of Resident Services
Health Facilities Management
Sikeston, Missouri

Donna Morgan
Social Services Director
North Cities Health Care
Coon Rapids, Minnesota

Jonathan Musher
Medical Director
Bethesda Rehabilitation and Nursing Center
Chevy Chase, Maryland

Barbara Perticarini
Director of Nursing
Bell Nursing Home
Belmont, Ohio

Ronald G. Thurston
Executive Vice President
Maine Health Care Association
Augusta, Maine

Elllen Tishman
Director, Professional Development
American Health Care Association
Washington, D.C.

Fred Watson
President
Georgia Health Care Association
Decatur, Georgia

CONTENTS

WELCOME

Dear Student

Welcome to the American Health Care Association's *How to be a Nurse Assistant Career Training in Long Term Care*. This program consists of three components: a student textbook, a workbook, and an instructor's manual. This program has been specially designed for work in long term care and meets the 75-hour federal requirement for nurse assistant training. You will learn through textbook content, written take-home exercises, and various classroom and clinical experiences directed by your instructor. This program will prepare you for your state's nurse assistant competency and evaluation text.

The textbook has 25 chapters. In chapters 1-9, you will be introduced to general information and caregiving concepts. In this section you will develop a basic understanding of residents, long-term care and your role. In chapters 10-18 information will be bridged to practical caregiving themes and technical skills. In chapters 19-24 concepts and approaches from the earlier sections will be applied to residents requiring advanced care. Chapter 25 combines the program's themes with time management, prioritization, and methods to keep motivated so that you are ready to begin your first day on the job.

In this program you will learn how to balance the art of caregiving with the science of nursing. That is, you will learn not only the tasks (such as eating, bathing and dressing to name a few) involved in caring for residents, but you will also learn the importance of maintaining each resident's dignity and individuality as you assist them with various tasks. It is our goal that after you are trained with *How to be a Nurse Assistant: Career Training in Long Term Care,* you will have the necessary skills to begin your career as a nurse assistant.

The content of this program is based on the author's philosophy of "mindful" caregiving, derived from the writings of Ellen Langer in her book <u>*Mindfulness*</u>. With this program, you will learn how to be a mindful caregiver. With a mindful attitude, resident's activities of daily living will not become routine but will be growing experiences where resident autonomy and individuality are encouraged. By following the themes of caregiving (communication, autonomy, respect, safety, infection control, observation, and time management) in this program you will have a positive influence on those residents in your care.

Best wishes for a successful career!

Introduction to Long Term Care

I f you ask 10 people what makes life worth living, you will get 10 different answers. One may say, "Life is worth living when I am with my family," while another might say being able to travel makes it all worthwhile. Although the dictionary defines living as the condition of being alive, to each person that means something different. You may define living and what makes life worth living differently from a resident of a long term care facility. You may share some common words or ideas, but what holds true for one person may not be true for another.

As a nurse assistant, you need to understand and respect how residents define living. What a resident feels makes life worth living does not change when he or she enters a long term care facility. This textbook's focus is on how you can help keep life worth living for residents in a long term care facility, but first you must understand what a long term care facility is.

This chapter focuses on long term care facilities. You will learn why people enter long term care and what services they receive. You will learn about the other members of the health care team and one way services are managed.

WHAT IS LONG TERM CARE?

Long term care is a part of our health care system. This system includes many different types of facilities, such as hospitals, home health agencies, clinics, mental health centers, hospices, and alcohol/drug addiction facilities. Long term care facilities are becoming an even more important part of the whole system because of the increasing elderly population in this country, a growing study of aging (gerontology), and the need for different ways to provide care due to the growing costs of health care. More nurse assistants than ever now work in long term care.

A long term care facility is sometimes called a nursing facility, nursing home, convalescent home, assisted living center, rehabilitation center, or residential care facility (Fig. 1-1 and Fig. 1-2). It may be a separate building, a unit in a hospital, or a converted home that provides special services to people with special needs, such as nursing services that cannot or should not be given in the person's home. The person usually needs the services for *long term*. Some residents will receive care for the rest of their lives. Others may live in a long term care facility for a long time even though care focuses on the person's eventual return home.

Most facilities have residents with different needs. Special units or wings may give specific types of care. Other specialty facilities offer specific types of care for certain populations of residents, such as the following:

▶ **Alzheimer's Disease Unit/Facility** provides care primarily for residents with a diagnosis of Alzheimer's disease, which causes memory loss. Residents often wander, so safety is a major consideration. These facilities are structured with the wandering, forgetful resident in mind.

▶ **Pediatrics Unit/Facility** provides care for children, often with severe disabilities, from birth to 22 years of age.

▶ **Traumatic Head Injury Unit/Facility** provides care for people, often young adults, with traumatic head injuries, focusing on rehabilitation.

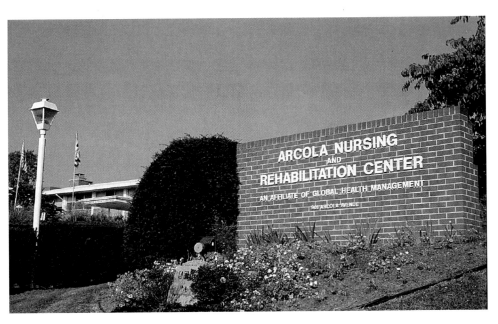

Fig. 1-1. Arcola Nursing and Rehabilitation Center.

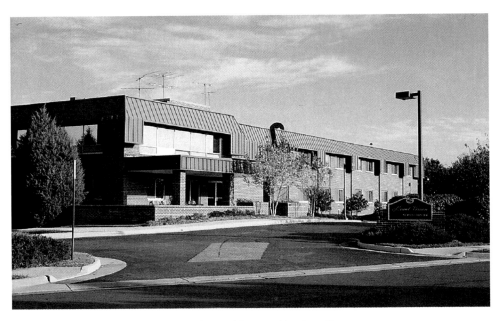

Fig. 1-2. Mount Vernon Nursing Center.

▶ **Rehabilitation Unit/Facility's** primary goal is restoring residents to their optimal level of functioning. People usually come directly from hospitals for a set period.

▶ **Subacute Unit/Facility** provides care to residents needing high levels of nursing care, such as intravenous therapy, respiratory, cardiac, or wound management.

▶ **AIDS Unit/Facility** provides care for residents with the diseases that accompany HIV infection and Acquired Immune Deficiency Syndrome (AIDS).

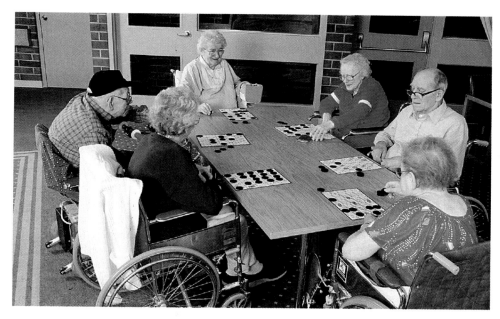

Fig. 1-3. Some residents enjoy establishing friendships with others at the facility.

WHY ARE PEOPLE ADMITTED TO LONG TERM CARE FACILITIES?

Each resident in a facility is a special individual with a long and unique history. The only thing that residents have in common is that they live in a long term care facility.

Some residents choose to live in a long term care facility because they want:

- Assistance with activities of daily living: meals, walking, dressing, bathing
- Security: knowing someone is just a call away if they fall, get sick, or just want to talk
- Friendships: being around other people with similar interests, concerns, and problems (Fig. 1-3)
- Independence: not having to depend on their family

Some people think that residents are "dumped" into facilities by families who no longer care for them. This is not true for most residents. Most residents are there because they need the kind of care given in a long term care facility. The following are true of many but not necessarily all residents:

- There are more women than men, mostly because women live longer than men. (However, in some special facilities, such as veteran's facilities, residents are mostly men.)
- They may have many health problems and can no longer care for themselves.
- They can no longer be cared for by their families or have no family.
- The average age is 84. Even though most residents are elderly, some are younger.
- Short-term residents may need 24-hour care for a health problem but are not sick enough for a hospital (Fig. 1-4).

Residents who have families usually enter a facility only when the family can no longer care for them, either because of other family responsibilities or because the problems of a resident are more than they can manage.

The reasons a resident lives in a long term care facility can change. For example, a resident may come to a facility for minimal nursing support but then become ill, go to the hospital, and return needing rehabilitation services. But the goal of long

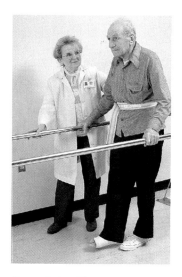

Fig. 1-4. Short-term residents, like those receiving physical rehabilitation, may need special care but are not sick enough for a hospital.

term care is always the same: to maintain or restore each resident's level of optimal functioning, to help all residents achieve their best.

In long term care facilities, residents receive one or more of the following types of care:

> **Rehabilitation:** Residents who need rehabilitation often stay for several weeks to several months. They may have had an illness or injury and need assistance to get back to their previous level of abilities before going home.

> **High Level Nursing Care:** This is care for residents needing subacute care involving both nursing and rehabilitation services. This care involves a team approach by many health professionals.

> **Continuous Supportive Care:** Most residents need ongoing assistance and support with basic needs such as eating, bathing, and movement. They also need basic health care, involving giving medications, monitoring their vital signs, and counseling. This care may include restorative care also. The long term care facility is their home, and you may become like family to them.

> **Respite Care:** Individuals may come to a facility for respite (temporary) care when family members who are the primary caregivers need a break or are temporarily away from home.

> **Hospice Care:** Hospice care is special care given to individuals who are dying. Not all long term care facilities have a hospice. A hospice is usually a special unit that is very home-like. Visitors may come anytime, meals can be prepared on the unit, and every effort is made to ensure each resident's comfort.

Some residents are active and independent, while others require more assistance. The units in facilities are often organized around how much care residents need. The level of care determines how a unit is staffed, including numbers of nurses and nurse assistants. Residents are often very involved in their care and help staff develop their care plans.

WHAT SERVICES ARE PROVIDED IN LONG TERM CARE?

The services residents receive depend on their individual needs. When they are admitted to the facility, their needs are assessed and a care plan is developed. Facilities operate under government rules and regulations. Because most facilities receive government Medicare and Medicaid funds, they must follow these regulations to receive reimbursement.

These rules and regulations are the minimum requirements in a long term facility. They help the facility clearly state service requirements and define staffing needs, and help residents know what to expect when they move into a facility. These regulations state the rights of all persons living in long term care facilities. They outline how a facility must determine a resident's level of care and work with each new resident to develop a plan of care. A facility must provide services all residents need to maintain at least their level of ability at the time of admission. For example, if a person enters a facility walking with a cane, every attempt must be made to help that person keep walking with a cane. If the person develops no other physical problems, he or she should not have to use a wheelchair or be confined to bed. Also, residents must be stimulated and motivated to stay alert. All staff must be aware of each resident's level of ability and work toward maintaining or improving that level (Fig. 1-5).

The Federal Rules and Regulations state that a long term care facility must provide the following services:

> **Nursing Services:** These services range from physical care, such as bathing, to restorative care, to psychosocial care, such as support at the time of death. They focus on all areas of health care, including health promotion, independence, and health maintenance.

> **Dietary Services:** Each resident receives a nourishing, well-balanced diet that meets his or her daily nutritional and special dietary needs. Food choices are based on each resident's preferences, always considering taste.

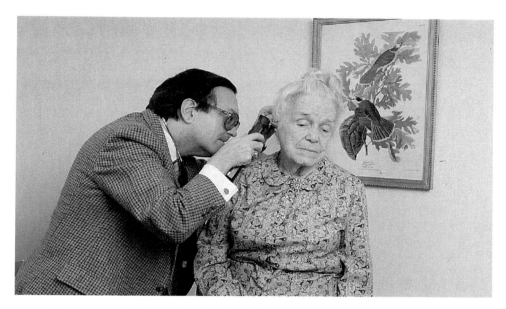

Fig. 1-5. Services provided by facilities require that staff develop a plan of care for each resident and work to maintain the resident's level of ability.

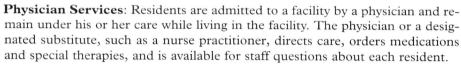
Physician Services: Residents are admitted to a facility by a physician and remain under his or her care while living in the facility. The physician or a designated substitute, such as a nurse practitioner, directs care, orders medications and special therapies, and is available for staff questions about each resident.

Specialized Rehabilitative Services: Physical therapy, speech-language pathology, occupational therapy, recreational therapy and activities, and health rehabilitative services for mental illness and mental retardation are available either on site or through local resources such as hospitals or health centers.

Dental Services: Facility staff assist residents in routine dental care. Emergency dental services are also available.

Pharmacy Services: The pharmacy provides routine and emergency drugs to residents.

Administrative Services: This department manages resources and helps all other departments run smoothly.

Social Services: This department coordinates admissions, discharges, and transfers of all residents, and provides financial guidance to residents and their families.

A facility is also required to have infection control and quality assurance programs, and recreational therapy and activities to encourage residents to stay active. The facility must protect the health and safety of residents, staff, and visitors. The state licensing body surveys all facilities every year to ensure that they comply with all rules and regulations.

The federal rules and regulations are a framework for facilities to make their own operations plans. These rules ensure that every resident receives the same high quality of care, regardless of how they pay for these services and whether they are able to request these services themselves.

WHO PROVIDES CARE IN A LONG TERM CARE FACILITY?

An interdisciplinary team cares for residents in long term care facilities. This means that staff from every department are directly or indirectly involved in each resident's care.

Each person is a member of the team. As in sports, effective team players respect each other and work together well. This is also important in the facility. As a nurse assistant, you will come in contact with people from every service. This may happen casually in the hallway and in more formal team meetings. The team approach helps give residents the highest quality care because information is shared, care is coordinated, and a comprehensive care plan is developed with each resident for his or her own needs. Following are all the team members and their general responsibilities:

- Each **resident** is always the most important person on the team. Each resident is the primary customer purchasing the service. All efforts must be made to meet individual needs and to maintain quality of life.
- A **resident's family** supports a resident in decisions about care and provides valuable information to the staff. If a resident is no longer able to make decisions about care, the family usually assumes the role (Fig. 1-6).
- **Nursing staff** are the largest staff in the facility and assist residents with the activities of daily living, personal hygiene, and monitoring and promoting health. Included are registered and licensed nurses and nurse assistants.
- **Physical therapists** work with the muscle groups to help residents maintain and increase their physical abilities, such as walking using assistive devices.
- **Occupational therapists** work with fine motor skills to help residents keep using their hands and arms for activities.
- **Speech therapists** work with residents who have difficulty with speech.
- **Physicians** are responsible for each resident's health and the treatment of illness and disease.
- **Social workers** counsel residents and families and arrange services such as Medicaid applications or home care services for residents who are discharged.
- **The activities coordinator** plans and carries out activities, such as shopping, going to plays or other outside events, and organizes games and discussion groups (Fig. 1-7).
- **The dietician or food supervisor** plans and prepares meals, assesses a resident's likes and dislikes, and ensures proper nutrition.
- **The spiritual counselor** provides spiritual guidance, coordinates religious services, and assists family members with counseling.

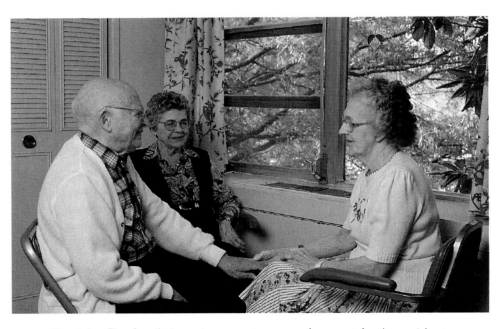

Fig. 1-6. The family is an important source of support for the resident.

▶ **The administrator** manages the entire facility.

Other important people provide additional functions in the facility. These people work in these departments:

▶ **Building maintenance:** Maintains the physical structure, including the grounds of the facility.

▶ **Housekeeping:** Keeps the facility clean at all times.

▶ **Personnel:** Hires all staff in the facility.

▶ **Bookkeeping:** Provides all accounting, payroll, purchasing.

▶ **Laundry:** Cleans and maintains all the linen and residents' clothing in the facility.

Each team member provides a special skill or knowledge. Together, residents and their families guide the team members' plan of care. For example, a person with a fractured hip is referred by his or her **physician** to the facility for rehabilitation services. The **family** and **resident** are met by the facility's **social service department** at the hospital. The referral is reviewed by the **social worker, physical therapist,** and **registered nurse.** The resident, family, physician, and other team members together make a plan for rehabilitation and discharge. Rehabilitation services are ordered by the physician and recommended by the **physical therapist,** and implemented by the **rehabilitation and nursing departments,** which includes you, and followed through on discharge by the **social worker.** All the departments work together to accomplish each resident's goals.

As a member of the team, you play a very important part. In fact, you will spend more time with each resident than anyone else. You will learn information and develop relationships that no other team member can match. You will be in a position to assist each resident to make life worth living in long term care. At this point you must be wondering how all these people and the care they provide are managed.

HOW DOES CARE GET MANAGED?

Working in a long term care facility is an important and demanding job. All the services and different people who work and live there add up to a busy and fast-paced environment.

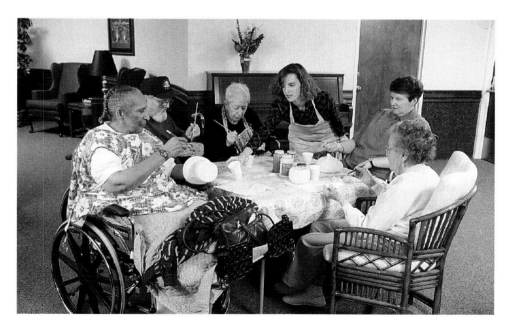

Fig. 1-7.   The activities coordinator may plan a project such as ceramics to give residents an opportunity to create.

Providing quality is everybody's job. Employees must do their very best work and work as a team to accomplish the goals set by each resident, resident's family, and staff (Fig. 1-8). This approach is called Total Quality Management (TQM). TQM is a way of thinking about your job and the work you do. It includes the following components:

▸ **Customer focus:** The key to quality is thinking of everyone as a customer and identifying how to meet or exceed their needs and expectations. Remember the customer is the person receiving, paying for, or requesting service. Instead of thinking of everybody you work with and work for as bosses or co-workers or family members, think of each as a customer. To see the importance of this, think about a bad experience you had as a customer. Maybe you had a bad experience grocery shopping. Maybe the items you were looking for were not available or not shelved where you expected, the selection of items was not good, and when you got to the checkout line, the cashier did not know the prices for the items you wanted to buy and the person bagging the items was sloppy. When you got home you found your eggs were broken! As a customer, you would be unhappy and dissatisfied. As a nurse assistant, you provide a valuable service to each resident, your customer. Remind yourself of what it feels like to receive poor customer service, and think of what kind of service makes you happy and satisfied. Now translate that type of service and approach to what you do as a nurse assistant. Treating everyone you come in contact with as a customer helps you treat them well and makes them more satisfied.

▸ **Process improvement:** A long term care facility is a busy, complicated place. If you break down each task into steps, you can see how complicated each actually is. These individual steps are the process, and there are millions of processes going on in the facility each day. As a nurse assistant, you can begin to look at those processes to see if there is a new or better way to accomplish the same task. If you suggest to your supervisor a better way to do something, it may save everybody time and effort and make the "customer" happier and more satisfied.

▸ **Measurement:** Quality can be measured. The TQM approach means that you learn about what your customer expects and how well you are meeting those ex-

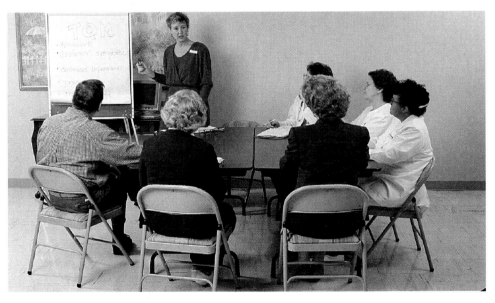

Fig. 1-8. Total Quality Management emphasizes working as a team to help employees provide quality care for residents.

pectations. This might mean that the facility you work in conducts a resident survey to identify how satisfied all residents are. It may mean that you collect information about a particular process — for example, how often residents get to their activities on time, or how long each doctor's visit lasts — so that you can determine how to improve the service you are offering.

▶ **Cross function:** Another key to TQM is a meeting of all the people with overlapping jobs to discuss how to improve processes. When everyone whose work overlaps gets together to discuss how the work gets done and how to make things easier and better, chances are your work will become easier and the customer will be more satisfied. For example, think about how many different people are involved in providing meals to each resident. A doctor orders a therapeutic diet, a nurse receives the order and documents and communicates it to the dietician, the dietician reviews the diet and establishes a meal plan and menu for this resident, the cook prepares the food as ordered, the dietary aides apportion the food and prepare and distribute the trays, and as a nurse assistant, you assist residents with eating their meals. All these people involved in the process can then discuss whether it meets the expectations of your co-workers, each resident, and other customers. This is an example of cross function.

▶ **Employee teamwork:** The TQM approach means that if the people who actually do the job are asked how to do it better, the processes can be improved and the facility will run more smoothly. As the expert in your own job, you need to offer advice and suggestions about how to meet and exceed your customer's needs.

▶ **Continuous improvement:** Enhanced quality does not happen overnight. Making each customer happy requires time and effort. Because your customers' expectations may change, you will constantly look for new ways to meet them. Success does not happen overnight, but you will see results if you are dedicated to quality.

These are the building blocks of the TQM approach. It may seem complicated at first, but this is really just a different way to look at your job, the people you work with, and the people you work for. How does this translate to your job?

1. Think about your job as having two job descriptions. The first job description is the one you are given when you come to work. It lays out all of your responsibilities and tasks for each day. The second job description has a single task. It reads, "Identify, share, collaborate, and explore ways to make your job better, more efficient, and more sensitive to the customers you serve."

2. Treat residents, residents' families, co-workers, guests, and visitors as customers. Identify what makes them satisfied and rate EVERY interaction with EACH customer as if it were your only opportunity to make him or her satisfied.

3. Work with other staff, residents, family members, and anyone you come in contact with as a customer. Think to yourself, "Do I know what my customer expects from me?" "Have I done all that I can to meet their expectations?" "What can I suggest ensure the customers are satisfied?"

4. Strive to do the best job you can and push yourself each day. Yours is an important and demanding job, critical for the exceptional care residents receive. By considering the components of quality, you will be more involved in working with residents and co-workers and improving the level of care.

IN THIS CHAPTER YOU LEARNED TO:

▶ define what makes life worth living

▶ describe a long term care facility

▶ give two reasons why people are admitted to long term care

▶ list the types of care offered in long term care facilities

▶ list and define the role of the members of the interdisciplinary health care team

▶ name all the services offered in a long term care facility

▶ explain total quality management

UNDERSTANDING EACH RESIDENT

Think about the things you consider important in your life, like being loved, looking your best, and deciding where you live and with whom you spend time. Remember significant events that have helped make you who you are, such as your parents praising you. You remember emotional highs, such as graduation from high school, birth of a child, or getting a job you really wanted, when you felt proud of what you had accomplished. Remember also the times of great sadness, such as the death of a loved one or the loss of a job or a home.

Now think about the people with whom you work: residents, other staff, families. Imagine how they have had similar experiences. Think about how everyone has to deal with good and bad experiences throughout their lives. Part of what makes these experiences positive or negative involves whether one's needs are met. All human beings have the same basic needs to keep their physical body safe and functioning properly and to nourish the social, spiritual, and sexual aspects of their personalities. Depending on one's own life experiences, we each have developed our own way to meet these needs. We all have the same needs, but how we experience or meet these needs is different. Your role as a nurse assistant includes helping to identify and meet each resident's needs while he or she is in your facility.

This chapter discusses meeting residents' needs and how people have to cope with changes in different stages in life. The psychological changes of aging are included, along with suggestions for helping residents adjust to these changes.

Understanding each resident also involves understanding his or her legal rights, related to how care is given in long term facilities. You must become familiar with these rights because you are accountable for protecting each resident's rights.

BASIC HUMAN NEEDS

A need is something you find necessary or desirable for life and well-being. All human beings have similar physical, social, sexual, and spiritual needs. The psychologist Abraham Maslow described basic needs in a hierarchy (Fig 2-1). This means that there is a natural order of priorities for how you meet needs.

1. *Physical needs* are things one needs to stay alive, such as oxygen and food. These needs must be met before one can focus on the next level of needs.
2. *Security needs* are the second level, involving both physical safety, such as a fear of bodily harm, and psychological safety, such as a feeling of security. This hierarchy means, for example, that if you were starving, you may risk your life to obtain food, but when your need for food is met, you will be more aware of safety and behave more cautiously to protect yourself from danger.
3. *Social needs* involve the approval and acceptance of others. Most people, once comfortable and safe in their surroundings, need to feel involved with others through friendships and group activities.
4. *Status needs* become important after one's social needs are met. Status involves recognition and respect from others. All people need to be treated with respect.
5. *Self-fulfillment needs* are the highest level. Self-fulfillment is the feeling of contributing and achieving goals, feeling satisfaction. Not everyone reaches this level, and few people function at this level all the time. Yet it is important to most people to make a contribution and to feel that they have achieved something in their lives.

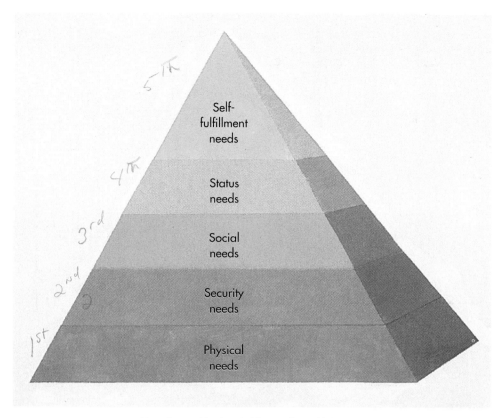

Fig. 2-1. Maslow's Hierarchy of Needs.

The following sections describe these different human needs as they relate to residents in long term care facilities, and your role in helping residents meet these needs.

Physical Needs

Physical needs are those things necessary for survival, such as food, water, oxygen, rest, and movement. Meeting one's own physical needs independently is important to everyone. Healthy people assume that they will get out of bed on their own, prepare their own meals, and take care of their own personal hygiene. As we grow older, however, physical changes may make us depend on others for help in meeting physical needs (Fig. 2-2). Have you as an adult ever had to depend on someone else to take care of you? It may seem pleasant for a while, but not being able to take care of yourself over a long time is frustrating and often leads to feelings of worthlessness and depression.

When you help each resident meet his or her physical needs, such as eating, turning over in bed, and bathing, do it in a way that helps him or her be as independent as possible. Offer help as needed, but avoid taking over tasks residents can accomplish for themselves. For example, you may need to open a milk carton for a resident and insert a straw, but let him or her hold the carton or glass while drinking. When turning or getting out of bed, a resident may move slowly but still can make the move, given time and support. Be patient. Do not do something for residents simply because you think it "takes too long" for them to do it themselves. Remember, it is easy to reduce independence by simply doing everything for them. This will over time increase their dependence and reduce their sense of self-worth.

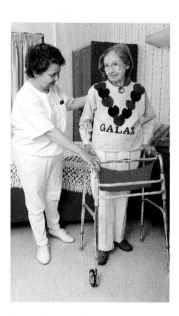

Fig. 2-2. Being able to provide for one's own physical needs is important; however, as we grow older physical changes may require others to help us meet those needs.

Safety Needs

Infants and children depend on others to keep them physically safe. Children are very vulnerable to physical and emotional abuse and neglect because they depend on others to meet their needs. Society tries to protect children through laws and agencies that protect children from abuse and neglect. As we become adults, we assume responsibility for ourselves, but laws still help protect our rights. As we grow older, the physical senses we need to protect ourselves—sight, hearing, touch—may diminish, causing us to become less independent, and we again become vulnerable to injury and abuse. We may have to depend on others to help us stay safe, which is often the reason elderly people become residents of long term facilities (Fig. 2-3).

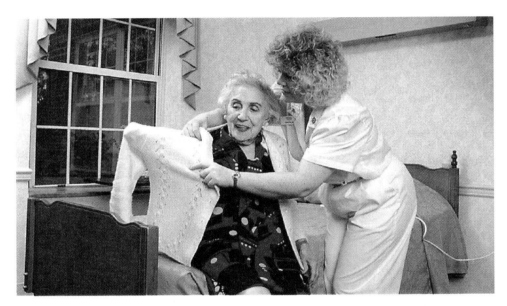

Fig. 2-3. When people are no longer physically able to protect themselves, long term care facilities can provide a safe and secure environment.

A resident may move into the facility only after a long struggle to stay independent. For example, an accident or fall may result from diminished eyesight or difficulty maintaining balance. After such an accident, family members fear for the person's safety and persuade him or her to move into the facility. This resident may have a serious medical problem that caused or resulted from the accident, but he or she may still have a desire to be fiercely independent. You may have to balance your concern for a resident's safety with the need for independence. Discuss safety with the person and work together to develop a plan that gives as much freedom as possible.

Social Needs

Social needs include interaction with others, recognition, and a feeling of belonging. Many people derive their personal identity from groups such as family, church, job. By interacting with others, we have a better sense of who we are. How we feel about ourselves depends much on how others react to us. When you wear a new outfit or a new hairstyle, how do you feel if family and friends do not notice? When you do a job well, think of the difference it makes whether someone else notices.

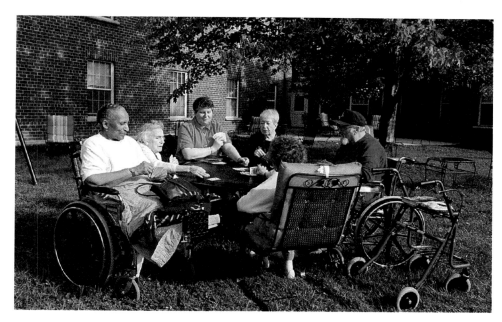

Fig. 2-4. Special activities can help residents fulfill their need for social interaction.

Residents have the same needs for interaction and recognition. A resident who has been removed from his or her usual support group needs your support for weeks and perhaps months after admission. A resident may need to establish new relationships, but may be reluctant to take the first step. Think about what it was like for you when you first came to a new school or job, or when you attended your first training class. Most people approach new situations cautiously, but everyone has his or her own way of dealing with new situations. You may go up to someone, introduce yourself, and start talking with the other person, while someone else may wait before comfortably joining in. Most people seek some common ground for relating to others, but many have trouble taking the first step in new situations.

Special activities in the facility help residents get together and start to know each other (Fig. 2-4). You can help bring residents together informally, such as at meals and while relaxing in common areas. You can bring together residents with similar interests, or you may help them attend community events.

Status Needs

Status needs involve recognition and respect from others. Being rewarded for what you do is important at this level of need. Recognition can take many forms: verbal praise, a positive nod, a letter of acknowledgement. Have you ever found yourself desperately needing someone's approval? As a child you looked to your parents for approval. As you grow older and have more life experiences, more people influence your need for recognition. School teachers, trainers, peers, bosses, co-workers, and spouses are just a few who influence recognition. Each person fulfills your need for recognition in very different ways, and the need for recognition from each can have different meaning.

As you begin to care for residents, you enter a resident's circle of people that influence his or her need for status. Consider recognition and respect of each resident in each caregiving activity. You can incorporate this consideration by simply calling each resident by his or her proper name, always asking permission, explaining care, knocking on a resident's door and waiting for permission to enter his or her room, respecting and acknowledging a resident's belongings, and recognizing achievements a resident has reached. Encouraging residents to get fully dressed and to always use their personal belongings will also assist in maintaining their status.

Self-fulfillment Needs

Self-fulfillment involves achievement, independence, and being all you can be. This is the highest level people can reach. Think of Maslow's hierarchy of needs as a ladder. To reach the top, you must have climbed past all prior needs. You will go up and down the ladder of needs based on what is going on in your life. The need to reach self-fulfillment is a lot like climbing the ladder; you have a goal, you put a plan in place to reach it, you take a few steps forward and a few steps backwards, but eventually if you keep focused you reach the top.

Asking your residents what is important will help you understand where they are in the need ladder and how you can assist each resident to reach his or her own goals. Encouraging residents to work at their independence is your primary focus. Remember that any achievement can mean self-fulfillment at different times. For example, a resident who has had a recent stroke may feel that being able to walk again would be a great achievement. This resident may focus all his or her energy on that goal. Once it is achieved, his or her energy will shift to a new level. You can encourage residents to set new goals and new achievements to assist them in being the best they can.

Sexual Needs

The need for sexual expression is both a physical and a social need. Sexual needs involve warm, loving, caring feelings shared between people. Sexuality may also involve feeling masculine or feminine. Sexual needs are not limited to sexual acts such as kissing, intercourse, or masturbation. Sexual needs are also met through close physical contact with another. Our culture often views sexuality as something for the young and ignores the needs of the elderly. Many people find this a difficult topic to discuss. But people do not lose their need for close physical contact or interest in sex just because they have passed age 50—or any later age (Fig. 2-5). Studies of healthy adults show that most seniors are sexually active or interested in having sex into their 80's and 90's. However, our society often treats older people as though they are not supposed to have sexual needs and feelings. Many seniors tend to accept society's views and feel guilty about their feelings or give up opportunities for meaningful sexual experiences.

The physical changes of aging require some change in sexual activity. Men may take longer to develop an erection and may have difficulty maintaining it. Women often experience vaginal dryness, which if not treated can lead to painful intercourse. However, older residents can compensate for these changes if they know how. Chronic illness and physical decline may make sexual expression uncomfortable or even unsafe without modifications.

A resident's more limited privacy often interferes with the expression of sexual feelings. Most residents have roommates, so time alone with a spouse or intimate friend is hard to arrange. You can help by planning alternate activities for the roommate during such visits. Let other staff know that they are not to enter the room until the resident or spouse requests. Frail and very ill residents may have difficulty balancing sexual expression with their needs for safety and supervision. Some staff may also be uncomfortable at the thought of residents having sex in the facility.

Many older people have difficulty expressing their sexual needs after losing a spouse through death or divorce. Since women usually live longer than men, single women far outnumber single men in older age groups. But sometimes residents who meet in the facility develop close, loving relationships. As long as both partners consent and there are no safety concerns, they have the right to privacy together. Residents' family and staff may find such relationships embarrassing or undesirable. Help everyone be more accepting by encouraging residents, family, and staff to talk

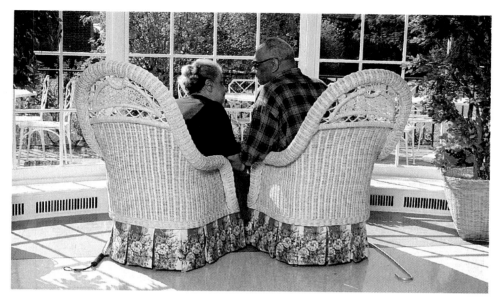

Fig. 2-5. The need to express loving feelings is both physical and social. Intimacy achieved through physical contact exists at any age.

about their feelings and say how they would like to be treated. The key consideration is mutual consent.

Masturbation is a normal outlet for meeting sexual needs, but this makes some people uncomfortable. Many people do not talk about it openly, and some older people may have grown up with the idea that it is wrong. If you are aware that a resident uses masturbation as an outlet, respect the person's needs and provide privacy. Because of confusion or other factors, a resident may express sexual feelings in places that make others uncomfortable, for example, masturbating or exposing himself or herself in a group setting. This behavior usually makes other residents uncomfortable, and you need to act to preserve all residents' privacy and dignity. You may need to move this resident to a private place or distract him or her with some other activity.

Spiritual Needs

Spirituality is much more than religion, although many people meet their spiritual needs through religion. Spirituality can help a person meet security, social, and self-fulfillment needs. Spirituality involves finding meaning in life, a search for a sense of relatedness to something greater than ourselves. In addition to religious rituals, a person may express spirituality through prayer, meditation, and reading. Residents, like all people, find spirituality in different ways. Respect each resident's ways, do not pass judgment, and never impose your beliefs on a resident. Typically, as people grow older, they tend to look more to their spiritual or inner selves to find meaning for their lives. They benefit from reflecting on their lives, remembering life events and working through losses, guilt, and regrets. They are not just "living in the past," but are developing their present self-esteem. You can encourage this process by listening and asking questions of a resident about his or her past. You can also help residents validate experiences. For example, if a resident says, "I wish I could have done more with my wife before she died," you can say "Tell me what you and your wife did." Then, "It sounds to me like you did quite a bit together and that you were always there." This can help this resident look at the experiences he had with his wife and maybe go beyond any regrets that he may not have done enough.

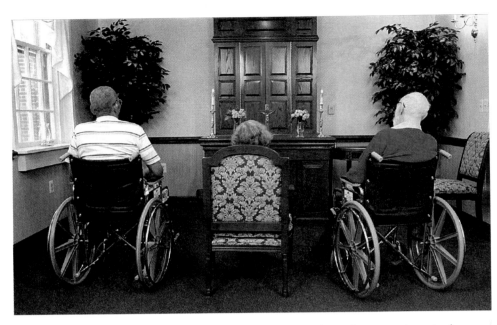

Fig. 2-6. For many people religious practice is an important part of life. Fulfilling spiritual needs provide residents with a sense of comfort and help them cope with concerns about their own death.

Religious practices often provide spiritual comfort, especially when one is coping with major life changes, such as the loss of a loved one or facing one's own death. Rabbis, priests, and ministers can help when a resident questions, "What has my life meant?" You can assist residents to attend the facility's place of worship for residents (Fig. 2-6). Notify the clergy if a resident requests a visit. Provide privacy when the clergy is visiting. Residents or family members may ask you to pray with them. If you are comfortable with this, join in the prayer. If you are not comfortable, you can stay quietly with the resident or ask another to take your place.

Many religious and ethnic groups celebrate their own religious holidays, often marked by special ceremonies and traditional foods. Find out what special days your residents observe and assist them in continuing rituals that have meaning for them. You can also help them to teach others about their rituals and share religious ceremonies. Facilities often plan special activities for common holidays such as Christmas, Easter, Rosh Hashanah, and Yom Kippur. Remember that some people do not celebrate these particular holidays, and respect their right to choose not to be involved in the celebrations.

Meeting Different Needs

Basic human needs occur on a continuum. Needs change, and one moves through different needs up and down these levels. You may move back and forth between levels many times. For example, you probably get hungry several times a day. When you are hungry (or tired, or physically ill), you tend to focus on getting food (or rest, or medical treatment), and you pay less attention to other things around you. When you have attended to the physical need, then you can again attend to safety and social needs.

Often we meet more than one need with the same activity. Many social celebrations involve food: family reunions, recognition banquets, funerals. In these you meet your most basic need for food, but at the same time you meet needs for interactions with others, a feeling of belonging, and recognition of your accomplishments. Depending on one's experiences, everyone has a different emphasis for dif-

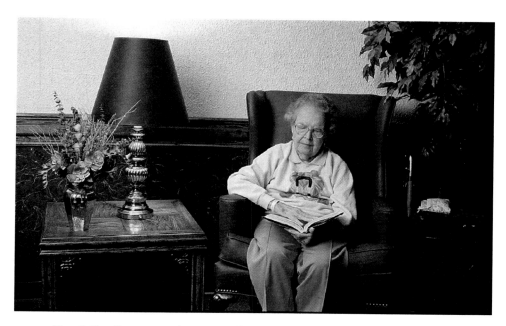

Fig. 2-7. Getting to know residents' personal preferences and their needs allows you to adjust your care accordingly.

ferent levels. For example, for some, being with people is important to their sense of well-being. For others, time alone to read or pursue other solitary activities is essential to emotional stability.

As you work with residents, remember this idea of a continuum. Needs change from moment to moment. What is important for a resident when feeling well physically may be different from what is important when he or she is experiencing severe physical pain. This is why it is so important for you to get to know the residents in your care (Fig. 2-7). You can then see changes in their needs and adjust your care accordingly.

What Do You Have in Common With Residents?

All human beings have the same basic needs. Just because a person is older does not mean that his or her needs have changed. Most people approach meeting their needs in the same way all of their lives. In the following descriptions of three different people, look for the basic needs that are the same for all three, and notice also the different ways they meet these needs.

Ellen is a 32-year-old single mother of three children, who works as a nurse assistant in a long term care facility in her home town. After a divorce two years ago, she had to rely on public assistance and food stamps to give her children food, clothing, and housing. She enrolled in a nurse assistant course and later got her job. Although she has a large family, she has little daily contact with them and receives little financial or emotional support from them. Her primary social outlet is her church.

Bruce is a 25-year-old disabled veteran, confined to a wheelchair since a car accident three years ago on active duty in the Army. He was in military hospitals for 18 months for acute care and rehabilitation. He receives a military pension that lets him live in his own apartment with a paid companion. His parents live in the same city and will help in emergencies, but he prefers to take care of himself. Before his accident he was active in sports, and he had trouble accepting his present limitations. He now has joined a support group for people with spinal cord injuries and is training for wheelchair athletics.

Maureen is a 67-year-old resident in a long term care facility in the city where her oldest daughter lives. She is a diabetic, has had a below-knee amputation of her right leg, and has mild dementia. She was admitted to the facility six months ago after her children realized her husband could no longer care for her. Her husband now lives with the oldest daughter and visits every day for several hours. Maureen is alert and is often fully oriented to her surroundings. She insists on doing everything she can for herself, and she prefers that her husband help her with those things she cannot do herself.

What do you have in common with these three people? Do they remind you of anyone you know? Are their needs different from yours, your family's, or those of the residents in your care? All have the basic human needs in common: to eat, to be safe, to be as independent as possible, and so on.

Can you identify the basic needs in each example? Most people react to new situations in ways that have worked in the past. This is true also for residents in your facility. A resident who has always looked forward to new situations will more easily cope with moving into the facility than a resident who always hated change and has lived in the same house for 50 years. Did you notice that each person wanted to stay independent?

The need to be with other people also remains much the same throughout life. Being with others helps meet both safety and social needs. Being with others may also cause conflict and frustration, however, for others do not always behave as you want. Some people try to avoid conflict by avoiding others. Respect the different ways people relate to other people. You may relate well to someone who is outgoing and talkative, but how should you change your approach with someone who is quiet and shy?

Your basic patterns of behavior stay much the same at work, at home, and in social situations with friends. Become aware of how you relate to others and what situations make you uncomfortable. Are you uncomfortable with someone who is crying? What about someone who is angry? You will encounter people like this in your job, and you will need to give them thoughtful care. When you are involved in a situation that is hard for you, seek help from peers or your supervisor.

SOME THINGS DO CHANGE WITH AGING

Aging is not a disease but a natural process that starts at birth and cannot be stopped or reversed. Human beings growing older have declining function in most of their organs and tissues, but aging does not automatically mean illness or "senility." The changes caused by aging are the same for everyone, though they occur at different rates. Cultural stereotypes of "old people" just do not fit many seniors today. Some myths people believe are:

- All people over 65 live in long term care facilities
- All older people are sick
- All older people are confused and miserable
- You cannot have sex if you are over 65
- All old people are deaf and have no teeth
- You cannot teach someone old new information

None of these statements are true. In fact, no one description is true for everyone. You must consider each resident as an individual. Be sure to ask the charge nurse if you are not sure about something concerning older people.

For some, the years after raising children and career are a time to slow down and enjoy the good things in their lives. They may accept that the past cannot be changed and focus on the present. Retirement gives the chance to explore activities they never had time for before. They enjoy their friends and participation in social groups with common interests (Fig. 2-8).

Some changes are more difficult to cope with. Chronic illnesses often develop and limit physical abilities even more. Accepting physical changes requires adjustment. People who defined themselves through their appearance and strength may

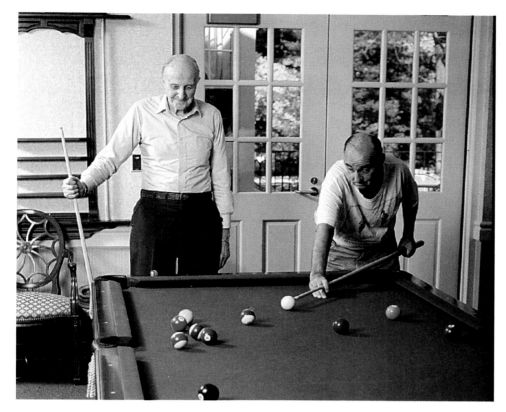

Fig. 2-8. Retirement gives people the opportunity to enjoy the activities they didn't have time to do before.

have difficulty coping with aging. As we grow older we also experience losses of significant others, family, and friends. Depression, hopelessness, and feelings of uselessness are common reactions to such losses. Even "loss" means different things to each of us. Although some see retirement as a chance to try things they never had time for while working, others view it as a loss of identity and purpose in their lives. Retirement may also be a loss of financial security for some.

All human beings face some common aspects of aging. The three R's of growing old are reality, responsibility, and rights.

▶ Accepting reality includes inevitable changes and adapting one's expectations and life-style because of these changes. This includes physical adaptations, financial adjustments, new relationships. It may mean accepting the death of a spouse or partner and one's own imminent death (Fig. 2-9).

▶ Fulfilling one's responsibility means planning for the rest of one's life and resolving past issues that may now have a different value.

▶ Exercising rights means one continues to participate fully in life, making choices and asserting one's rights to be involved in decisions about one's life.

REACTIONS TO MOVING INTO A LONG TERM FACILITY

Consider the following descriptions of some residents of nursing facilities.

Mrs. Thomas is a 70-year-old widow. Her three children live in different states, all long distances from her home. She has been active in church work and has enjoyed volunteer work since her retirement five years ago. She has lived alone since her husband's death two years ago. Her diabetes is controlled by diet and oral medication. Her vision is impaired by cataracts, and two months ago she fell and suffered a broken hip. After recuperating from surgery in an acute care hospital, she entered a long term care fa-

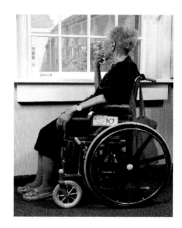

Fig. 2-9. Inevitable changes occur with aging. It is important for people to be able to accept these changes and adapt one's expectations and life-style.

cility for physical rehabilitation. She expects to return home with help from a home health agency.

Mr. Morton is an 82-year-old bachelor, a retired carpenter who has lived alone all of his adult life. Neighbors noticed a gradual decline in his functioning, and one of them called Adult Protective Services to check on him. The case worker found him confused and his home unkempt. After he was hospitalized for treatment of high blood pressure and malnutrition, he was admitted to a long term care facility. He is diagnosed as having Alzheimer's disease, and he is very confused and has a tendency to wander (Fig. 2-10).

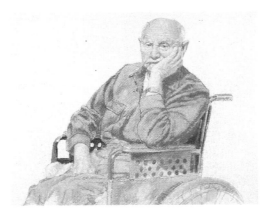

Fig. 2-10. Diagnosed with Alzheimer's disease, Mr. Morton, who wanders frequently, was admitted to a long term care facility.

Mr. Everett is a 72-year-old man who lived with his wife of 54 years in their home for 40 years. He is a retired engineer and enjoys gardening and home workshop. Since he retired 10 years ago, he and his wife enjoyed traveling to visit children and friends. He had no serious health problems until he suffered a stroke three months ago. He has left-sided paralysis. He is depressed and easily frustrated with his inability to communicate. His wife comes to the facility every day and stays with him most of the day (Fig. 2-11).

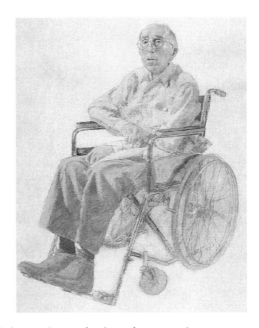

Fig. 2-11. Admitted to a facility after a stroke, a once very active Mr. Everett has become depressed.

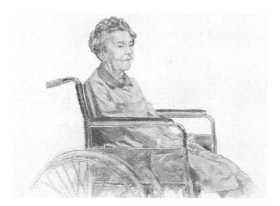

Fig. 2-12. Diagnosed with terminal breast cancer, Mrs. Cortez informs the staff that she is "ready to go," but her family requests that all efforts be made to keep her alive as long as possible.

Mrs. Cortez is a 68-year-old married housewife who was living with her husband of 50 years. Four of their seven children live only a few blocks away. Mrs. Cortez has focused her energy on taking care of her family and her home. She was admitted to the nursing facility two weeks ago with terminal breast cancer that has spread to other organs. Several members of her family are with her almost all of the time. They have requested that all efforts be made to keep their mother alive as long as possible. Mrs. Cortez has told facility staff that she is "ready to go," and wishes her family could let her go (Fig. 2-12).

Mrs. Lewis is an 85-year-old widow who has lived with her son's family for the last 20 years. She kept house and cooked for the family until two years ago, when she suffered a mild stroke that left her with left-side weakness. She then lived at home, cared for by her granddaughter. She has suffered a gradual physical and mental decline, with incontinence and increasing confusion. She entered the facility after the family became "just worn out" caring for her. Family members are having a hard time dealing with their feelings about placing Mrs. Lewis in the facility, and their visits are infrequent and brief (Fig. 2-13).

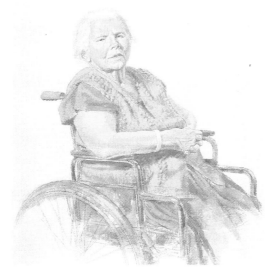

Fig. 2-13. Having problems with the decision to put Mrs. Lewis in a facility, her family's visits became infrequent and brief.

Although these residents are different in many ways, they have some things in common. For example, moving into the facility was a big change in life-style for all of them.

Moving into a long term care facility is often only one of many changes a resident has had to cope with. As you learned in Chapter 1, people enter a facility because they need help with care. Being dependent on someone else to meet one's basic needs is often the most difficult part of aging. One loses the ability to control one's life. Moving into the facility also means giving up many personal possessions and familiar routines and people. Living in a group situation means losing privacy and having to accommodate other people's needs and demands.

You may not know what other changes or losses a resident has experienced before or by coming to the facility. Some losses at first may not seem much to you, such a weekly bridge game, but to the person this may be a loss of a valuable support group and recognition. Only the person experiencing a loss can know its true significance.

Remember that everyone has developed his or her own way of dealing with change. Residents react in many different ways to moving into the facility. Some residents may act happy for the family but be withdrawn in their room after the family leaves. Others may complain bitterly to the family about being "put in this place," then cheerfully join in activities with peers after the family leaves. Some will simply accept the change and make the best of their new home.

Your interaction with residents influences how they adjust to the move. Let residents know you care. Spend time with them, listen to them, and assure privacy when giving care. Encourage residents to assume as much control as possible over decisions that affect them. Even simple things like deciding when to take a bath and choosing what to wear can help residents feel in control. Encourage independence by letting residents do as much as possible for themselves. For example, even though it sometimes may take longer, let residents feed and dress themselves if they can. Encourage participation with other residents in activities such as meals, games, parties, and discussion groups. Give residents time alone when they want it.

RESIDENT RIGHTS

Rights are both human privileges and legal protections. Residents have the same rights as you: to be treated with respect and dignity, to pursue a meaningful life, to be free of fear. They also have the legal rights of all U.S. citizens, including the right to vote and freedom from discrimination on the basis of age, sex, race, religion, ethnic group, or disability.

All residents also have the right to the same high quality of care, regardless of how their care is paid for. A resident whose stay is funded by Medicaid is entitled to the same care and caring as a resident who pays for care with personal funds. The facility and staff are legally responsible for protecting and promoting each resident's rights. Violating a resident's right is breaking the law, and punishment could include being fired and being fined or sent to jail by a court of law.

A 1987 federal law guarantees residents of long term care facilities other rights. This law was passed because studies showed rights were not being protected in all places for all residents. Violations lead to serious legal penalties, and staff are responsible for actions and failures to act. This law, The Omnibus Budget Reconciliation Act (OBRA), begins with the statement, "The resident has a right to a dignified existence, self-determination, and communication with and access to persons and services inside and outside the facility. A facility must protect and promote the rights of each resident...." The facility's first responsibility is to inform all residents of their rights both orally and in writing. Rights are explained to each resident on admission and must be posted in writing in the facility, often in the lobby or entrance to the facility. This is often called the "Residents' Bill of Rights" (Fig. 2-14).

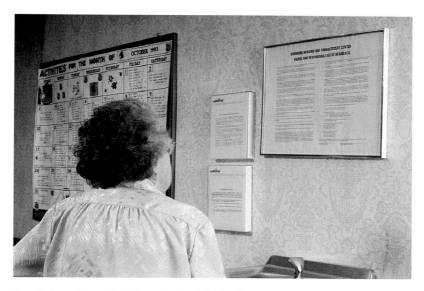

Fig. 2-14. The "Residents' Bill of Rights" must be posted at every facility.

The law also requires an ombudsman program to protect residents' rights. Each state must appoint an advocate, called the ombudsman, to investigate complaints by residents or others about violations of rights. The ombudsman has authority to solve problems for a resident. If the ombudsman cannot resolve the problem, he or she may represent a resident, negotiate a solution, or file a lawsuit. The facility must inform its residents how to contact the local ombudsman program.

Ombudsmen also monitor state regulations and help strengthen laws that protect each resident's rights. As well, ombudsmen help educate the public and train volunteers to assist residents and their families.

Residents have many specific rights. They are grouped here under the following headings to make it easier to remember them:

1. Rights to exercise one's rights
2. Rights to privacy and confidentiality
3. Rights to information
4. Rights to choose
5. Rights to notification of change
6. Protection of residents' personal funds
7. Grievance rights
8. Transfer and discharge rights
9. Rights to be free from restraint and abuse

Exercising One's Rights

▷ Each resident has the right to exercise his or her rights as a resident of the facility and as a citizen or resident of the United States.

▷ Each resident has the right to be free of interference, coercion, discrimination, and reprisal from the facility in exercise of his or her rights.

▷ If a resident is judged incompetent under the laws of a state, the rights of a resident are exercised by the person appointed by the state to act on the resident's behalf.

How to Assist Residents With Their Rights

What all does this mean? You encourage residents to exercise their rights by giving them choices and an opportunity to be heard. For example, help them vote using an absentee ballot if they are unable to go to a regular voting place. If they are not mentally competent to make their decisions, an appointed person acts for them legally. Cooperate with residents to enable them to exercise their rights.

 ### Rights to Privacy and Confidentiality

> Each resident has the right to confidentiality of his or her personal and medical records. A resident may approve or refuse the release of personal and clinical records to anyone outside the facility, except when a resident is transferred to another facility or when release is required by law.

> Residents also have the right to privacy in their accommodations, in written and telephone communications, during medical treatment and personal care, when meeting with visitors, and in meetings with family and others.

 ### How to Protect Residents' Rights to Privacy

Do not discuss residents' personal or medical information with anyone without a legitimate need to know. Do not talk about residents' personal information with other residents, with relatives and friends of a resident, with visitors, with the news media, or with your own friends. Discuss residents with other staff only in a private place and only about information needed to provide care for a resident. Do not gossip.

When you assist a resident with care, always provide privacy by knocking and announcing yourself, pulling a curtain, closing the door, and draping a resident's body appropriately. You may have to explain to visitors or other residents to leave the room.

Assist a resident when needed to read and write letters, but never open mail addressed to a resident unless a resident requests you to. If your facility does not provide a phone in each resident's room, provide for private phone conversations using a phone booth or a cordless phone in a resident's room (Fig. 2-15).

Give residents time alone with visitors, and help them find a private place for visits, especially visits with spouses or significant others. If needed, engage a resident's roommate elsewhere to protect a resident's privacy in the room (Fig. 2-16).

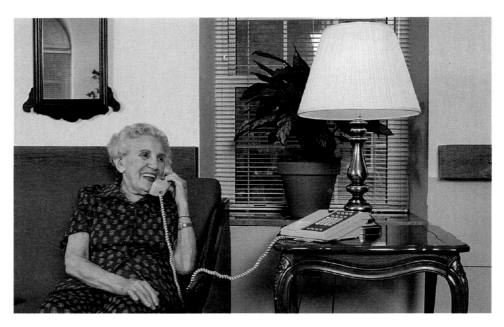

Fig. 2-15. Residents should be provided with areas for having private phone conversations.

Encourage residents and families to join groups such as a Resident Council or Family Support Group. Staff often attend such meetings to answer questions and help solve problems. These groups may also ask to meet without staff, as is their right.

Information Rights

▷ Each resident has the right to see his or her personal and medical records within 24 hours of requesting them. If requested, a resident must receive a copy of such records within two working days.

▷ Residents have the right to be fully informed, in a language they can understand, of their total health status.

▷ Residents must be informed of services for which they cannot be charged and all other services and the charges for them. Residents must be informed of any change in these services. Residents have a right to see their financial records and to have everything explained to them.

▷ Residents must receive a written description of their rights, including their eligibility status for Medicaid benefits.

▷ The facility must post the names and addresses of client advocacy groups and the ombudsman program.

▷ Residents have the right to read the written report of the most recent survey of the facility by federal or state surveyors, and to see the facility's plan for correction of any deficiencies noted in the report.

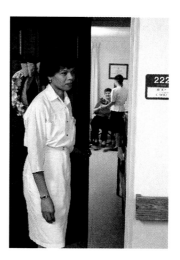

Fig. 2-16. Privacy is an important right for residents and their families.

Your Responsibilities for Providing Information

Most of this information is given to residents and their families at the time of admission. This is a lot for anyone to remember, and a resident or family may later ask you questions about rights. You need to know where to find the information or where to go for answers. If a resident asks to see his or her records, for example, tell the charge nurse immediately. Other information is posted in the facility for residents and staff. Procedure manuals at the nurses' station contain the facility's policies for protecting specific information rights. As stated earlier, you are likely to see the "Residents' Bill of Rights" posted prominently in the facility. Instructions for contacting the ombudsman and other advocacy groups are usually posted where residents and their families are most likely to gather, such as in the lounge areas and dining rooms.

When residents ask questions, actively help them find the answers. Read a copy of resident rights with them or to them when needed. Go with them to the areas where information is posted. With questions about their medical condition or treatment plan, ask the charge nurse or doctor to talk with them, and inform the nurse or doctor about a resident's specific concerns. Chapter 6 on Communication discusses ways to discuss rights with residents with special communication needs.

Rights to Choose

Residents have the right to choices about their living arrangements and their medical care, as long as those choices do not interfere with the rights of other residents (Fig. 2-17).

▷ Each resident has the right to refuse a treatment and to refuse to participate in experimental research.

▷ Each resident has the right to choose a personal attending physician, to participate in planning his or her care, and to be informed in advance about changes in care or treatment that may affect his or her well-being.

▷ Each resident has the right to perform voluntary or paid services in the facility, but cannot be required to work.

▷ Each resident has the right to keep and use personal possessions, within the limits of space and safety considerations.

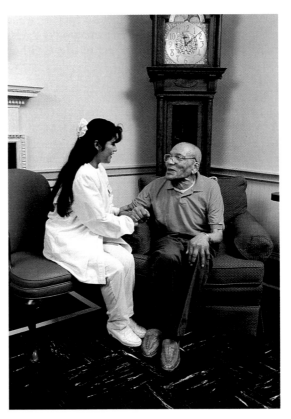

Fig. 2-17. Residents have the right to voice opinions and give input about their medical care.

- Each resident has the right to share a room with his or her spouse, if both live in the facility and both consent.
- Each resident has the right to self-administer his or her own medication, if the treatment team deems it safe.
- Each resident has the right to activities, schedules, and health care according to his or her own interests and needs.
- Each resident has the right to interact with members of the community both inside and outside the facility.
- Each resident has the right to meet in resident and family groups, for which the facility must provide space and support staff.
- Each resident has the right to have the facility reasonably accommodate individual needs and preferences.

How to Assist Residents in Exercising Their Right to Choose

An important service you can provide is to make sure residents are aware of their choices. Inform them about activities in the facility. Find out what their interests are, and help them keep doing what they enjoy. Some residents may want to help out with tasks in the facility, such as watering plants and making their own beds. Residents may also want to help other residents, such as assisting at mealtimes; however, they cannot feed residents. No resident has to perform such tasks, but some feel more useful and increase their self-worth if they do things for themselves and help others. Later chapters give you other ideas about encouraging and protecting residents' choices about their care and their environment.

If residents want to stay active in their community, encourage their continued contact with organizations and attendance at meetings if their health allows. Try to think of ways to personalize life for residents in the facility. Avoid doing things by routine for your own convenience, and encourage residents to set up their own routines as much as possible.

A resident's choices may have to be limited when they interfere with other residents' rights. To prevent such problems facilities have rules ensuring fair treatment of all residents. Staff should always attempt to meet the needs of all residents with limiting a resident's rights.

Rights to Notification of Change

- Each resident, family, and physician must be informed of any change in a resident's physical, mental, or psychosocial status, including any accident that causes injury.
- If treatment must change because of a resident's changed status or resources, the resident must be notified.
- Each resident must be notified in advance of a planned change in his or her room or roommate.
- Every resident must be informed of any changes in resident rights.
- The facility must maintain an updated record of the address and phone number for residents' legal representative and interested family members.

When to Notify Residents of Change

If you must change the way you have been doing something for a resident, such as the time for performing a treatment, notify the resident in advance and when possible ask his or her preferences for rescheduling.

If you witness an accident that injures the resident, tell the charge nurse so that the physician and family are notified. If a family member gives you a new address or phone number, be sure to record it in that resident's record.

Even in simple things like a delayed meal, notify residents and give a time to expect service. A resident is always included in a decision to change rooms or roommates. Remain with the resident to be sure he or she is comfortable with the decision.

Protection of Residents' Personal Funds

- Residents have the right to keep and manage their own funds or to have a private party do so. If a resident wants the facility to manage his or her funds, the facility must hold and safeguard these funds and provide quarterly statements as requested by a resident or legal representative.

Your Responsibility Regarding Residents' Funds

All staff must help safeguard each resident's personal belongings. If you know a resident is keeping a large sum of money or is not managing money appropriately, report this to the charge nurse, family, or legal representative so that they can protect the resident's interests. The facility must try to prevent theft of residents' belongings, including money.

Grievances

- Each resident has the right to voice complaints without fear of retaliation or discrimination.
- The facility must take prompt action on complaints.
- Federal law requires each state to have an ombudsman program to investigate complaints from residents and family members and act as their advocate. The facility must notify residents and their families about this program (Fig. 2-18).

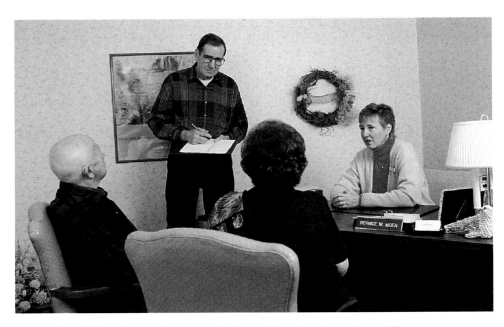

Fig. 2-18. The ombudsman is the resident's advocate and the person who investigates complaints and grievances from residents and family members.

Your Responsibility Regarding Resident Grievances

You can encourage residents to become involved in resident councils. You can offer written information to residents about the formal grievance procedure. If a resident complains to you, you must tell the charge nurse or administrator. You must not let the complaint negatively affect how you care for a resident. For example, if a resident complains that you have been rude, you must not argue with him or her about what you said but keep assisting with care with respect and concern.

No matter what the complaint is, the facility must investigate to determine if it is valid. This means that if a resident complains about you, the charge nurse must investigate. This does not mean that the people you work with think you did something wrong. The investigation is made to determine the facts for your protection as well as the resident's.

If a resident or family member continues to complain or feels the facility has not done enough regarding the complaints, refer the family to the charge nurse or social worker.

Protecting a Resident's Right to Voice Complaints

A resident may complain to you about another staff member, and you should report this to the charge nurse or another supervisor. The facility will follow up on your report. If you do not think the facility is addressing a resident's complaint, you may contact the ombudsman yourself.

Transfer or Discharge Rights

Transfer and discharge are the movement of residents to a location inside or outside the facility. A resident can be involuntarily transferred or discharged only:
- In a situation threatening the life of a resident or others
- With advance notice so another place can be found
- When a resident no longer needs the services of the facility

▶ When a resident has failed to pay for services after reasonable notice
▶ When the facility ceases to operate

When a transfer or discharge is planned, enough advance notice must be given to ensure the process is safe and orderly.

Your Role in Transfers and Discharges

If a resident is unhappy or frightened about a move, listen to his or her concerns (Fig. 2-19). Do not discount a resident's feelings with comments like, "Don't worry about it. Everything will be all right." Help him or her understand why the change is needed, and be sure he or she has time to adjust.

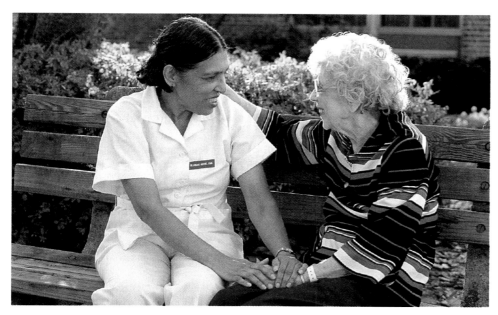

Fig. 2-19. Listening to a resident who is being transferred or discharged will help that resident adjust.

The Right to be Free from Restraint and Abuse

▶ Each resident has the right to be free from any physical or chemical restraints imposed for discipline or convenience.
▶ Each resident has the right to be free from any verbal, sexual, physical, and mental abuse, corporal punishment, and involuntary seclusion.
▶ The facility must have and follow written policies to prohibit mistreatment, neglect, and abuse of residents or their property.
▶ Alleged violations of these rights must be reported to the administration and other officials as required by state law. The facility must investigate thoroughly all alleged violations and report its findings.

What You Can Do to Prevent Resident Abuse

The first thing you must do is understand what these terms mean:
▶ *Physical restraints* are any mechanical devices that restrict a resident's movement, such as bed rails, a vest restraint to keep a resident in bed or in a chair, limb restraints to limit use of arms or legs, or geri-chair or lap pillow to prevent standing or walking.

- *Chemical restraints* are medications used to sedate a resident or slow muscle activity.
- *Verbal abuse* includes using profanity, calling a resident names, yelling at a resident in anger, making oral or written threats, and teasing a resident in an unkind manner.
- *Physical abuse* is any action that causes actual physical harm, such as handling a resident too roughly, performing the wrong treatment on a resident, and any hitting, pushing, pinching, or kicking of a resident.
- *Neglect* is failing to do something you should have done, and this may also be physical abuse. Neglect includes failing to carry out proper hygiene, to turn a resident to improve circulation, and to provide food and water regularly.
- *Negligence* is failing to act as a reasonable person with the same training would act in the same circumstances. Gross negligence refers to actions that show no concern for the well-being of others.
- *Sexual abuse* is not limited to specific sexual acts but also may include touching residents in an intimate or suggestive manner, making sexual comments, and allowing another resident to do such acts.
- *Mental abuse* is any action that makes a resident fearful, such as threatening him or her with harm or threatening to share something he or she doesn't want others to know, or actions that belittle or make fun of a resident.
- *Corporal punishment* means physical punishment, such as spanking or slapping.
- *Involuntary seclusion* is the isolation of a resident against his or her will, such as locking a resident in a room alone.

You are not allowed to place a resident in a physical restraint just because it is more convenient for you or other staff. A doctor's order is required, and you or the charge nurse must document the reasons for restraint according to the facility's policies. Residents can be restrained only for their personal safety or the safety of others. For example, a resident may be placed in limb restraints if he or she pulls out tubes required for a medical treatment he or she has agreed to or if he or she is trying to hit other residents and this behavior has not yet been assessed; usually the reason for hitting is found and the cause can be removed. As nurse assistant you may be the one who discovers why a resident feels threatened enough to act this way.

When a resident is restrained, you must check that the restraint is used properly and check often to prevent circulatory problems. If a resident seems to be overmedicated, such as is sleeping all the time or has unusually slurred speech, report this to the charge nurse. Chapter 19 provides many good ideas for working with residents to avoid the use of restraints.

Theft of a resident's belongings is another form of abuse. Help prevent theft by marking belongings with the resident's name, listing belongings on an inventory record, and helping residents keep belongings in the same place. You may suggest that family members take home items of monetary value. Also protect items of sentimental value.

Obviously you must not commit patient abuse yourself, but you must also report any abuse you observe, no matter who the abuser is. Another staff member, another resident, or a family member may abuse a resident. If you do not report abuse you see, you are as guilty of abuse as the actual abuser. If you feel uncomfortable about reporting abuse to someone in the facility, you may call the ombudsman instead.

Laws severely punish those who abuse residents, including fines, imprisonment, or both. You can be charged with assault for threatening to harm a resident. The charge of battery can be brought against anyone who causes physical harm. The law requires the facility to have procedures to protect residents. You must protect residents who are vulnerable to abuse from other residents or others outside the facility. Whenever abuse is alleged, the facility must investigate and report its findings to state agencies. During the investigation you may be asked about your actions.

This does not mean that you have done anything wrong, but the facility must act seriously to protect residents.

If a charge is brought against you, you have a right to ask for a hearing and may even want to hire a lawyer. Sometimes it is not your fault even if you have been charged. Remember that you are innocent until proven guilty.

A nurse assistant found guilty of resident abuse not only loses her or his job but is reported to the state nurse aide registry. Facilities are not allowed to hire anyone who has been found guilty of neglecting or mistreating residents or who has been reported to the state registry for abuse, neglect, or mistreatment of residents or misappropriation of their property.

The Importance of Your Role in Protecting Residents' Rights

The legal penalties for violating a resident's rights are serious. They show you the importance of your role in ensuring residents' health and well-being. Residents are vulnerable because of physical and psychological frailties. You must provide a safe environment for them. Treating them with dignity and genuine respect for them as unique individuals helps ensure their basic rights. Do your job in a caring way and you do not have to worry about compromising someone's rights.

Look back again at the descriptions of the facility residents earlier, and think about how you could ensure that their basic rights are protected. Do you think any of them needs to have someone appointed to make decisions for him or her? What would you do in such a case? How would you provide residents with privacy to be with their spouses? Mr. Morton's wandering increases, and the staff feels he needs to be restrained while they prepare a safe place for him to wander. What is your facility's procedure to guarantee each resident's right to be free from unnecessary restraint? Mrs. Cortez tells you she does not want any more tube feedings because they are just prolonging her death, and she is tired of fighting. Does she have a choice in this? How do you communicate to her physician and her family that she has made this choice?

These are just some of the issues for these residents. You may think of many more. Never stop thinking about the rights of residents you assist. You are their first advocate.

IN THIS CHAPTER YOU LEARNED TO:

▸ define basic human needs

▸ list ways to meet residents' needs

▸ describe how residents' basic needs are similar to your own

▸ describe at least two changes that occur with aging

▸ state how to protect residents' rights

3

RESIDENTS AND THE AGING PROCESS

The body is made of different systems. We usually study each system separately to better understand it, but all the systems work together for our bodies to live. Think of an appliance you have in your home. What happens if any one part breaks? The appliance doesn't work very well, and sometimes it won't work at all. The same is true for the body. Each part of a body system must work by itself, and each system must also work with other systems, for the body as a whole to work properly. For example, the cardiovascular and respiratory systems work together as the heart and lungs work. The heart pumps the blood, which has received oxygen from the air breathed through the lungs, through the body. Then the blood carries carbon dioxide back to the lungs so that the waste can be breathed out.

Each system of the body ages. There is no one pattern of aging for everyone, and different systems age at different rates, but there are general characteristics of aging. These changes:

▷ Reduce the functioning of the system
▷ Take place gradually
▷ Happen naturally
▷ Happen to everyone

Aging often scares people, but the aging process actually begins at birth. Aging is a natural process that happens to everyone (Fig. 3-1). Many factors influence aging, such as how a person lives and his or her family history. These factors affect how a person ages, but not the fact that aging will occur eventually. For example, the sun influences how the skin ages. Everyone's skin eventually wrinkles with age, but wrinkling occurs faster if you have spent much time in the sun.

Always be careful not to judge someone by the way he or she looks. Just because someone looks old doesn't mean that person doesn't think clearly or have feelings like you or other younger people. Never confuse aging with poor health. And never should anyone feel that old age takes away the ability to live happily. The key to aging well is to be positive about the changes.

Understanding the normal structures and functions of the body, and the changes that occur with aging, will help you to identify signs and symptoms of a problem in any body system. A sign is something that you can observe: what you see—a resident is sweating, smell—a resident's breath has a foul odor, hear—a resident is coughing, or touch—a resident is very warm. A symptom is something a resident feels inside and tells you about such as a complaint of aches and pains.

Carefully observe residents to watch for, recognize, and note any changes. Report these changes to the charge nurse. You will learn to use all your senses to observe changes and recognize any abnormalities. Think about someone you know well: a co-worker, your child, or a friend. How can you tell when they are sick or not feeling well? Don't you use your senses to compare how they appear now with their normal appearance? You may notice they are pale, sound hoarse, or feel warm.

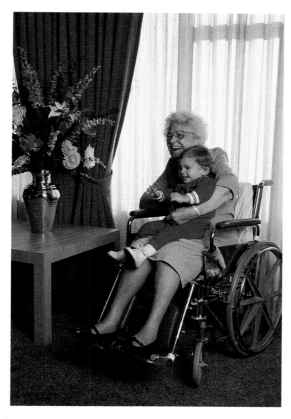

Fig. 3-1. Aging is a natural process that begins at birth, and although many factors influence aging, it occurs with everyone.

The same is true as you get to know residents. When you observe something different about a resident, look for other signs to find any reason for this change. For example, a person who is flushed and sweaty might be ill, or maybe just finished exercising. You will learn to observe each resident carefully and report information about any changes.

This chapter describes each system of the body. For each, you will first learn the main organs of each system—the anatomy. Then you'll learn the function of each system—the physiology (what it does). How each system ages and the results of aging are described. Finally, you will learn signs of abnormal changes you should watch for as you care for residents.

As you review each system, think about your own body. Can you observe changes that have happened to you over the years? What changes would you consider to be normal, abnormal, or unusual? How do you feel about these changes? Some people may view aging as a loss of function and others may view it more positively. What matters is how an individual resident feels about the changes (Fig. 3-2). Ask questions like:

▷ Do your limitations with walking cause problems for you?

▷ How does it feel to be stiff in the morning?

▷ What do you do to start your day off better?

By asking questions, you can better understand the psychological effects of aging on a resident and the development of abnormal signs and symptoms.

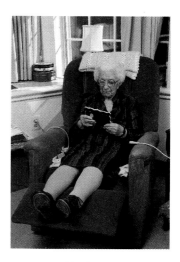

Fig. 3-2. Each resident is affected differently by changes caused by aging.

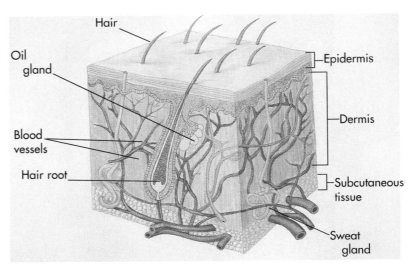

Fig. 3-3. Structures of the integumentary system.

INTEGUMENTARY SYSTEM (SKIN)
Structures

The skin is made up of two layers (Fig. 3-3):
- The epidermis is the top layer you can see and feel.
- The dermis is the thicker layer underneath the epidermis.

Beneath the two layers of skin lies a cushion called subcutaneous tissue. This cushion is made up of fatty tissue and helps give the skin a smooth look. Five structures within the layers of skin help the skin stay healthy and help protect the body:
- The oil glands help keep the skin moist.
- The sweat glands help the body get rid of heat and waste products.
- The hair roots and hair over parts of the body add to the appearance of the person and help protect the skin.
- The melanocytes are cells that give color to the skin.
- The blood vessels nourish the skin and help control body temperature.

The three extensions or outgrowths from the skin are:
- Hair
- Fingernails and toenails
- The mucous membranes that line the inside of the nose, mouth, and other body openings

Functions

The skin is very important to an individual's health because it covers the entire body and protects the body in two ways:
- It prevents germs in the environment from entering the body; it is the first line of defense against infection.
- It helps control body temperature by sweating when it is hot and by shivering when it is cold. When it is hot, the blood vessels to the skin dilate (expand) to let heat out; when it is cold, blood vessels constrict (narrow) to keep heat in.

Aging Changes

The skin often shows the signs of aging sooner than other body systems because of its life-long exposure to sun, wind, cold air, and drying soaps. Table 3-1 lists the changes that occur in the skin, hair, and nails as a person ages.

TABLE 3-1. Integumentary System

Change	Result
Decrease in oil production by the sebaceous (oil) glands	Dryness of the skin and hair
Thinning of the underlying dermis layer of the skin	Wrinkling of the skin
Decreased elasticity of the skin	Sagging skin
Shrinkage of the hypodermal (subcutaneous) layer of the skin, due to loss of fatty tissue	Difficulty with adjusting to heat loss, especially on the face and backs of hands

Abnormal Signs and Symptoms

▷ Change in color or size of any skin growth such as a mole, freckle, or wart, etc.
▷ Bleeding
▷ Rash (red bumps on skin)
▷ Reddened areas
▷ Open sores
▷ Bruises
▷ Cuts
▷ Flaking skin
▷ Complaints of itching or pain
▷ Very hot skin
▷ Cold, damp skin

Questions to Consider

▷ What does this resident's skin normally look like?
▷ Is a growth new, has it changed, or has it always been there?
▷ Has this resident done something new, such as started a new medication, tried a new skin lotion, or worn new clothes, that might have caused a rash?
▷ Does the reddened area go away when you change the resident's position?
▷ What has the weather been like? Is a resident's skin dry and flaky because of the weather?
▷ Does a resident have any concerns about the appearance of his or her skin?
▷ Has a resident's attitude about personal hygiene changed?
▷ Should this change be reported to the nurse?
▷ How does the change affect the resident's well-being?

MUSCULOSKELETAL SYSTEM

Structures

The musculoskeletal system is made up of bones, muscles, tendons, ligaments, and joints (Fig. 3-4).

▷ Bones provide a frame for the body.
▷ Muscles allow the body to move.
▷ Tendons attach muscles to bones.
▷ Ligaments attach bones to other bones.
▷ Joints are where two or more bones come together.

Functions

The musculoskeletal system helps give the body its shape and enables it to move. Movement is important for one to get around and be active.

Aging Changes

As a person ages, changes take place in the musculoskeletal system. Table 3-2 lists those changes.

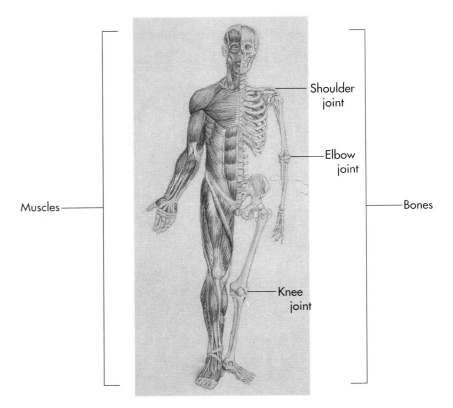

Fig. 3-4. Structures of the musculoskeletal system consist of bones, muscle, tendons, ligaments, and joints.

TABLE 3-2. **Musculoskeletal System**

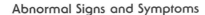

Change	Result
The spinal column shortens	Loss of height; loss of minerals from bones
Increased risk of breakage	Loss of muscle mass
Loss of strength	Loss of elasticity of muscles; muscle stiffness

Abnormal Signs and Symptoms

▶ Swollen, reddened joints
▶ Bumps or bruises on arms and legs
▶ Complaints of increased stiffness, inability to move, or pain (Fig. 3-5)

Questions to Consider

▶ Is a resident favoring a certain position?
▶ Is the resident's position being changed often?
▶ Is the resident getting up and moving or walking enough? Does he or she need help?
▶ Does the resident have problems moving in the morning or after sitting for any length of time?
▶ Does the resident favor one arm or leg over the other?
▶ Do the resident's shoes and/or assistive devices fit properly?
▶ Can you do anything to promote and support the resident's ability to move (offer your arm, move things out of the way)?
▶ Should the change be reported to the nurse?
▶ How does the change affect the resident's well-being?

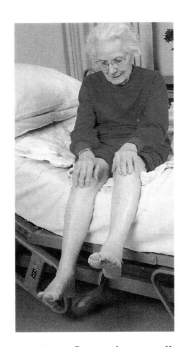

Fig. 3-5. Discomfort or stiffness in the joints is an indication of abnormalities in the musculoskeletal system.

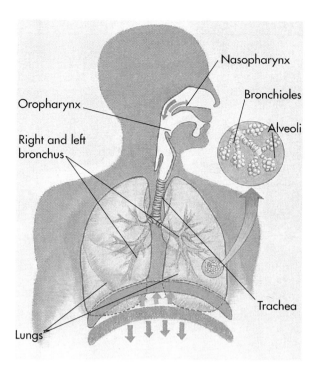

Fig. 3-6. Structures of the respiratory system.

RESPIRATORY SYSTEM
Structures

The main structures of the respiratory system are (Fig. 3-6):
- The nasopharynx is the nasal passage.
- The oropharynx is the mouth and oral passage.
- The trachea connects the mouth and nose to the lungs.
- The lungs take air in, move oxygen into the blood, and remove carbon dioxide from the body.

The air passages inside each lung almost look like an upside-down tree:
- The right and left bronchus enter each lung as the trunk of each tree.
- The bronchioles are branches of each bronchus.
- The alveoli (air sacs) look like hundreds of blossoms on the bronchioles.

Function

The respiratory system takes in oxygen through the nose or mouth as we breathe in (inhale or inspire) air and passes it through the bronchi, bronchioles, and finally, into the alveoli.

The oxygen then passes into the blood vessels and is carried by the blood to all the body parts. The blood exchanges oxygen for carbon dioxide. The air that we breathe out (exhale or expire) gets rid of the carbon dioxide from the body. The heart and lungs work together to oxygenate the blood.

Breathing (respiration) is the exchange of oxygen and carbon dioxide in the lungs. This is one of the most basic and important of all body functions.

Aging Changes

The two most important changes in the lungs that gradually occur with normal aging are described in Table 3-3.

TABLE 3-3. **Respiratory System**

Change	Result
The chest wall and lung structures become more rigid	There is not as much room for air in the lungs and it is more difficult to take deep breaths
There is a decrease in the amount of air that is exchanged with each breath	During exercise, illness, or stress, a person has to breathe faster to get enough oxygen in and carbon dioxide out

Abnormal Signs and Symptoms

▶ Bluish-gray color around the lips, nail beds, and mucous membranes
▶ Gasping for breath or simply labored breathing
▶ Rattling or gurgling noise when breathing
▶ Foul-smelling breath
▶ Very fast or very slow chest movement
▶ Very cold or very hot skin
▶ Needing to sit up to breathe
▶ Pain with breathing
▶ Resident complains of shortness of breath, unusual color sputum, or funny taste in their mouth.

Questions to Consider

▶ Has the resident's breathing changed?
▶ What do the resident's lips, nail beds, and skin usually look like? Are they different?
▶ Is the resident sitting upright? Is it difficult for the resident to lie flat?
▶ Do you hear strange sounds when the resident breathes?
▶ Does the resident take frequent rest periods?
▶ Is the resident complaining of shortness of breath, difficult breathing, or less ability to do things?
▶ Is the resident coughing up unusual sputum (lung secretions)?
▶ Should the change be reported to the nurse?
▶ How does the change affect the resident's well-being?

CIRCULATORY SYSTEM
Structures

The heart and blood vessels working together make up the circulatory system. The heart is located underneath the ribs between the two lungs; the largest part lies in the left side of the chest. The heart is a muscle with four chambers (Fig. 3-7).

The heart pumps blood through the blood vessels to every body part. Every time you count a resident's pulse, as you will learn to do, you are counting how fast the heart pumps blood to the body. Three types of blood vessels carry blood to and from the heart and organs throughout the body:

▶ Arteries carry oxygenated blood from the lungs and heart to the organs.
▶ Capillaries, tiny blood vessels, connect arteries and veins and exchange oxygen for carbon dioxide inside the organs.
▶ Veins carry unoxygenated blood from the organs back to the heart and lungs.

Functions

The circulatory system carries oxygen from the lungs and other vital nourishment to all the cells of the body. It also carries waste products to some body organs for the body to get rid of them.

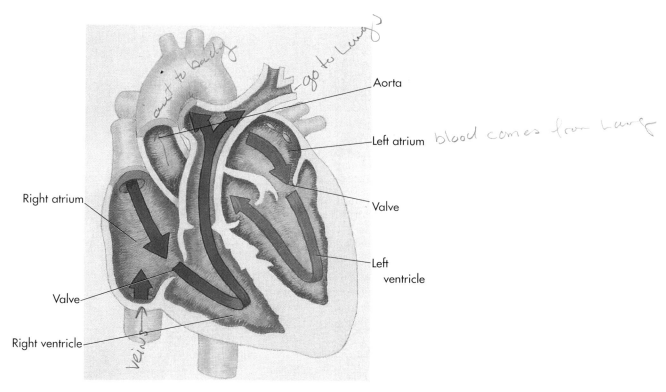

Fig. 3-7. The heart muscle works with blood vessels to make up the circulatory system.

Let's trace the blood through the heart. First, the body returns unoxygenated blood (the oxygen has been used by the organs) to the right atrium. The blood passes through an opening (valve) into the right ventricle, is carried by blood vessels to the lungs where the blood is oxygenated, and is returned to the left atrium. The blood then passes through a valve into the left ventricle and is pumped out of the heart into the largest blood vessel, the aorta.

The aorta branches off to the upper and lower parts of the body and connects with smaller blood vessels that carry oxygenated blood to every organ and cell in the body.

Aging Changes

Table 3-4 describes normal changes in the heart and blood vessels that occur with age.

TABLE 3-4.   Circulatory System

Change	Result
The heart muscle pumps with less force	The heart has to work harder to pump the same amount of blood
	The heart can become overworked during strenuous activity, forcing the older person to take more frequent rest periods
The blood vessels become more rigid and stiff	The heart has to work harder to pump blood through rigid vessels; blood pressure is higher

Abnormal Signs and Symptoms

▶ Swollen extremities, especially the legs and feet
▶ Shortness of breath
▶ Poor color in feet
▶ Weight gain or loss
▶ Complaints of chest pain or indigestion
▶ Increase or decrease in blood pressure
▶ Cold, damp skin
▶ Increase or decrease in pulse, irregularity in pulse

Questions to Consider

▶ Is there any puffiness or swelling in the resident's feet or ankles, or the sacrum in bed-ridden residents?
▶ Has the resident suddenly gained weight?
▶ Is the resident suddenly unable to do things he or she could do before (walk to the dining room, climb stairs)?
▶ Is the resident's heart rate regular? Is the resident's blood pressure normal?
▶ Is the resident complaining of dizziness?
▶ Should the change be reported to the nurse?
▶ How does the change affect the resident's well-being?

DIGESTIVE SYSTEM
Structures

The main structures of the digestive system are (Fig. 3-8):
▶ The mouth takes in food and fluid. In the mouth, food is chewed and mixed with saliva, beginning the digestive process.
▶ The esophagus is a tube that passes swallowed food and fluid from the mouth to the stomach.

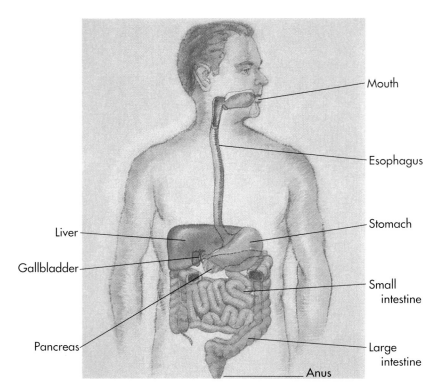

Mouth

Esophagus

Stomach

Small intestine

Large intestine

Anus

Liver

Gallbladder

Pancreas

Fig. 3-8. Structures of the digestive system.

- The stomach is a sac-like organ that mixes food and fluid with digestive juices, preparing it for absorption.
- The small intestine is a long tube-like structure where most absorption of nutrients takes place.
- The gallbladder is an organ that stores bile, used in the digestion of fatty foods.
- The liver produces bile.
- The pancreas produces digestive juices, which continues the breakdown of foods for nutrients for the body, and insulin, which regulates the body's blood sugar level.
- The large intestine is a long tube-like structure that moves the remaining food and waste through the body to the rectum and out of the body through the rectum. The large intestine absorbs fluids the body needs.
- The anus is the opening from which food wastes, in the form of a bowel movement, come out.

Function

The function of the digestive system is to provide the body with a continuous supply of nutrients and fluid and to remove waste products.

Aging Changes

Many changes that would affect digestive function occur normally in the digestive system of older persons (Table 3-5).

TABLE 3-5. Digestive System

Change	Result
Food passes through the digestive system more slowly The amount and effectiveness of digestive juices are decreased	Constipation: decrease in the frequency of bowel movements; decreased ability to tolerate food or large meals Decrease in specific nutrients being absorbed

Abnormal Signs and Symptoms

- Loss of appetite, food left on tray
- Decrease in bowel movements reported in the resident's record
- Increase in bowel movements, especially if they are watery
- Change in color of bowel movement: bright red (blood), black, green
- Change in texture of bowel movement: watery, sticky, rock-like, slimy, loose
- Foul odor of bowel movement
- Complaints of feeling bloated
- Excessive straining when moving bowels
- Nausea, vomiting, or pain
- Swollen abdomen
- Abdomen feels firm or is tender to touch
- Loss of control of bowels (incontinence)
- Weight loss

Questions to Consider

- Do I know the resident's normal eating habits?
- Do I know the resident's normal bowel pattern?

> Is the resident getting enough exercise, fluid, fiber?
> Is the resident gaining or losing weight?
> Does the resident enjoy meals?
> Should the change be reported to the nurse?
> How does the change affect the resident's well-being?

URINARY SYSTEM

Structures

The urinary system is one of the most important systems in the body because it helps maintain fluid balance (the amount of water in the body) and eliminate liquid wastes. The urinary system is made up of four major structures (Fig. 3-9):

> The right and left kidney maintain the fluid balance of the body by filtering out waste products and producing urine.
> The right and left ureters are tubes that carry urine from the kidneys to the bladder.
> The bladder is a sac-like muscle that stores the urine until it is eliminated.
> The urethra is a tube that carries the urine from the bladder to the outside.

Functions

The urinary system eliminates waste materials from the blood and reabsorbs the proper amount of water and salt.

Aging Changes

Significant changes in the kidneys and bladder gradually occur with normal, healthy aging (Table 3-6).

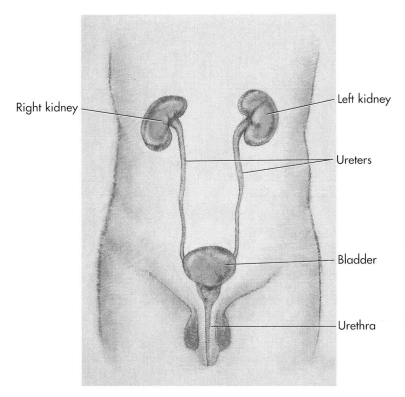

Fig. 3-9.   Structures of the urinary system.

TABLE 3-6.   Urinary System

Change	Result
Decreased size of kidneys	Slowing of kidneys' ability to filter the blood
Decreased bladder capacity	More frequent urination
Decreased muscle tone of the bladder	Decreased ability to empty bladder: residual, left over urine will be present right after urination

Abnormal Signs and Symptoms

▶ Very dark yellow urine
▶ Very small amounts of urine
▶ Bloody or orange urine
▶ Cloudy urine
▶ Complaints of burning or stinging on urination
▶ More frequent urination
▶ Very strong odor in urine
▶ Loss of urine control (incontinence)

Questions to Consider

▶ Is the resident getting adequate fluids?
▶ Are the intake and output equal?
▶ Is the resident emptying the bladder completely?
▶ Is the female resident wiping the urethral area correctly, moving from front (near pubic bone) to back (towards anus)?
▶ Am I responding to call lights fast enough to meet the resident's elimination needs?
▶ Does the resident have good hygiene?
▶ Should the change be reported to the nurse?
▶ How does the change affect the resident's well-being?

NERVOUS SYSTEM
Structures

The nervous system has three major parts (Fig. 3-10):

▶ The brain is located in the protection of the skull. Messages are received and interpreted in the brain, the human body's communication center. Information is processed and stored. All of our thinking, reasoning, and judgment is a function of the brain.
▶ The spinal cord contains nerves that control movement. These extend down the back. It is protected by the spine, or vertebral column.
▶ The nerves are fibers that extend from the spinal column to all parts of the body. The nerves carry messages in both directions between the body and brain: information received from the outside world is processed in the brain, and travels back to the body for a response.

Function

The nervous system is like a communication center. This system helps you make sense out of the world. The nervous system works with the sensory and endocrine systems to direct all the other body systems.

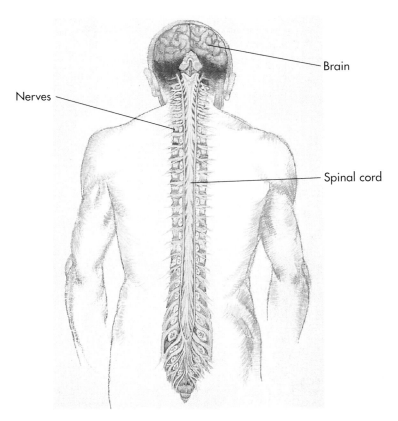

Fig. 3-10. The nervous system has three major parts: the brain, the spinal cord, and the nerves.

Aging Changes

Table 3-7 describes changes in the nervous system that occur gradually with normal aging.

TABLE 3-7.   **Nervous System**

Change	Result
Slowing of nerve impulses	Longer time for residents to learn new information
	Response time to normal situations slows, which may result in injury
Decrease in blood flow to certain areas of the brain	Decrease in short-term memory ability

Abnormal Signs and Symptoms

▷   Loss of interest in learning, confusion, isolation, memory loss
▷   Impatience
▷   Complaints of not remembering where things are
▷   Complaints of not being as quick to react as in the past
▷   Paralysis
▷   Reduced sensation
▷   Involuntary motions
▷   Tremors

▶ Unsteady walking
▶ Speech problems

Questions to Consider

▶ Have I reinforced recently learned behavior?
▶ Do I take every opportunity to go over new information with the resident?
▶ Is the resident able to move without assistance?
▶ Does the resident have any tremors or weakness?
▶ Is the resident steady on his or her feet?
▶ Should the change be reported to the nurse?
▶ How does the change affect the resident's well-being?

ENDOCRINE SYSTEM
Structures

The endocrine system includes many different glands. Glands are organs that make and release substances called hormones, which keep organs working correctly. The parts of the endocrine system are (Fig. 3-11A and 3-11B):

▶ The pituitary gland, located in the brain, secretes hormones and regulates other glands such as the ovaries and testes. It is often called the "master gland."
▶ The adrenal glands, located on top of the kidneys, secrete hormones that regulate metabolism. They also help regulate sodium, water, and potassium in the body. Adrenal glands release hormones that increase blood sugar, control blood vessel constriction, and help us to react in emergency situations.
▶ Cells called the Isles of Langerhans, located in the pancreas, secrete insulin, which controls the breakdown of carbohydrates (sugars) in the body.
▶ The thyroid and parathyroid glands located in the neck secrete hormones that help regulate metabolism, the ability to produce energy.
▶ The female ovaries, located in the pelvic area, secrete hormones controlling sexual function and involved in becoming pregnant.
▶ The male testes or testicles, located in a sac behind the penis, secrete a hormone controlling sexual function and sperm production.

Functions

The endocrine system makes hormones that help the body work properly. Some vital functions of these hormones are the regulation of body energy, the breakdown of sugar for energy, and the ability to have children.

Aging Changes

Table 3-8 describes some of the changes in the endocrine system as a person ages.

TABLE 3-8. Endocrine System

Change	Result
Glands slow down the rate of releasing hormones	This change affects blood studies in the resident, but should not affect the overall health of the resident
Decrease in insulin production	The body takes longer to process sugar; there may be a reduction in energy
Dramatic decrease in the amount of hormones produced by the ovaries	Monthly menstrual cycles will stop, along with the ability to have children. This process is known as menopause
Male hormone production will decrease but not stop	May decrease sexual response

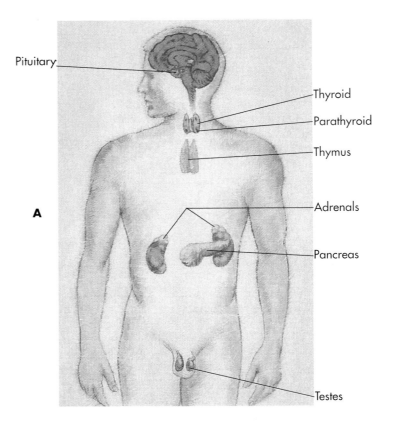

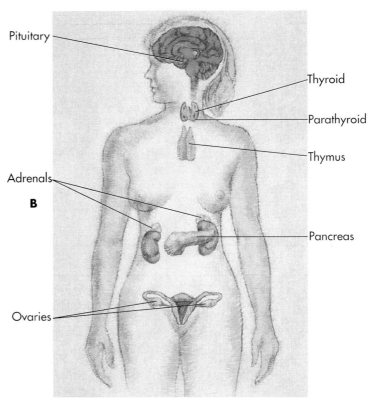

Fig. 3-11.   A, The endocrine system of the male. B, The endocrine system of the female.

Abnormal Signs and Symptoms

▷ Excessive thirst (drinking large amounts of fluids)
▷ Dramatic increase in urine output
▷ Increase in the amount of food eaten
▷ Complaints of feeling tired or cold

Questions to Consider

▷ Has there been a dramatic increase in the resident's requests for water?
▷ Is the resident going to the bathroom more than normally?
▷ Have I seen the resident eating lots of food?
▷ Is the resident lethargic?
▷ Should the change be reported to the nurse?
▷ How does the change affect the resident's well-being?

SENSORY SYSTEM

The organs of the sensory system are the eyes, nose, ears, tongue, and skin. The sensory system gives us information from the world outside the body. The senses receive and send information to the brain. Aging influences the function of the senses. Sight and hearing are most commonly affected by aging.

The Eye
Structure

The eye is a round ball with several major structures (Fig. 3-12):
▷ The sclera is the "white" of the eye.
▷ The iris is the "color" of the eye and helps regulate the amount of light that enters the eye by controlling the size of the pupil.
▷ The cornea protects the iris.
▷ The retina is the back of the eye, where light images become nerve impulses to the brain. The brain interprets the impulses into pictures for processing.
▷ The lens, along with the iris, helps direct light to the retina.
▷ The pupil is the opening through which light passes to get to the retina.

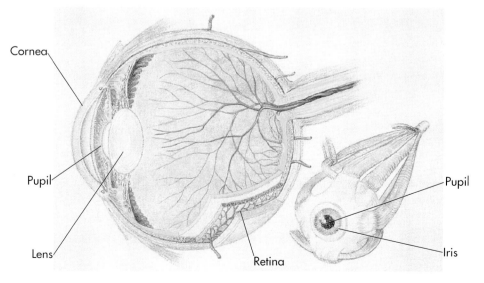

Fig. 3-12. Structures of the eye.

Function

Sight gives us knowledge about our surroundings that is important in being able to care for ourselves.

Aging Changes

The changes in the eye with age are described in Table 3-9.

TABLE 3-9.　Sensory System: The Eye

Change	Result
Lens becomes flattened	Decreased ability to focus at normal reading distances
Lens becomes more yellow	Greens and blues are difficult to see, reds and oranges easier to see
Lens becomes more rigid	Objects can only be seen clearly at a greater distance
The pupil size becomes smaller	Because less light reaches the inner eye, it is more difficult to see in the dark or in poorly lit areas

Abnormal Signs and Symptoms

▶ Discharge from the eyes
▶ Excessive watering
▶ Inability to find things, bumping into things
▶ Complaints of not being able to see well, inability to focus clearly, or burning
▶ Complaints of eye pain

Questions to Consider

▶ Does the resident have enough light?
▶ Is the resident wearing eyeglasses? Are they clean and the correct prescription?
▶ Am I leaving things where the resident can find them?
▶ Am I addressing the resident directly?
▶ Is the resident concerned about loss of sight?
▶ Is the resident having trouble distinguishing colors?
▶ Should the change be reported to the nurse?
▶ How does the change affect the resident's well-being?

The Ear
Structure

The ear has three areas (Fig. 3-13):
▶ The inner ear
▶ The middle ear
▶ The outer ear

Each area has special structures related to hearing. Sound enters the outer ear and is transmitted through the middle ear to the inner ear. Nerve impulses from the sound go from the inner ear to the brain for interpretation. Special structures inside the ear also help the body maintain its balance. If these structures are not working properly, a resident may feel dizzy.

Function

The ear lets us hear. Hearing, like vision, helps us to be aware of the world around us, giving clues to danger as well as pleasure.

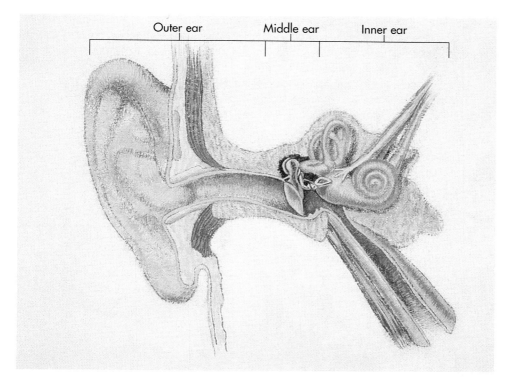

Fig. 3-13. The ear consists of three areas: the inner ear, the middle ear, and the outer ear.

Aging Changes

There are two main changes in the ear with age (Table 3-10).

TABLE 3-10. Sensory System: The Ear

Change	Result
Hearing structures of the ear become stiff	Loss of hearing of high-frequency sounds
Soft wax production decreases	Hard, dry wax builds up in the ears and can cause a hearing loss

Abnormal Signs and Symptoms

▷ Isolation or anger
▷ Discharge from the ear
▷ Continual tugging or scratching of the ear
▷ The resident yells when talking
▷ The television or radio is very loud
▷ Ringing in ears
▷ Dizziness or unsteadiness

Questions to Consider

▷ Am I speaking directly to the resident?
▷ Am I lowering the tone of my voice?
▷ Am I speaking clearly?

▷ Are the resident's ears being checked for wax?
▷ Is the resident using a hearing aid? Is it clean and operating properly? Does the resident know how to use the hearing aid? Is the battery working?
▷ Does the resident avoid group activities?
▷ Is the resident withdrawing or seeming fearful?
▷ Should the change be reported to the nurse?
▷ How does the change affect the resident's well-being?

The Other Senses
Aging Changes

Table 3-11 lists changes that occur in the other senses as a person ages.

TABLE 3-11.   **Sensory System: The Other Senses**

Change	Result
Smell	
The ability to identify or detect odors decreases with age, more commonly in men than in women	Resident may not be able to detect harmful odors, like chemicals or smoke from a fire
Taste	
There may be a decrease in the ability to taste salt and sweet tastes	Resident may request more seasoned foods
Touch	
Decreased sensitivity in the skin of the hands	Resident may not be able to tell how hot items are, which could cause a burn

Abnormal Signs and Symptoms

▷ Inability to taste or smell food, or complaints that the food is bland
▷ Burns on skin

Questions to Consider

▷ Does the resident like the type of food served?
▷ Is water temperature adjusted correctly?
▷ Is the resident checking water temperature with the inner part of his or her wrist?
▷ Should the change be reported to the nurse?
▷ How does the change affect the resident's well-being?

REPRODUCTIVE SYSTEM
Structures
Male

The main structures of the male reproductive system are (Fig. 3-14):
▷ The penis is used for sexual intercourse and urination.
▷ The testes are two oval-shaped glands that manufacture sperm cells. The testes are sometimes called the sex glands or gonads, and produce the male sex hormone testosterone.
▷ The scrotum is the sac holding the testes outside the body.
▷ The prostate gland secretes one of the fluids in semen. Semen is produced by the seminal vesicle.

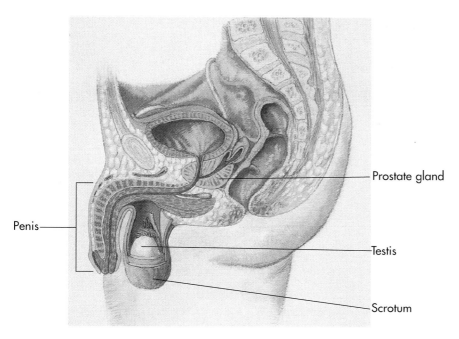

Fig. 3-14. Male reproductive system.

Female

The main structures of the female reproductive system are (Fig. 3-15):

▶ The fallopian tubes are two tubes that carry the egg cells from the ovaries to the uterus.

▶ The ovaries are two almond-shaped glands located in the pelvis. The ovaries hold the eggs and produce hormones called estrogen and progesterone.

▶ The uterus is the muscular organ that holds the fetus during pregnancy and sheds its lining during menstruation.

▶ The vagina is the muscular canal used for sexual intercourse, childbirth, and passage of menstrual flow.

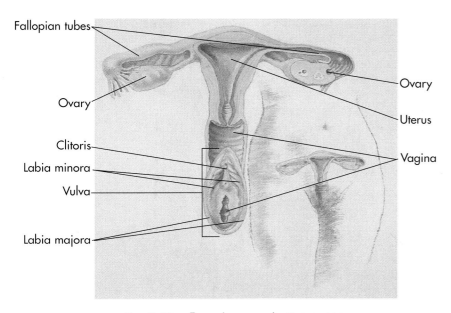

Fig. 3-15. Female reproductive system.

▶ The vulva is the external structure of the female sex organs. It is made up of the labia majora and minora, which are the skin flaps located on either side of the vagina, and the clitoris, which gives sexual pleasure to females.

Functions

The reproductive system provides sexual pleasure and the reproduction of human life.

Aging Changes

Table 3-12 describes the changes that occur in the reproductive system as a person ages.

TABLE 3-12. Reproductive System

Change	Result
Dramatic decrease in the amount of hormones produced by the ovaries	Monthly menstrual cycles will stop, along with the ability to have children.
Decrease in vaginal lubrication	Dryness in vaginal walls
Male hormone production will decrease but not stop	May decrease sexual response

Abnormal Signs and Symptoms

▶ Foul smelling discharge from vagina or penis
▶ Vaginal itching
▶ Bleeding
▶ Difficulty with sexual intercourse
▶ Mood changes

Questions to Consider

▶ Have I considered the resident's need for physical intimacy?
▶ Have I considered the resident's need for privacy?
▶ Should the change be reported to the nurse?
▶ How does the change affect the resident's well-being?

4

THE ROLE OF A NURSE ASSISTANT

Nurse assistants work in long term care for many reasons. Some want to become nurses, and working as a nurse assistant is great experience for future employment. Others like working with the elderly. Many have cared for family members in their homes and want to continue to care for others. What are your own reasons? You should answer that question for yourself. Your understanding of your own reasons will help you think about your role, ask for guidance from other staff members, plan for your continuing education, and keep you motivated.

For example, if you plan to become a registered nurse, you may pay more attention to the relationship between nurse assistants and the charge nurse. You may choose to develop skills to include in your style as a nurse assistant and later as an R.N. If you love to learn about people, you can ask questions about a resident's past experiences while providing care. Learning about a resident's past helps you learn about who he or she is now. The key is to understand your own special reasons for working as a nurse assistant. This key will help unlock many opportunities for you as a nurse assistant (Fig. 4-1).

This chapter introduces you to the roles of a nurse assistant in long term care. It has three sections:

▷ *Providing Care:* Here you will learn about the philosophy of caregiving and how to develop a trusting relationship. You will learn how values and culture influence care you give.

▷ *Job Functions:* This section includes a typical nurse assistant job description. You will learn your responsibilities and tasks for the care you will give.

▷ *Taking Care of Yourself:* Here you will learn about managing stress, ethics, assertiveness, and getting feedback.

PROVIDING CARE

What does it mean to provide care? Everyone has his or her own style of caregiving. As a nurse assistant, you will develop your personal caregiving style.

Nurse assistants assist with about 80 percent of all residents' care. Other team members help guide this care. For example, physicians write orders for specific treatments, and the charge nurse shows you how to follow these and the plan of care. Yet you have more contact with residents than any other member of the health care team. You will be closer to each resident than anyone else in the facility. This is a very privileged position.

If you (or someone you love) were ill, how would you want to be cared for? If you were with one person more than anyone else, what would you want that person to be like? This person, the person you rely on the most, is usually the nurse assistant. The best way to think about how to care for residents is to think about how you would like to be treated as a human being and as a customer of a service, as you learned in Chapter 2.

Providing the Best Care Possible

You have already learned that a long term care facility is a place where people live and receive organized care. The care you give should involve balancing the science (skills) of nursing, which is the task you must perform, and the art of caregiving, your personal caregiving style (Fig. 4-2). These two must go hand in hand. Without either, you can not provide quality care.

For example, a nurse assistant who focuses only on skills may be efficient, but also may seem cold and uncaring. A nurse assistant who focuses only on the art of caregiving may be caring and compassionate, but may be slow and inefficient. Both skill and art are important in themselves, but if you balance both you will be the best caregiver. Then you will be caring for residents in a thoughtful, efficient way—mindfully.

You can often balance skill and caregiving by doing both at the same time. Below are two examples of this:

▶ While helping Mrs. Smith prepare for breakfast, you ask about her plans for the day. Ask her how she's feeling, what she would like to wear today, and if she is expecting any visitors. You show you care about Mrs. Smith as much as about getting your job done.

▶ Mr. Wong is sitting in his chair while you make his bed. You say something like, "While I'm making the bed, why don't you tell me about your children who came to visit last night?" If it is evident to Mr. Wong that you are really listening and truly interested while making the bed, he will feel that you are paying attention to him (Fig. 4-3).

While you do your day-to-day duties, remember to act mindfully and balance the science of nursing with the art of caregiving. This will help you give the best care possible.

Mindful Caregiving

What is mindful caregiving? It means paying attention to details, looking at situations openly, being observant, and mostly, being willing to change. When you are

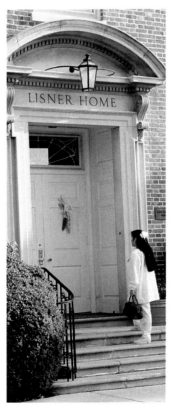

Fig. 4-1. Understanding your own reasons for choosing work as a nurse assistant will provide you with many opportunities.

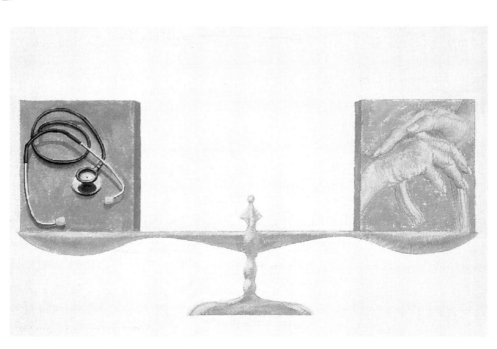

Fig. 4-2. Providing quality care requires a balance of the science of nursing and the art of caregiving.

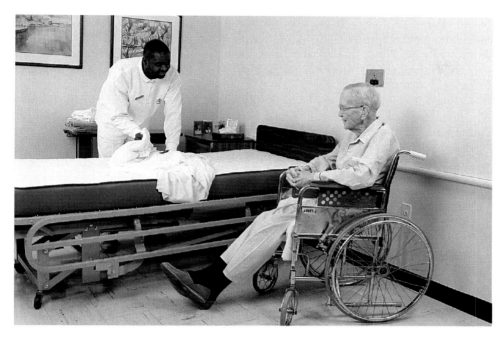

Fig. 4-3. Listening while making the bed gives balance to skill and caregiving at the same time.

caring every day for the same residents, you may start to expect that everything will always be the same. Your actions might become automatic, with poor results. Consider the following situation:

You have been caring for Mr. Jones for the last month. You know he likes to eat breakfast, then shave, and then bathe and dress. Every day is the same. Today, you go in to get his breakfast tray and prepare his shaving supplies. Later, you return to put away his shaving equipment and start preparing for his shower. You help him take his shower and dress. Then suddenly you notice that he did not shave.

Today, Mr. Jones found that his son was very ill and had been admitted to a hospital. He is so unhappy that he did not bother to eat or shave. You mindlessly assumed that today was the same as every other day. You didn't even notice at first that he hadn't eaten his breakfast or shaved and that he was quieter than usual. You are the person Mr. Jones spends the most time with. To Mr. Jones, you are a friend, but today you were so busy, or mindless, you didn't even notice him. How would you feel if the person you spend most of your time with didn't notice your unhappiness? You might feel that person doesn't care for you after all. See why you should not let routine activities become routine?

In a long term care facility, you will care for a number of residents. You must pay close attention to all your actions. Let's look at the case of Mr. Jones again. One of your daily goals is to help Mr. Jones shave. What should you have noticed that would tell you something was wrong?

In this situation, you had two opportunities to notice something was wrong. First, the change in Mr. Jones's eating habits should have made you question: "Mr. Jones, you didn't eat your breakfast today. Is there something wrong?" If you missed this, you should have noticed that Mr. Jones, who usually cares how he looks, didn't shave. Simply paying attention to the process of a resident's routine and noticing any changes in that routine can help you be a better caregiver by picking up signals when something is wrong. This is part of mindful caregiving.

You could also miss important signs and symptoms by not paying attention as you go about your job. Consider the same example. Mr. Jones might have skipped his breakfast and shaving because he was feeling ill rather than depressed. If you did not really look at him but just automatically removed his tray and shaving equipment, you would miss that he was flushed and his skin felt hot. This information is very important and should be reported right away. Mr. Jones could have a serious infection.

In both situations, you missed important signals from this resident. In the first, Mr. Jones needed you to listen to him, and in the second, to notice his condition and report it.

Being mindful when you provide care and never letting routine care, such as eating, bathing, and dressing, become "routine" helps prevent this situation (Fig. 4-4). Residents have a right for you to meet their needs. A nurse assistant who mindlessly cares for residents strips residents of their independence and dignity and misses important clues and signals.

Understanding Residents' Routines

Nurse assistants often ask, "How do I know what a resident likes or dislikes?" One of your responsibilities is to understand how residents and their families want to be cared for.

The best way to learn about residents is by asking questions (Fig. 4-5). You can ask a resident, family, and other health care workers (especially the charge nurse). You can also review residents' care plans and medical records to learn more about their preferences. Below are questions you can ask residents:

1. How do you like to begin your day?
2. Do you like to be up and ready for breakfast?
3. How do you like to bathe?
4. What do you need help with?
5. What can I do to help make you more comfortable?
6. What do you do in your spare time? Read? Watch television? Walk? Visit with friends?

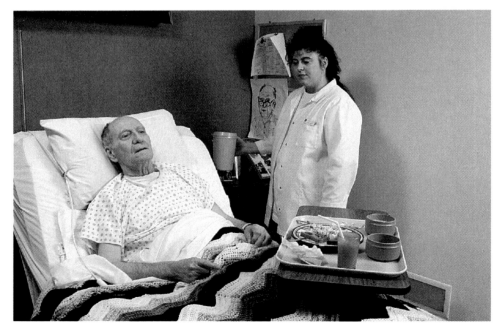

Fig. 4-4. Always be attentive to the resident's needs. Don't allow care to become "routine." Residents have a right to the best care you can give.

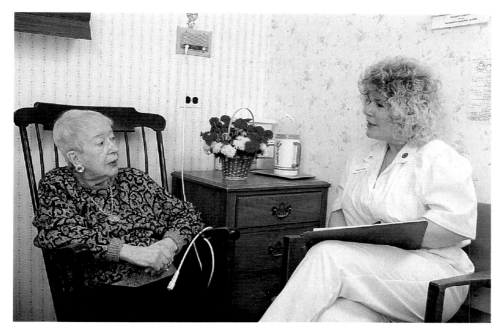

Fig. 4-5. Learning about residents can help you understand how they want to be cared for.

7. Describe the typical kind of day you like.
8. Do you like to nap during the day?
9. What gives you the most trouble when dressing?
10. How much would you like me to help with your personal care?

Try to think of other questions you would want asked by someone trying to learn about you. With such questions, you learn that all residents have their own preferences for their care. Every resident you ask may want to be treated respectfully, but each may define "respect" differently. For example, one resident feels that privacy is very important and that questions about his or her family are disrespectful. Another may want you to be interested in his or her family. Remember, no two people are the same. Everyone has different habits, beliefs, and wishes.

Asking questions is important also as you and residents work together to create a daily routine. Routines are patterns of activities you and each resident establish individually, including dressing, bathing, and grooming. Think about your own morning routine. Do you drink coffee first, or brush your teeth, or take a shower? You probably have your own routine that you've followed for years. Now think about times when your routine has been disrupted. The coffee maker is broken, or you missed your bus, or one of your children is sick. At such times you realize what a comfort your personal routine is. The same is true for residents. They too like to do certain things at certain times of the day and in certain ways. Remember that a change in routine can be very disruptive and upsetting. You may think it's easier if you set the routine for residents, but that would take away their individuality and their choice. Routines relate to residents' personalities and should be an individual matter.

Values and Culture

Values are beliefs people have about what is important or of value to them. Values guide people in choosing how to live their lives. Everyone's values are individual and very personal. Values come from a person's family, religion, friends, education, and individual experience. Following are examples of values:

- Being healthy and active
- Respecting authority, parents, teachers, policemen
- Being able to take care of oneself
- Making a lot of money
- Practicing religious beliefs
- Being useful
- Having close friends

Try to understand the values of each resident you care for. Although this takes time, it's worth it. Residents' values help you understand what gives meaning to their lives and why they act as they do. For instance, a resident who doesn't visit with other residents or take part in social events may value privacy over friendships. You may feel the person is lonely because you would be lonely if you spent so much time alone. But that reflects your own values, not this resident's. A resident may simply enjoy his or her time alone.

To learn a resident's values, ask questions like these:

- What is important to you?
- What did you do for a living?
- Did you do a special kind of work?
- Did you go to religious services?
- Is family important to you?

Sometimes a resident's values may be very different from the values of his or her friends or family members, your own values, or society's (Fig. 4-6). This does not mean one person's values are right and another's wrong. Values are not right or wrong.

A strong influence on values is our culture. Culture involves the customary beliefs, social forms, and material traits of a racial, religious, or social group. Culture influences one's food preferences, personal care practices, clothing choices, and family relationships. For example, in some cultures, a "laying on of hands" is believed to cure illness. Some cultures expect women to dress in a certain way. Other cultures have rituals for personal care, such as cutting hair or bathing. Remember that your own values and culture might influence the care you give, just as residents' values and culture affect their preferences for care. Instead of acting only on your own values and culture, learn each resident's values to provide quality care for that resident.

Ethics

There are no right or wrong values, although sometimes a decision must be made that favors one value over another. A decision involving values is a matter of ethics. Ethics is the study of good and bad, right and wrong, and moral duty. Ethical dilemmas often concern how someone values quality of life. One may value life in various ways and make different ethical decisions based on those values, as in the examples in Table 4-1.

Most decisions about care do not involve conflicting values. A resident and family usually make ethical decisions about care along with the physician without a conflict of values.

Developing Trust

It takes time to learn about residents. Some openly tell you who they are and what they like and don't like. Others are slow to share this with you. You should develop a trusting respectful relationship with all residents, but for some this takes a little longer. Trust is the basis for any relationship. A relationship cannot grow without trust. To develop a trusting relationship with a resident, follow these guidelines:

- Make sure residents feel safe. Support them when walking. Help them when they ask you. Answer their call bells.

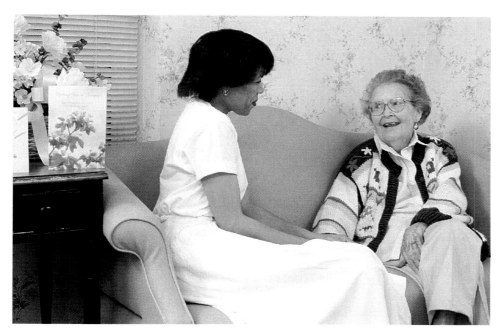

Fig. 4-6. Understanding a resident's values may explain why they might act a certain way.

TABLE 4-1. Examples of ethical decisions based on individual values.

Value	Ethical Decision
Life is worth living only when one has the hope of being able to take care of oneself.	To choose not to be resuscitated if a cardiac arrest should occur, if one is bedridden with severe contractures and is in much pain To choose not to have a feeding tube if one can no longer eat To choose to remain in the facility if seriously ill and not be moved to a hospital
Life is worth living no matter whether there is hope of ever taking care of oneself.	To choose to be resuscitated if a cardiac arrest should occur, regardless of one's functional ability or amount of pain To choose to have a feeding tube if one can no longer eat To choose to go to the hospital for treatment of a serious life-threatening illness

▷ Listen to what residents want you to do and how they want things done and follow their exact instructions.

▷ Be clear about what you can and cannot do for residents.

▷ Be courteous at all times.

▷ Be honest and open with residents. If a resident calls you for assistance when you are on your way to help another, ask if he or she can wait 10 minutes until you finish helping the other. If the resident can wait, be sure to come back in 10 minutes as you promised. Always be reliable.

▷ Be consistent. Assist each resident with A.M. care at the same time each day based on each resident's preferences. Remind residents who you are by giving

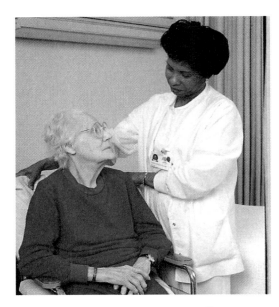

Fig. 4-7. Treating all residents with respect will increase resident satisfaction.

your name and saying what you're going to do. Treat each resident respectfully (Fig. 4-7).

▶ Dress professionally. Dressing well conveys your respect for residents. Being well dressed also helps residents feel that if you do a good job of taking care of yourself, you will also do a good job of taking care of them.

An important part of gaining a person's trust is keeping his or her confidence. When caring for and talking with a resident, you learn many personal things about him or her. You must keep this information confidential. Do not talk about residents with other residents or with anyone not connected with a residents' care.

If you feel uncomfortable or embarrassed about certain kinds of care (like assisting with toileting), tell the charge nurse about your feelings. You may even talk with residents, who may have the same feelings as you. If you do not discuss your feelings openly, you may send mixed messages to a resident. For example, when a resident asks for assistance with toileting, you may frown even though you try to answer positively, and the resident will see this. Work to overcome feelings of discomfort or embarrassment to avoid reacting in ways that hurt the trusting relationship you are building with residents. More about nonverbal communication is covered in Chapter 6, Communication.

JOB DESCRIPTION

As a nurse assistant, you are a member of the nursing team. You work closely with other nurse assistants and the charge nurse. Chapter 11, Working with the Nursing Staff, covers in detail these relationships.

Your facility usually gives you its personnel policies, including your job description. This is usually a description including the following information:

▶ Department
▶ Title
▶ Overview of the job
▶ List of responsibilities
▶ Specific functions
▶ Qualifications

Carefully read your facility's job description for nurse assistants. You can then discuss with your charge nurse any questions or concerns you may have.

NURSE ASSISTANT JOB DESCRIPTION

Department:_____

Date of Hire:_____

GENERAL PURPOSE:

To perform nonprofessional direct patient care duties under the supervision of nursing personnel and to assist in maintaining a positive physical, social, and psychological environment for the residents.

QUALIFICATIONS:

▶ State Registered Nurse Assistant in good standing according to all applicable federal and state certification requirements or in training to become a State Registered Nurse Assistant.

▶ At least 18 years of age.

▶ Ability to read, write, and follow oral and written directions, and have successfully completed elementary education.

▶ Speak and understand English.

▶ Have positive attitude toward the elderly.

ESSENTIAL JOB FUNCTIONS

A. PERSONAL CARE FUNCTIONS

Duties:

Assist residents with daily bath; dressing; grooming; dental care; bowel and bladder functions; preparation for medical tests and exams; ear and eye care; and positioning in and out of beds, chairs, bathtubs, etc.

Physical and Sensory Requirements:

Walking; reaching; bending; lifting; grasping; fine hand coordination; pushing and pulling; and ability to distinguish smells, tastes, and temperatures.

B. NURSING CARE FUNCTIONS

Duties:

Provide nursing functions as directed by supervisor, including daily perineal care; catheter care; change dressings; turn residents in bed; sponge baths; measure and record temperature, pulse, and respirations; weigh and measure residents; perform restorative and rehabilitative procedures and observe and report presence of skin breakdowns; review care plans daily; report changes in resident conditions to supervisor; and record all necessary charting entries and report all accidents and incidents.

Physical and Sensory Requirements:

Bending; lifting; grasping; fine hand coordination; ability to communicate with residents; ability to distinguish smells, tastes, and temperatures; and ability to hear and respond to resident pages.

C. FOOD SERVICE FUNCTIONS

Duties:

Prepare residents for meals and snacks, identify food arrangement and assist in feeding residents as needed, record food and fluid intake, and perform after-meal resident care.

Physical and Sensory Requirements:

Lifting; grasping; fine hand coordination; ability to distinguish smells, tastes, and temperatures; and ability to write or otherwise record intake.

D. RESIDENTS' RIGHTS FUNCTIONS

Duties:

Maintain resident confidentiality; treat residents with kindness, dignity, and respect; know and comply with Residents' Rights rules; and promptly report all resident complaints, accidents, and incidents to supervisor.

Continued.

CDC ? ᵒ

NURSE ASSISTANT JOB DESCRIPTION—cont'd

Physical and Sensory Requirements:

Ability to communicate with residents and ability to remain calm under stress.

OTHER JOB FUNCTIONS

A. SUPPORT FUNCTIONS

Duties:

Assist as directed in proper admission, transfer, and discharge of residents; inventory resident possessions and report food articles and medications found in resident rooms; and report defective equipment to administration.

Physical and Sensory Requirements:

Ability to communicate with residents and ability to read and write in English.

B. SAFETY AND SANITATION FUNCTIONS

Duties:

Understand and use CDC Universal Precautions, OSHA Blood Borne Pathogen Standard, and follow established infection control, hazardous communication, and other safety rules; ensure cleanliness of assigned residents' rooms; properly maintain and record resident restraints; and promptly report all violations of safety and sanitation rules to supervisor.

Physical and Sensory Requirements:

Walking, bending, lifting, grasping, fine hand coordination, ability to read and write, and ability to distinguish smells.

C. STAFF DEVELOPMENT FUNCTIONS

Duties:

Attend and participate in orientation, training, educational activities, and staff meetings.

Physical and Sensory Requirements:

Ability to understand and apply training and in-service education.

D. ALL OTHER DUTIES AS ASSIGNED

I understand this job description and its requirements; I understand that this is not an exclusive list of the job functions and that I am expected o complete all duties as assigned; I understand the job functions may be altered by management without notice; I understand that this job description in no way constitutes an employment agreement and that I am an at-will employee.

_____
Date

_____
Employee

_____
Supervisor

Be sure you understand your job responsibilities and what is expected of you every day. Learn the typical 24-hour routine in the facility to understand what happens during each shift: the day shift (usually 7 a.m. to 3:30 p.m.), evening shift (3 to 11:30 p.m.), and night shift (11 p.m. to 7:30 a.m.). In all, care is provided to residents 24 hours a day, 7 days a week, all year.

Your responsibilities to residents and your employer include the following:
1. Recognize residents as individuals:
   ▶ Find out residents' likes and dislikes.
   ▶ Ask how they want things done. Get to know their routine.
   ▶ Learn about residents' cultures.

▶ Find out if they have cultural preferences related to their care, and follow their preferences.

2. Promote autonomy (self-determination):
   ▶ Be knowledgeable of residents' rights.
   ▶ Be sure to respect residents' rights when giving care.
   ▶ Encourage residents to maintain their optimal level of functioning.
   ▶ Support residents' choices in personal care (Fig. 4-8).
   ▶ Encourage residents' participation in all decisions about their care.
   ▶ Maintain privacy.

3. Provide mindful caregiving:
   ▶ Balance skills and the art of caregiving (Fig. 4-9).
   ▶ Observe residents closely.
   ▶ Watch for any changes in residents' attitude or behavior.
   ▶ Encourage and support residents to determine their routines.
   ▶ Report any changes to the charge nurse.

4. Be a good employee:
   ▶ Be reliable.
   ▶ Be healthy: get enough sleep, eat a balanced diet, exercise.
   ▶ Be considerate of others.
   ▶ Cooperate with other team members.
   ▶ Be efficient with your time and supplies.
   ▶ Follow all personnel policies.
   ▶ Dress appropriately: neat and clean.
   ▶ Pay attention to personal hygiene.
   ▶ Do not use drugs or drink alcohol during work hours or before coming to work.

Tasks Nurse Assistants Commonly Perform

Assisting with personal care for residents:
▶ Bathing
▶ Oral hygiene

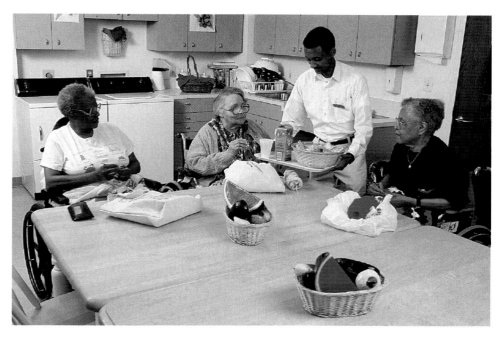

Fig. 4-8. Respecting residents' rights includes supporting their personal choices.

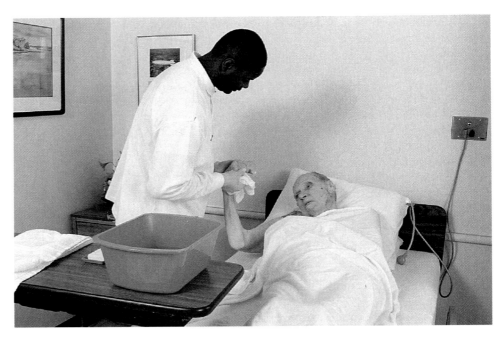

Fig. 4-9. In providing the best service to the resident, balance the art of caregiving with nurse assisting skills.

▶ Grooming (hair and nail care)
▶ Dressing and undressing
Assisting residents with mobility (Fig. 4-10)
▶ Walking
▶ Positioning
▶ Range-of-motion exercises
Assisting residents with meals:
▶ Transporting to dining room
▶ Preparing the environment
▶ Preparing residents
▶ Feeding residents
Providing comfort to residents:
▶ Back rubs
▶ Fluffing pillows
▶ Holding hands (if a resident desires)
▶ Gentle touches (if a resident desires)
Providing emotional support for residents:
▶ Listening carefully
▶ Working with family
▶ Holding a resident (if he or she desires)
▶ Being with residents when bad news is given
▶ Sharing experiences
Maintaining each resident's environment:
▶ Practicing infection control procedures
▶ Cleaning residents' rooms
▶ Making residents' beds
▶ Preventing injuries (Fig. 4-11)

TAKING CARE OF YOURSELF

To do your job well, you need to feel well. This means taking care of yourself both physically and emotionally. Your work can be very demanding at times. You

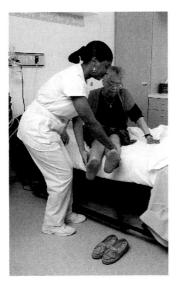

Fig. 4-10. Help residents maintain mobility.

may feel you have too much to do and residents demand too much. You may feel stress.

Coping with Stress

Sometimes coping with stress is difficult. In addition to demands at work, you may have personal concerns about your children, your spouse, money, or many other things. Following are some ways to cope with stress:

▶ Make a list of what you need to do, starting with what is most important, and cross off each item as you finish.

▶ Explain to a resident if you are not able to fully listen to him or her by saying something like, "Mr. Jones, I want to hear what you are saying, but right now I have a lot to do. May I come back a little later? Let's set a time."

▶ Make time daily to do something relaxing for yourself, like reading, taking a walk, or spending time with a friend.

▶ Talk to a friend or spouse about your feelings and stresses. It always feels good to know someone understands you or has gone through the same problems.

In cases of extreme stress, such as stress caused by a death in your family, marital separation, or any situation when you feel stress is interfering with your work, discuss your situation with your supervisor. If necessary, ask for a leave of absence.

Coping with Your Emotions

Some residents you care for may become like family, and if they get sick, move home, or die, you may feel sad and miss them. To help you cope with your feelings, you may want to:

▶ Talk about your feelings with co-workers or your family.

▶ Take some time to think about why you miss that person and what he or she meant to you.

▶ Let yourself feel sad. This is a normal reaction to the death of someone you care about.

▶ Sometimes when you're feeling sad or stressed, you need to walk away from the situation, or be alone to cry or scream.

In your job you will not have to decide about resuscitating residents, starting tube feeding, or sending residents to the hospital. Even so, you will feel whether these things should be done or not, based on your own values. Sometimes you may be uncomfortable with a decision or feel it is wrong. To manage your feelings of discomfort, you can:

▶ Talk to your supervisor, who may give you information that helps you better understand the decision (Fig. 4-12).

▶ Talk to your minister, priest, or rabbi about your feelings.

▶ Remember that although you need to talk about your feelings about a situation, each resident also has a right to privacy. Once the decision has been made, do not try to talk a resident into changing his or her mind.

Evaluating Your Work: Learning to Grow

How do you know you're doing everything that needs to be done? You need feedback from residents, their families, co-workers, and your supervisor about your work. Feedback tells you much about how well you are doing. It helps you improve your work, and it lets you know when you're doing a good job.

Supervisors often consider questions like the following when deciding how good a job a nurse assistant is doing:

▶ Does the nurse assistant complete all the work assigned?

▶ Does the nurse assistant ask questions?

▶ Do all residents that the nurse assistant is caring for state that they are comfortable?

▶ Does the nurse assistant check on all residents frequently?

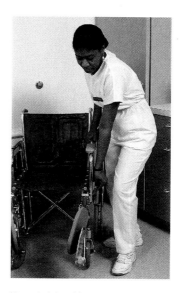

Fig. 4-11. Maintaining each resident's environment, such as locking the wheelchair, will help prevent injury.

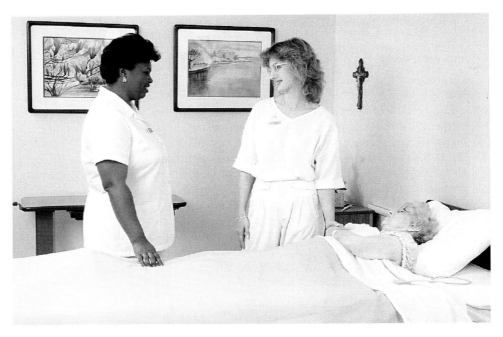

Fig. 4-12. Communicate with your supervisor any concerns you may have.

▷ Does the certified nurse assistant report changes in residents immediately?
▷ How do the certified nurse assistant's co-workers feel about the nurse assistant's work?
▷ Is the nurse assistant a team player?
▷ How do residents and their families respond to the nurse assistant?

If you find yourself feeling that you could do a better job, talk with your supervisor, and ask questions like these:

▷ "Did you check my work today? How did I do?"
▷ "Can I show you how I do this, to see if it's the best way?"
▷ "I seem to have a problem in this area. Can you help me?"

Open communication with other staff helps you grow as a nurse assistant. You will feel more satisfied with your work if you seek feedback. Check with residents also. Ask questions like these: "Have I met all your needs? Is there anything else I can do for you?" Ask family members if they see improvement in the resident. Do they like the schedule you and the resident have worked out for routine care and other activities?

Most important, accept the feedback you get positively. Change what you can, and get help in more difficult areas.

Assertiveness: How to Accomplish What You Think Is Important

Assertive behavior is taking steps to do what you think is important without hurting other people. You are assertive when you speak up for yourself or say no when asked to do something you don't feel comfortable with. In your work you need to communicate assertively every day. You need to be assertive to do what is best for both residents and yourself. Do you ask for what you want, instead of expecting others to read your mind? Can you say no without feeling guilty if someone asks you to do something you can't do? Do you look for solutions to problems instead of complaining about them (Fig. 4-13)? These are types of assertive behavior. Being assertive is different from being aggressive. Aggressive behavior hurts other people or makes them angry, and you usually don't accomplish what is important.

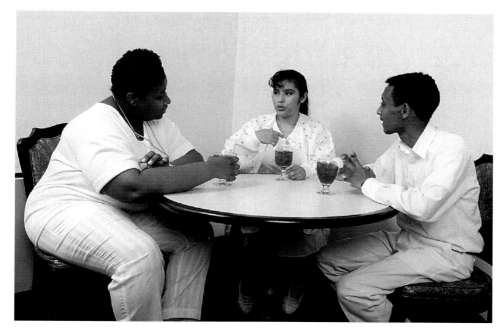

Fig. 4-13. Sharing your thoughts with other staff members and looking for solutions to problems are good examples of assertive behavior.

However, you are being passive if you don't say anything at all, keeping your feelings and needs inside. If you do not speak up for yourself, you miss opportunities. For example, you are asked by the charge nurse to do a task you have not been taught. The following are three different responses.

Assertively you would say, "I am not familiar with that skill. If you show me how, maybe I can do it the next time."

Passively you would say something such as, "If you really want me to, I will try to do it."

Aggressively you might say, "No way. That's not my job."

Remember also that, even if you act assertively, you still may not get what you want. Others may still say no. Your supervisor may not let you work on another shift, or a resident may not want your help. The important thing is to stand up for yourself and be responsible for seeking what is important to you.

5

WORKING WITH FAMILY

Have you heard the expression, "You can attract more flies with honey than with vinegar?" It means being kind and positive is more successful than being brusque and negative. This old saying still holds true. Think about how every day you interact with many people. The quality of our relationships with others depends much on how well we interact and work together. Think about how you like others to treat you. Don't you respond more favorably to someone who is kind and considerate? How do you react when someone is demanding or rude, or ignores you?

In the same way you need to work well with a resident's significant others. These are the family members and others most important to a resident. How you relate to them reflects your caregiving and the facility as a whole. Being friendly, caring, and professional helps you gain the family's trust and begins a positive relationship. Being defensive or cold, however, hinders the relationship. How you treat a resident's family shows your respect not only for the family but for the resident. It also shows your commitment to TQM. You can work more effectively with family if you are genuinely pleasant with them. Family are also considered customers.

You will spend a lot of time with residents' significant others. Consider them members of the health care team. Often they know the resident best and can give you valuable information and guidance to help in your caregiving (Fig. 5-1).

This chapter discusses how the loved one's moving into the facility impacts family and friends. You will also learn how to help these others cope by involving them in care activities.

WHAT IS FAMILY?

People are an important part of our lives. Think about the special people who matter the most in your life—your family and friends. They are important to you and you care about them. Think about why they are so important. Can you imagine what life would be like without them?

Significant others affect us emotionally through their personalities and their actions. They influence us in many ways. They help bring meaning into our lives as we share experiences.

Nursing home residents may have a few or many significant others in their lives, such as their spouses, brothers and sisters, nieces and nephews, children and grandchildren (Fig. 5-2). Significant others also include friends, a special person of the opposite or same sex, neighbors, and former co-workers. Because of their special bond, significant others are often very important to residents. Since there is no real difference in this respect between family and others, this book will use the one word "family" to describe all significant others.

WHY IS FAMILY IMPORTANT?

Think of family as an extension of a resident. Residents identify with family members because of their past experiences and special memories. Their relationships are personal and often have developed over many years. Family members usually know a resident better than anyone else. In addition:

▶ Family is familiar in a facility that is unfamiliar for residents.

▶ Family can bring comfort to a resident.

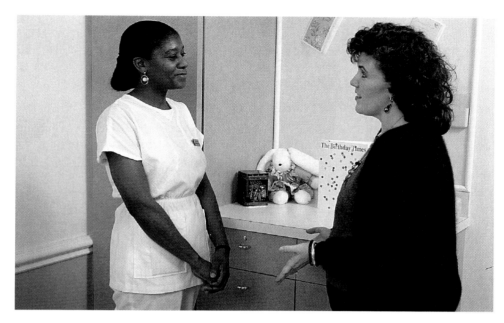

Fig. 5-1. Spend time with residents' family members because they can be valuable additions to the health care team.

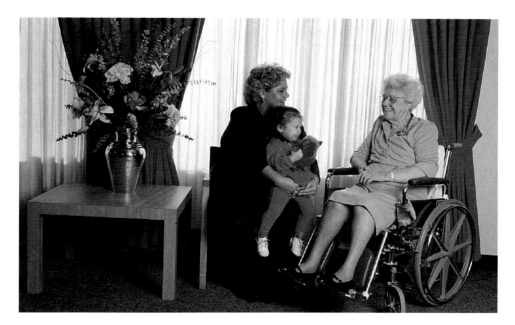

Fig. 5-2. Residents may have many significant others that bring meaning into their lives.

▷ Family can offer knowledge about a resident.
▷ Family can provide assistance in caring for a resident.
▷ Family provides financial support for some residents.

To give good care for residents, consider who is important to them and how they value the relationships. Residents who have been close to family all of their lives want to keep these relationships. Think about how you feel when you are away from someone close to you. Do you feel hurt, angry, or sad?

Not all families are the same. Each resident has a unique relationship with his or her family. Some have strong family relationships. Others are more distanced. Some have difficult or strained relationships. Always be careful not to impose your own family values. Continue to support each resident and his or her family whatever their relationship may be, even if you don't agree with it or find it hard to understand.

WHAT HAPPENS WHEN RESIDENTS GET ADMITTED?

Admission of a family member to a facility is usually stressful for the family because many changes are happening (Fig. 5-3). Changes related to moving into the facility affect each resident physically or emotionally, and these changes impact the family. Family roles and responsibilities may shift or be reversed. Families who cared for their loved ones are turning that responsibility over to you and others who at first seem like strangers to them. The family may feel they have a secondary role as you become the primary caregivers. Often for the first time, sons and daughters find themselves in the uncomfortable position of having to make major decisions for their parents.

Role changes and reversals can dramatically affect families who were comfortable with the way things used to be. The family must make new decisions. This has begun even before admission, as the family had to find the right facility and tend to their loved one's financial and property matters. Family members may disagree or argue about some things. Relationships among themselves or with the resident may change and cause more stress.

Family members may have different feelings when their loved one enters the facility. Many find it difficult to admit they can no longer care for their loved one or that he or she is no longer independent. It may be hard to accept these changes and that the resident may never come home.

Rarely does a family place a loved one in a facility because they don't want to care for the person. It is often hard for families to care for elderly or ill relatives. In many families, both partners work and cannot stay home to give care. Caring for one's parents is especially challenging for people also caring for their own children. These partners can feel torn between the needs of their children and their parents.

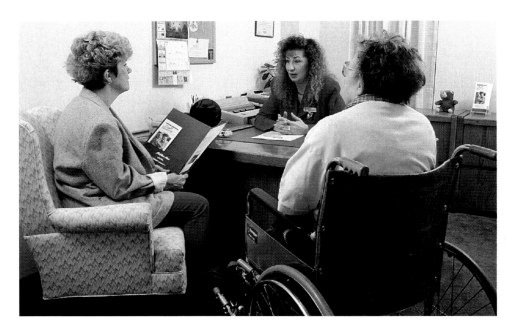

Fig. 5-3. Admission of a family member to a facility may be a stressful time for the family.

Any family trying to care for a sick or elderly relative at home feels stress. Most try their best to care for elderly family members at home as long as they can. Most families place their loved one in a facility only as a last resort after they have exhausted themselves and community services. By this time the family often is suffering from chronic stress. Families can feel "burned out" after caring for their loved one for a long time. They are physically and mentally exhausted. You will encounter many families suffering from chronic stress.

Think about your current situation and what it would be like to care for a dependent family member in your home. How would you manage? Could you find time for everything you would need to do? Would it cause you stress? Maybe you are caring for someone in your home and know how stressful it is.

The Adjustment Process

Like residents, families must also adjust before they can feel comfortable with their loved one living in a facility. Adjustment occurs gradually over time. It also takes time for the family to develop a trusting relationship with you (Fig. 5-4). Some families may need six months or more to adjust to the facility. During this time family members may have many different reactions. Typical family emotions are described in the following sections.

Try to watch for and recognize these feelings because they affect how the family behaves toward both you and their loved one. These feelings are a normal part of the adjustment process and may last a long time. Family members may react differently at different times. Accept that this period lasts until everyone is comfortable and a trusting relationship develops.

Guilt

Often family members feel guilt when they place their loved one in a facility. Some feel they are abandoning the person, no matter how difficult it would be to keep caring for them at home. Some families may have promised their loved one that they would always stay at home but had to break this promise because of a change in the person's condition. They may feel very guilty and try to make it up

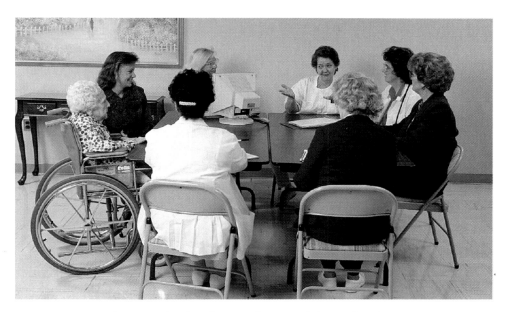

Fig. 5-4. It may take family members a while to develop a trusting relationship with facility employees. Team meetings with residents and family members may help you gain insight into their adjustment.

by visiting often and becoming heavily involved in care and decision making. Helping them stay involved and feel useful builds trust, and often their attention is helpful for their loved one and provides continuity. Help families relieve their guilt by saying, "You made the right decision. Your mother will get the best care possible." Giving the best care possible then helps the family resolve their guilt.

Anger

Some family members may feel anger about losing control of care for their loved one. They may resent the staff who they feel are replacing them, especially if they think the facility is giving better care then they did. They may also be angry because of family disagreements about placing the loved one, particularly if the decision had to be quick decision because of a crisis. Typically, angry family members may be critical of you or other staff. They may seem demanding. These family members may be the most challenging for you. Sometimes a social worker or other staff member can help you and the family work together.

Uncertainty

Some families feel uncertain about their decision. They are not sure what to expect from the facility and worry whether they made the right decision. They may be nervous and tense. The facility is unfamiliar to them, and they may be afraid. They worry about their loved one and want him or her to get the very best care. These families may be very emotional when visiting. They may check on staff to make sure that their loved one is being cared for as they want. You can help them feel confident that you do care about their relative and will do your best.

Sadness

Some families will be very sad. They may have a hard time coping with being separated from their loved one if they lived together or cared for them. They may grieve over the person's increased dependency or declining health. Even though they visit, they feel a tremendous sense of loss. These family members may cry often when visiting or seem distraught. Their visits may become less frequent or stop because the situation upsets them. Listen to their distress and help them talk about their feelings. Sometimes you can find a way to lighten the situation with a little laughter together after the tears.

Loss of Control

Many family members who cared for their loved ones for a long time feel a loss of control or responsibility as you and other staff take over the caregiving. Sometimes family members' main role in life was to care for the loved one, and now they feel they have nothing left to do. These family members may try to regain some control by becoming involved in care and decision making.

Relief

Finally, some family members feel relieved when their loved one enters a facility. Taking care of the person at home can be stressful and tiring, especially for those with other responsibilities. These families are relieved by the "respite," or rest, from caring for their loved one.

Your Relationship with the Family

From the moment you meet them, consider the family part of the team caring for each resident. Family members can share information about a resident, interact with him or her, and help with care. You can help families feel comfortable in this role.

When a resident is admitted, take this opportunity to begin to know the family. Comfort them by welcoming them and introducing yourself. Explain how you will assist with care. Get to know them by name and their relationship with resident.

If the family has not yet seen the facility or unit, let the charge nurse know so that they can tour the facility. Orienting families helps them to become comfortable with an unfamiliar place (Fig. 5-5). Introduce them also to other members of the health care team who will help care for their loved one. Help them meet the families of other residents too. Other families can give much support to each other.

You need to let the family know about special policies and upcoming events. Show them the posted calendar of events, and explain the different activities. Find out what their family member's customary daily routines were at home and consider these for the resident's care plan. Let them know when he or she will have meals, therapy sessions, and recreational activities. Families are interested in their loved one's activities. Encourage visits and family participation.

Families need to feel important and useful. Help the family decide if they want to be involved in their loved one's care. If so, what would they like to do? If not, that is OK. Encourage the family to bring favorite things or foods. The family can help motivate a resident who seems down or is upset by illness or therapy. Family members often make the best cheerleaders.

You will work with the family as long as you care for their loved one. Be involved with families of residents who have been there as well as for new families. How the family feels about the care being given their loved one affects their attitude toward staff. If the family feels their loved one is well cared for, they will have a positive feeling for you and other staff. They will be able to trust you. But if they feel their loved one is unhappy or not cared for properly, they will react negatively and have a hard time adjusting. Because you spend much time with each resident, you can get to know family members, understand their feelings, and help adjust as easily as possible.

INVOLVING THE FAMILY IN CARE

Some family members want to help care for their loved one. They may have cared for the person already for years and need to feel useful. Yet families often are

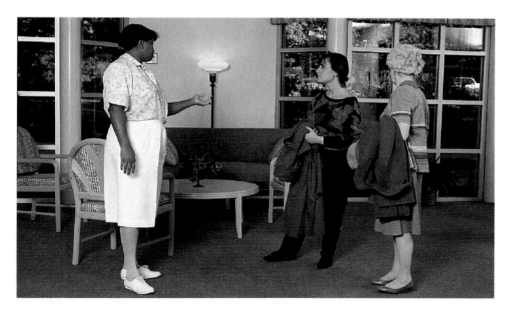

Fig. 5-5. Orient families with the resident's new environment, introduce them to other members of the health care team, and help them meet families of other residents.

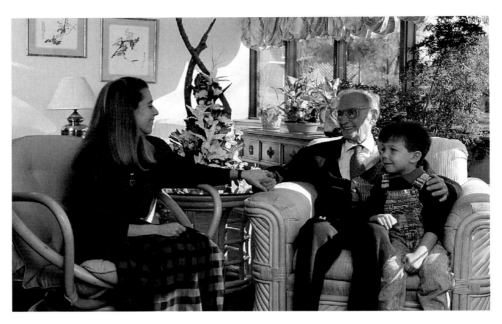

Fig. 5-6.   Families can play an important role in caregiving. Encourage family involvement with facility activities.

unsure how they can help and do not want to seem "pushy" or interfere with staff. Try to actively find out what role they want to play instead of waiting for them to offer on their own.

Family members can participate in resident care in many ways. They can do all or part of personal grooming at bath time. They may want to help their loved one eat and drink. They can be good companions during physical therapy sessions. They may want to join him or her for a special activity such as crafts, music, or games. Family can also participate by shopping for clothes or special items. Your facility may have special events that encourage family involvement. All of these activities encourage family members to participate in important ways (Fig. 5-6).

Encourage family members also to join in resident care conferences (Fig. 5-7). They often have valuable information about the person. Family members can become involved in the family council and influence facility policies for all residents' benefit. Both are good opportunities for families to participate in resident care and feel satisfied with their contributions.

You will find it very helpful to have families involved in their loved one's care. Recognize and acknowledge their contributions with positive feedback and thanks. Just as you like to know that you are appreciated and doing a good job, families need to know this. Positive strokes help to keep families motivated to stay involved. But be careful not to take advantage of their help or take it for granted. Some families may try to do all the care because they are afraid to let go. You can help them by making them feel confident of your care.

Sometimes you may be uncomfortable having family members help care for a resident. You may be used to doing things a certain way and the family member may do it differently. Or you may feel the family member is looking over your shoulder or trying to do your job. Family members sometimes give you directions for how to care for the person. Always listen to what family members are saying. They may know that he or she prefers care in a certain way. Consider their suggestions. If you are uncomfortable with the suggestion or manner of a family member, discuss it with the charge nurse.

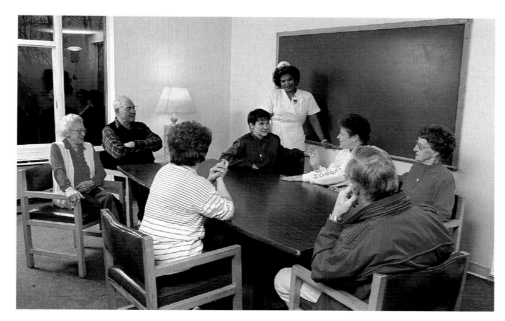

Fig. 5-7. Family council meetings allow families to participate in facility policies.

Communicating Effectively with Each Family

Families can tell you much about a resident. They can share his or her medical history, habits, and likes and dislikes. They can share stories about his or her life before they entered the facility. This information helps you and other staff understand a resident better and give better care. Feel comfortable asking the family for this information. Let the family know that by helping you, they are helping their loved one.

To work well with the family, you need to communicate with them effectively. Use the skills described in Chapter 6 on communication. Good communication begins with the family knowing who you are and you knowing who they are. Make yourself available to talk with the family during visits or on the telephone. Let them see you interacting with their loved one.

Often the family will ask you for an update on a resident's condition. They may ask about his or her progress and how he or she has been feeling or acting. Feel comfortable answering these questions. You can also ask them for advice about what to do if their loved one behaves in certain ways. Remember that the family cares about the well-being of a resident and will look to you for support and guidance.

Talking with the family about a resident openly and supportively is important. Demonstrate your support by really listening to what the family says. Do not let anything distract you, or the family member may feel you are not really listening. If a family member asks to speak to you when you are busy, try to arrange a later time when you have finished the task. Find a quiet spot so you can both relax and talk. This helps develop a positive relationship.

Always take care not to judge what a family members say or do. Be objective and do not agree or disagree with their opinions, especially if they are angry or frustrated. If family members disagree with each other or with their loved one, you should not take sides. This would only cause more problems.

To be sure you understand what a family member is feeling, let the person know what feelings, questions, and concerns you are hearing. This helps clarify exactly what the family member is saying. When you let them know you understand their feelings, they will be reassured that you have been listening to them.

Never try to hide anything from the family. If you are uncomfortable discussing some things with them, or they ask questions you cannot answer, ask them to talk to the charge nurse or the social worker. The charge nurse should be the one to report any change in a resident's condition to the family. Keeping the family informed of any changes is better than surprising a family member during a visit.

Families need to feel they are not cut off from their loved one. Look for and remove any barriers to communication. Be sure residents have access to the telephone and writing paper so that they can contact family members. By encouraging family to visit, making their visits comfortable, and involving them in care, you enhance a residents' relationship with their family.

Family Visits

Most families try to keep a close relationship with their loved one in the facility. They stay in contact with visits, telephone calls, cards and letters, and outings outside the facility. Most residents look forward to interaction with their families, and you should encourage it as much as possible.

During family visits residents can talk about old times and share their feelings and experiences with the people who matter to them most. This is a personal time. Ensure residents' privacy with their visitors, with no interruptions if possible. Families may bring in photos, special foods, or gifts for their loved one. They may take him or her to the chapel or for a walk outside. They may simply sit and hold hands.

Some family members visit regularly and frequently. A husband may come every day at lunchtime to eat with his wife. A daughter may bring her children to visit their grandmother every Saturday. Family members may come in groups or pairs. Some may come alone. Most visits are unannounced. Assist each resident in any way he or she may want to be prepared for such visits.

If a resident cannot communicate or is in failing health, visits can be difficult for family members. Always continue to support the family.

When Families Express Distress

Sometimes family members express their distress in ways that make you uncomfortable. Usually these have not yet adjusted to their loved one being in the facility. They may have unresolved emotions about the situation or some other stress in their life. They may be demanding, critical, or hostile to you and other staff. Do not take their comments personally. Be as supportive and nonjudgmental as you can. Report the situation to the charge nurse. Sometimes families have a well-founded criticism. Then the staff must recognize it and work hard to better meet the loved one's needs.

Other families may not visit or call very often. Others may seem to have little interest in a resident, or they may be upset by contact. They may have difficulty accepting changes in the person's physical or mental state. They may live far away or be busy with their jobs, family, or other responsibilities. A resident may feel this lack of attention and make the family feel even more guilty when they do visit. To help family members who feel uncomfortable visiting, greet them warmly and by name and tell them you are glad they came. Get them something to drink and sit with them for a few minutes. Encourage their loved one to tell them what he or she has been doing. If a resident cannot communicate, you should do so. You may need to remind a resident with memory loss of the names of family members. Be sure to reinforce the family's visit by thanking them for coming.

Often a family support group or the facility's family council can further help. Families having difficulty adjusting may find emotional support from others feeling the same way. Encourage the family's participation and give them information about these groups: when and where they meet and who to contact. Sometimes the social worker can help families work through their feelings. Families need to know these resources exist and where to find them. You can provide a necessary link.

YOU AS A FAMILY MEMBER

You may have more contact with some residents than they do with their own families and even than you have with your own family. Some residents may rely on you more and even trust you more than their own family. You may be the most consistent and caring person they see daily. A close, caring relationship may develop between you and a resident. You should enjoy this special relationship and appreciate the person's trust. But don't let these feelings interfere with your work or care of other residents. Any relationship needs some give and take.

Because you are a primary caregiver, you are a tremendous resource and support for families. Many family members openly appreciate your efforts and thank you. In some cases, you may find yourself becoming attached to a resident's family. This often happens when a resident cannot communicate and you do most of the communication with the family yourself.

IN THIS CHAPTER YOU LEARNED TO:

▶ define family

▶ state why family is important

▶ define the adjustment process

▶ described how to make the resident's family feel part of the health care team

▶ explain how to develop relationships with families

6

Sept 30, 1996

COMMUNICATION

A big part of your job as nurse assistant involves communicating with residents. Our culture emphasizes words in all forms: newspapers, magazines, books, radio, television, movies, lectures, and conversations. But communication is more than just words. Communication occurs through symbols, such as traffic lights and road signs. You learned very young that red means stop and green means go. Another symbol for stop is a hand held up, palm out. Words and symbols help give our lives structure, safety, and comfort.

Body language is also communication. We learn very young to "read" the body language of others around us. Remember how your mother looked when you tracked mud on the floor? She probably used words too, but they weren't as powerful as her look.

All of these aspects of communication are very important in your role as a nurse assistant. Communication involves both sending and receiving messages. We send and receive messages through words (verbal communication), through our body language (nonverbal communication), through touch, and through listening.

WHY IS COMMUNICATION SO IMPORTANT?

All people need to feel they are being heard. Moving into a long term facility often makes residents feel isolated and lonely. They are surrounded by strangers on whom they depend to help them meet their most basic needs. Having someone listen helps lessen the feelings of loneliness and isolation (Fig. 6-1).

When you show a resident you understand his or her feelings, you have started a relationship. Seeing things from another person's perspective is called empathy.

Residents who feel you understand them are more likely to share their feelings and needs. A trusting relationship can develop when they feel cared for and know what to expect.

Effective communication is important in many ways:

▶ It helps you understand each resident's needs
▶ It helps you develop a trusting relationship with residents.
▶ It makes your job easier and more enjoyable.
▶ It improves each resident's quality of life.
▶ It helps you gain cooperation from residents.

HOW WE COMMUNICATE
Verbal Communication

Verbal communication uses spoken or written words. Sounds simple enough, doesn't it? But words can have many different meanings, depending on one's culture and education. Take the word "frequently," for example. To a health care worker it may have a very specific meaning related to a health condition. A physician who hears that a resident is frequently thirsty may immediately view this as a symptom of a health problem. But the resident who said he is thirsty frequently today may be referring simply to the hot weather leading him to drink just a little more than usual. One person does not automatically know what meaning of a word is being used. As a nurse assistant, you use your communication skills to clarify meanings when giving care.

We all learn to use words in particular ways by listening to friends and family. In the same way you can learn the meanings of residents' words by listening to them speak. You can then use words familiar to them, to be sure they understand. Avoid medical jargon or slang, which many residents do not understand.

Your tone of voice, the speed at which you speak, and the clarity of your words often tell the listener much more than just the words you use. You can make it easier for others to understand what you are saying:

▶ Speak clearly and slowly.
▶ Look directly at the person you are talking to.
▶ Keep your hands away from your mouth while you are speaking. Do not talk with food or gum in your mouth.
▶ Reduce or eliminate other sounds such as radio, TV, and housekeeping equipment, by turning down the volume or closing the door to the room.

If you do not speak a resident's primary language, you must find someone to translate, such as a family member or staff member. You show real caring if you try to learn some words in this resident's language. You can post these words in the resident's room to help other caregivers communicate with the person. If your primary language is not English, and a resident you care for speaks only English, remember to speak only English with him or her. Workers who speak to each other in a language residents do not understand are confusing to residents who may be already having difficulty understanding what is going on around them. Speaking in another language may also give the impression that you do not want them to understand what you are saying.

Much of the official communication to residents about their rights and about the facility is given to them in writing. A resident may have difficulty reading this because of visual problems or "legalese" writing that needs explanation. You can help residents understand this information in your caregiving. For instance, you notice Mr. Smith has valuables in his room. Although he received the facility's policy about safeguarding valuables, do not assume he decided carefully to keep them with him. Say you are concerned that his things could be lost or stolen. Explain the facility's service for safeguarding his valuables, and encourage him to let you take care of his things.

Avoid medical terms or explain their meaning if they are routinely used in the facility. For example, instead of saying, "I need to check your vital signs," say, "I need to check your temperature, pulse, respiration, and blood pressure." When a resident is NPO, explain this means he or she cannot eat or drink anything, and explain why and for how long.

Nonverbal Communication

Nonverbal communication involves communication not done through words. Body language includes how you hold your head, arms, hands, and whole body, as well as your expressions and movements. For example, hands on the hips or arms crossed on the chest convey anger (Fig. 6-2). Eye contact shows attention and caring. Moving quickly communicates that you are in a hurry. Sitting down to talk with someone says that you are interested in him or her and care enough to take the time to talk (Fig. 6-3). Facial expressions convey many feelings, including happiness, humor, concern, pain, or sadness.

Consider the following interaction:

> Cheryl and Kate are talking about an experience Cheryl had earlier in the day.
> Cheryl: Boy, Mrs. Peacock sure was mad when I told her I would have to take the salt from her tray.
> Kate: What did she say?
> Cheryl: Oh, she didn't say anything. She just slammed her fork on the table and glared at me.

We often watch others' facial expressions to see if they received the message we tried to communicate. For example, if you explain something to someone and you see a wrinkled brow, you can guess he or she did not understand you. Often we are unaware of the nonverbal messages we are sending to others. Even if you don't intend to send a message nonverbally, such messages occur. Although people may try to use words to mask their feelings, their nonverbal communication often conveys the true feelings. That is why most people pay attention to the nonverbal messages others give them—to get the real message.

Think about some task you have to perform but don't really have time to do. For example, a resident with very long hair asks you to help wash and braid her hair. It

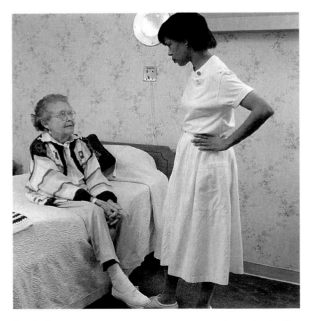

Fig. 6-2. Body language can convey many things, including anger.

is a busy day for you, but you know her family is coming to visit in the evening and she wants to look well. You know that you will be tied up for an hour if you agree to help. You may say, "Yes, I'll be glad to help you." But did you take a deep breath before you answered? Did you look at your watch and cringe? Did you hurry to towel-dry her hair and accidently pull it a bit? The resident may not say anything. She may even be quieter than usual. But think of the messages she receives from your nonverbal behavior. How might this affect your future relationship with her?

Pay close attention to what messages you are sending to residents when your verbal and nonverbal communication do not match. When a resident asks you to do something you cannot easily do now, instead of saying yes and then frowning, try discussing alternatives with him or her. Together you can come up with a plan good for both of you. Residents too may send different messages with nonverbal and verbal communication. For example, a resident may tell you he or she is not in pain, but you may see facial expressions of pain. When you are assisting a resident with care you should watch for nonverbal messages as well as listen to the verbal communication.

Touch

Touch is an important kind of nonverbal communication. Some people use their hands when talking, and to them touching another person is natural. Others are not comfortable being touched, and to them touch is an invasion of personal space. Hugs are for many people a common way of saying hello between friends or family members, and a means of communicating congratulations or condolences. For some, hugs and kisses are reserved for intimate relationships, and offering them outside such relationships is just not done.

Learn what each resident prefers regarding touch. Remember that each individual has his or her own comfort level for touching. Be aware how you feel yourself about giving and receiving touching. Some find it easier to give than to receive.

The old saying, "A picture is worth a thousand words," captures the meaning of nonverbal communication. What one sees is often much more important than what one hears.

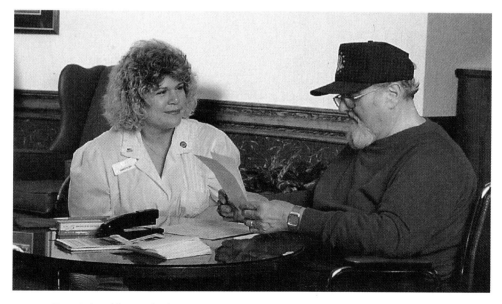

Fig. 6-3. Nonverbal communication often reveals our true feelings even though we may be unaware of it. Simply listening or making eye contact while talking with someone shows you care.

Listening

The more you know about another person, the better you can communicate with him or her. You have many chances to learn about residents in your daily, caring contact with them. The skill you need most is listening (Fig. 6-4).

Listening takes time. But you can listen while you help residents with care. You can learn much about their likes and dislikes, activities before entering the facility, and family relationships. But also take time just to sit and talk with them to show you are interested in them and they matter to you.

Being relaxed and unhurried when you talk with residents helps put them at ease. Convey your interest by making eye contact, leaning toward them, and nodding as they talk. Whenever you can, put yourself at the same height residents by sitting, squatting, or kneeling close to the bed or chair. Allow silences to occur as residents talk; do not try to hurry them.

If you do not understand something a resident says, ask him or her to repeat it. If you still do not understand, ask someone else for help. Do not pretend to understand if you don't, as trust depends on honesty and understanding. Residents need to trust you to communicate their real feelings and needs to you.

To let residents know you understand what they are saying, you can ask, "Is this what you mean?" This technique is called reflection. You restate in your own words what the other person said. Use this also to encourage a resident to continue talking. You might say something like, "It sounds like you have difficulty talking to your grandchildren about your feelings." If your interpretation is correct, this shows you understand the person's feelings. If your interpretation is not correct, this gives the person a chance to clarify what he or she was trying to say.

Your body language also helps you listen well. If you say you want to listen but your attention is on a task you are doing, you are not communicating real interest in what the person is saying. Maintain an open posture, with your arms comfortable at your sides or in your lap, not crossed in front of you. Touch residents from time to time on the shoulder or arm, if you and the individual are comfortable with that. Sit close enough for the person to see you clearly, but not so close that you threaten anyone's sense of personal space.

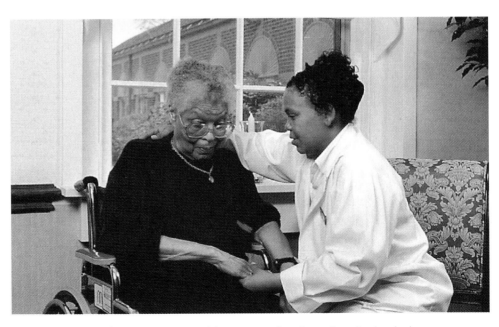

Fig. 6-4. Listening to a resident can take time, but it also helps you learn more about her or him.

Validating Communication

How do you know if a resident receives exactly the same message you meant to send? You need to validate, or check out, whether the other person understands your message as you intended. If you are giving instructions, you can ask the other person to repeat what you said or to perform the activity. To communicate a feeling, you might ask, "What did you hear me say?" Sometimes you know the person heard you correctly because he or she does what you requested. If you watch the other person's body language closely, you can also get strong clues about what he or she has heard: nodding or shaking the head, open or puzzled facial expression, and posture all communicate much (Fig. 6-5).

Promoting Effective Communication

Much of what you have learned about protecting residents' rights also promotes effective communication. The following are guidelines for promoting effective communication:

▶ Show respect for residents by calling them by their title and surname (Mrs. Jones). Never use nicknames such as "sugar" or "honey."

▶ Always ask residents if it is OK to do something. Explain procedures. Plan activities with them, and always keep your word (Fig. 6-6). If you cannot do something you promised, tell the resident and explain why.

▶ Respond to every resident's call light or call for help as quickly as possible. If a resident cannot ask for help or is hesitant, check on him or her frequently. Try to anticipate needs. For example, if a resident does not like to ask for help going to the bathroom but cannot go safely on his or her own, don't wait for him or her to ask but offer to help at appropriate times.

▶ Respect a resident's feelings. If a resident says he or she feels sad, use a reflective response, such as, "You feel discouraged right now?" Do not minimize his or her feelings by saying things such as, "Things aren't all that bad" or "Don't talk like that. It's going to be fine."

▶ Give hope, but not false reassurances. Instead of saying, "You'll feel better tomorrow," say, "I know you're having a tough time. But I think you will be more comfortable if we . . ."

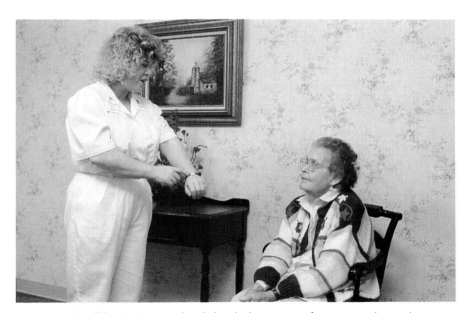

Fig. 6-5. Watch the resident's body language for strong clues about what the resident heard.

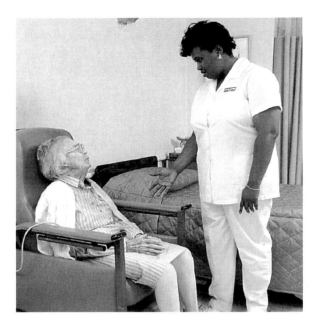

Fig. 6-6. It's important to keep your word when planning activities with a resident.

▶ Always assume that a resident can hear you. Even if the person is unresponsive, continue to explain who you are and everything that you are doing.

▶ Attend to each resident's personal care needs as quickly as possible. If clothing or bedding becomes soiled, putting the person in clean clothes and changing the bedding right away will show respect and concern.

▶ Offer residents choices in all daily activities. Look for ways to encourage residents to keep control over their lives. Ask them what they want to wear, when to take a bath, and when they want care. When possible, teach residents or family members how to do personal care by themselves, if they wish.

▶ Ask open-ended questions that encourage residents to talk, rather than asking "yes" or "no" questions. Try "How do you feel about this?" or "Tell me about that."

▶ Respect residents' privacy by not sharing personal information about them except to staff who have to know. If one resident asks something personal about another, give only general information, and encourage the person to talk to the other to share personal information.

Problems of Ineffective Communication

What happens if communication is not effective? If you are not communicating effectively with residents, you may not be able to meet their needs because you do not understand them fully. They may not tell you about a change in their condition that could lead to a serious medical problem. They may not report small complaints, leading to problems not being corrected. A resident or family member who is not comfortable talking with you may go instead to an outside agency for a problem that your facility could have solved. Residents may withdraw, feeling that no one is interested in them, and miss opportunities for relationships with other residents. You may become frustrated and discouraged in your work if you feel you do not have a helping relationship with the residents you care for.

ENDING A CONVERSATION

Communication is important, but so is getting your work done. How do you end a conversation when you must leave to do something else? You want to end the conversation with the person feeling good. You can simply say, "I really enjoy talking to you. Can we continue this conversation after dinner? I have to check on some other residents now." When you start a conversation, you can say, "I have about 10 minutes before I have to do something else. Could we talk for a few minutes?" When the time is up, you can say, "I have to go now, but I would like to continue our talk later." Set a time for this if you can, and be sure you come back. Never make a promise you can't keep.

SPECIAL COMMUNICATION NEEDS

Some residents may develop a child-like dependency on staff and family after entering the facility. Use your communication skills to encourage their independence in daily activities.

Other residents have physical problems that make communication difficult, such as a hearing or vision loss, or an inability to speak clearly due to an illness, stroke, or ill-fitting dentures. Some residents may be depressed, creating other special communication needs. Memory loss can also make communication more difficult. These special needs are discussed in the following sections.

Helping Residents Do More for Themselves

Encourage residents to do all they can for themselves. Staying physically active helps maintain good muscle tone and joint flexibility. Emotionally, being independent helps one feel better about oneself. If residents ask you to do something for them that they can do themselves, you can answer, "You do as much as you can, and I will help you with the hard parts" (Fig. 6-7).

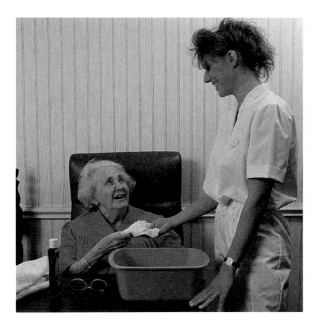

Fig. 6-7. Encourage residents to remain as independent as possible. The more they do for themselves the better they will feel emotionally and physically.

You and other staff can also develop a consistent approach for a resident who needs more encouragement. For example, if a resident goes from one staff member to another asking for help, the staff may pick one person to answer all his or her requests. Or the team may decide on one approach for all staff to use with this resident to be consistent.

When a resident starts taking responsibility for his or her care, give encouragement and praise. Say things like:

- "You did a good job. You should be proud of your accomplishment."
- "I'm glad to see you out of your room. I hope we will see you out more."
- "I'm glad you tried that. Tomorrow maybe you can do a little bit more."

Helping a Resident with Visual Impairment

With a resident who is blind or has impaired vision, follow these guidelines for more effective communication:

- Be sure the room is well lighted and sit where the person can best see you.
- If a resident has glasses, make sure they are worn and are clean.
- If a resident has another vision aid, such as a magnifying glass, encourage its use (Fig. 6-8).
- Be sure you always introduce yourself when you start talking to a resident, and keep talking to let him or her know what you are doing and where you are.
- Touch a resident to let him or her know where you are, and encourage a resident's own use of touch to locate objects in the environment. Keep items in the same place when you can so that the person can become familiar with their location. This also helps residents be independent in self-care.
- If a resident asks that you read mail or personal documents for him or her, by all means do so, but only when asked.

Helping a Resident with Hearing Impairment

Follow these guidelines for more effective communication with a resident with a hearing impairment:

- Minimize background noise.
- Since people with hearing impairments often neglect to use their hearing aids, encourage their use. Be sure the hearing aid is working properly.
- You may touch a resident to get his or her attention.
- Face a resident when talking so he or she can see your lips. Lip-reading helps residents understand what you are saying. Speak clearly, using your lips to emphasize sounds.

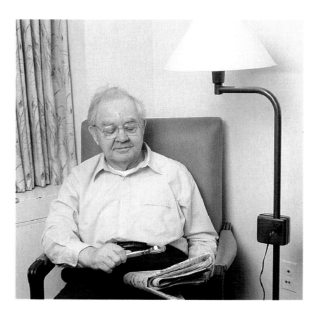

Fig. 6-8. If a resident is visually impaired, encourage them to use their glasses or any other visual aid.

- Use gestures or point to objects as you are speaking.
- Speak to the person's stronger ear if there is one.
- Restate what you have said if a resident requests. If needed, restate it again using different words.
- Be sure you have the person's attention and eye contact.
- In some cases you may need to use paper and pencil to write down what you are saying (Fig. 6-9).
- Always be patient.

Helping a Resident Who Is Depressed

Residents often experience depression and withdrawal because of the difficult transition into the facility. Use the communication techniques already discussed, and most important, be patient and persistent. Try the following ways to promote communication with a depressed resident:

- Spend some extra time just sitting with this resident, even if you get no verbal response.
- Invite a resident's participation in care activities and social activities in the facility. You might say something like, "I'll get a basin of water. While I'm doing that, I'd like for you to get your shaving cream and razor."
- Set goals for each resident with suggestions like, "Today we can just walk to the nurses' station and back. Tomorrow I would like for you to walk with me to the dining room."
- Ask family members and friends about the resident's interests in the past. Then you may be able to engage him or her in conversation about these interests.
- In all your efforts, keep trying. Your consistency may finally bring some response from the resident.

Helping a Resident with Cognitive Impairment

Some residents may be cognitively impaired and have much memory loss. Caring for residents with cognitive impairment is discussed in Chapter 22. Many residents may not remember recent events but can remember clearly things from their childhood. Encourage these resident to talk about the things they do re-

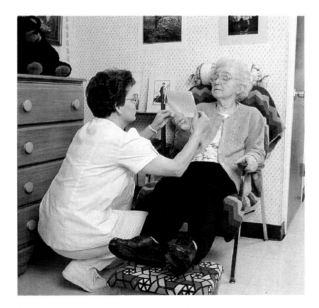

Fig. 6-9. In order to communicate with a hearing impaired resident you may need to write down what you are saying.

member. Follow these guidelines for those who have difficulty remembering things in the present:

▸ Keep your questions and your directions short and simple.

▸ Repeat information but try to understand the resident's feelings and his or her perceptions of the world.

▸ Use helpful visual reminders, such as calendars and clocks throughout the facility (Fig. 6-10). A wall chart in the room may help a resident remember daily routines, such as the steps in getting dressed or what time meals are served.

▸ Because of the memory loss, some things a resident says may not make sense to you. Never laugh at or make fun of this resident, who is trying hard to fill in the gaps in memory.

Helping a Resident with Speech Impairment

"Aphasia" is a medical term for difficulty putting thoughts into words. Stroke and other brain injuries often cause aphasia. Residents who have difficulty being understood may easily give up and become depressed. They may become withdrawn and stop trying to communicate. Once again, your time and patience can make a big difference. Try these ways to promote communication:

▸ Encourage a resident to use his or her hands, to point things out, to touch things as aids to understanding.

▸ Ask questions that can be answered yes or no.

▸ Since trying to make themselves understood can be frustrating, encourage residents to express their anger and frustration. If needed, sit quietly and let them cry for a while. Then keep trying to understand what they are saying.

▸ When you understand what a resident's particular sounds or symbols mean, let other staff know too so they can communicate better with this resident. You can put a chart on a resident's wall to tell others what the symbols mean. You can also make a list of common phrases, so the resident can simply point to what he or she needs.

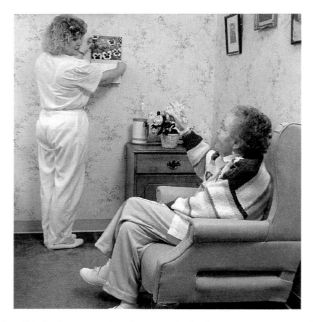

Fig. 6-10. Wall charts, calendars and clocks can serve as visual reminders to residents.

USING COMMUNICATION AS AN EFFECTIVE TOOL

Special communication needs arise with residents whose behavioral symptoms make you uncomfortable or are abusive, and with residents who are too demanding or rigid in their requests.

Responding to Sexual Advances

Sometimes a resident's or family member's behavior may make you uncomfortable. This may include sexual advances or comments. You need to communicate the fact that you do not like the behavior without being negative about the person. You might say, "That makes me very uncomfortable. Please don't do it again."

In some cases a resident cannot control his or her behavior. At times like these, the best thing you can do may be to distract this resident's interest to another topic or activity.

Some residents' behavior may make other residents uncomfortable, such as making sexual advances. If a resident is not competent to give consent, she or he must be protected from unwanted sexual advances. Often residents will tell staff when they see a resident making another uncomfortable. You will need to keep a close check on vulnerable residents, but you will find residents often protect the vulnerable resident and provide extra eyes you can use.

You must also protect others from unwanted sexual advances by an incompetent resident. You may have to physically move him or her from an area to prevent annoying or threatening other residents. Try to spend time alone with the person, and look for activities he or she might enjoy. Try to involve this resident in other activities to provide a diversion. Such activities may also encourage positive social contact to replace sexual advances that make the others uncomfortable.

Responding to Physical Abuse

Residents may also be verbally or physically abusive to you or other residents. You must protect others from harm, but you also must protect the abusing resident's rights. With verbal abuse, you can say, "You must feel very angry—can I help?" Often the person is just letting off steam, as we all do sometimes. With physical abuse, you must act to prevent harm to others, such as stepping between residents or removing an object a resident may use as a weapon. Those involved may need to move to separate areas for a cooling off period. Remember that other residents who see such a conflict may become anxious and need extra support and reassurance that staff will keep them safe.

In extreme cases a resident's aggression can cause an employee injury. A resident may express distress by hitting, kicking, head butting, biting, spitting, or throwing things, or by verbal responses such as yelling or cursing. Although it sounds simple, the best way to prevent this kind of aggression and possible injury is to know residents very well. What are they feeling and thinking, and why they are acting as they are? Constantly assess their moods, which can change with or without any reason you can see. Try to feel what they are feeling and then tailor your words and actions to meet their needs.

This assessment is not always easy. If a resident is on medication, depressed, ill, very tired, or in pain, his or her mind may not be working like yours. What makes sense to a resident may not make sense to you. But talk to this resident, watch facial expressions for changes, and pay attention to what the previous shift reports about the resident's actions.

Avoid surprising residents or being surprised by them. Never walk up from behind a resident and touch or startle him or her. Anytime you approach, be sure to smile, talk in a soft, friendly voice. Never order the person around. Use short sentences and simple yes-or-no questions. When the resident will not be surprised, gently touch him or her. This can be reassuring and help to let the resident know that you care.

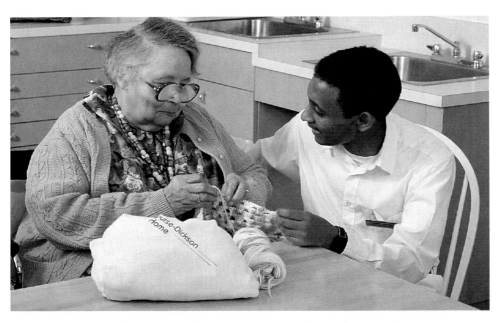

Fig. 6-11. Always be calm and patient with residents and reassure them that you care.

Remember two things when assisting each resident:
▶ Don't rush. Find out if it is a good time for the person. Allow plenty of time for him or her to hear and understand you. Give instructions using simple steps, and when needed repeat these using exactly the same words. Sometimes, because of your own frustration or a resident's, it may be best if you wait till later. Give the resident a hug or change the subject. Sometimes, if the situation becomes very tense, you may even need to leave the room.
▶ Even if the upset resident is looking at you when he or she begins this behavior, do not take these actions personally or consider yourself the cause. An aggressive resident may have an organic brain disease and isn't intentionally trying to hurt or annoy you. He or she is struggling with feelings or pain that are difficult to understand, and you just happened to be there when this resident simply could not cope anymore. Never, never argue with any resident no matter what he or she says. Always stay calm and patient (Fig. 6-11).

In situations involving resident aggression, try to be patient and understanding. Evaluate and communicate with this resident. If you consistently use this approach, both you and the resident will be aware of what's going on, and in that way you can avoid surprises and aggression-related injuries.

A resident who is abusive is often mentally impaired and cannot be held responsible for his or her behavior. Try to distract this resident to another topic or activity. Chapter 19 discusses when physical restraints may be needed.

Responding to Residents Whose Requests Feel Like Demands

You may meet some residents or family who are perfectionistic. They may insist everything be done a certain way and the same way every time. Some may demand that everything be exactly in the same place at all times. Others may have rigid standards for themselves and other people and difficulty bending rules. Usually these behaviors are learned in childhood. In stressful situations, such as moving into a nursing facility, these people may act this way as a means of coping with loss of con-

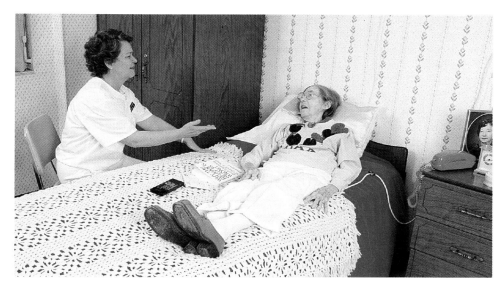

Fig. 6-12. One way to pull a withdrawn resident into conversation is to share an experience of your own.

trol. They are trying to control their environment, when everything feels out of control. Try to follow these guidelines:

▷ Remember that these behaviors are efforts to cope with stress, and try to respond in a nonthreatening manner.

▷ Do not take the behaviors personally.

▷ Encourage residents and family to have as much control as possible within reason and within the rules of the facility. For example, state how much time you have now and ask what he or she would like for you to do in that time.

▷ Use humor when you can. For example, if a resident or family member gives you a list of demands, you might say, "Whew! I'm good, but I don't know if I'm that good! Let's see if we can break that down into smaller parts."

COMMUNICATING ABOUT YOURSELF

As you talk to residents about their personal lives and families, you can share facts and experiences from your own life. This sharing often promotes communication. Be sure, however, to keep focused on the resident. You may, for example, share an amusing story from your family that is similar to a story the resident has told. This can be a good way also to engage a depressed or withdrawn resident in conversation (Fig. 6-12).

Like everyone else you will have bad days, but even then you must focus on residents' feelings rather than your own. Talk with your supervisor if you can't focus on your work because of a personal problem. If you notice that a co-worker has a problem like this, find a private moment and ask if you can help. Help could be as simple as listening for a few minutes or letting a supervisor know that another employee needs some extra attention.

A resident may ask about your family or children in a way that shows they want a give-and-take conversation about each other's problems. Use good judgment and talk to the charge nurse or social worker if you are unsure how to respond. Residents in their wisdom sometimes can help.

It is natural that you will react personally to things that happen on the job with residents or family members. You may become angry if a resident or family member criticizes your care for a resident. It is normal to feel defensive when criticized, but you make sure you don't express your negative feelings to residents. Talk to someone else about your feelings. A co-worker or supervisor may have had similar experiences and can suggest how to deal with your feelings. Sometimes just talking about the incident is enough. If needed, move away from the situation to cool off, making sure a co-worker or supervisor knows where you are and will care for residents during this time.

Tact is the art of saying the right thing at the right time. Few people can do this all the time, but you get better with practice. Take the time to get to know residents by listening and looking for clues in their body language. You can then respond more easily in ways that show you understand their needs and concerns. The more aware you are of your own needs and ways of relating, the more empathy and tact you will have for others.

7

PREVENTION AND CONTROL OF INFECTION

Did you ever think about why colds and the flu are more common in the winter? People used to think that being cold made it easier to catch a cold, but that has been proved wrong. Colds are more common in the winter because people tend to stay inside in closer contact with each other. Cold germs spread more easily among people in close contact. Someone in a weakened condition is also more likely to get a cold, because the body's natural defenses are not as successful in fighting off the infection. Still, anyone can catch a cold, since the microorganisms that cause a cold spread easily among people.

Fortunately, not all microorganisms are transmitted as easily as those that cause colds. Infections can be serious for residents in a long term care facility. But you as a nurse assistant and others in the facility work together to control and prevent the transmission of microorganisms. Some infection prevention and control measures are as simple as hand washing, but you will learn many other specific things you can do.

HOW MICROORGANISMS CAUSE INFECTIONS

Microorganisms are so small they can be seen only under a microscope. The most common types are viruses, bacteria, and fungi. People often call these microorganisms "germs."

Many microorganisms live naturally on the skin or in the intestine, vagina, mouth, or other parts of the body. These bacteria make up what is called our bodies' natural flora. In a healthy person, these microorganisms are in balance and cause no problems. However, if the natural balance is destroyed because of such things as illness, poor nutrition, stress, fatigue, or certain drugs, the microorganisms may cause infection. Also, microorganisms that live in one part of the body without causing problems can cause serious infection if they reach another part. For example, *Escherichia coli* bacteria (often referred to as *E. coli*) live normally in the gastrointestinal tract, but can cause urinary tract infections if they get into the bladder.

HOW MICROORGANISMS ARE TRANSMITTED: THE CHAIN OF INFECTION

You can think of how microorganisms are transmitted from one person to another as a chain with six links (Fig. 7-1). Each link must be present in the chain to make the chain complete and transmit an infection. The links in the chain are:

1. The microorganism that can cause infection
2. The reservoir where the microorganism lives
3. A route or portal of exit from the reservoir
4. A mode of transmission from the reservoir to a susceptible host
5. A route portal of entry into the susceptible host
6. The susceptible host

The Microorganism

The first link in the chain is the microorganism that causes the infection. Many types of viruses, bacteria, and fungi cause infections. Microorganisms that cause in-

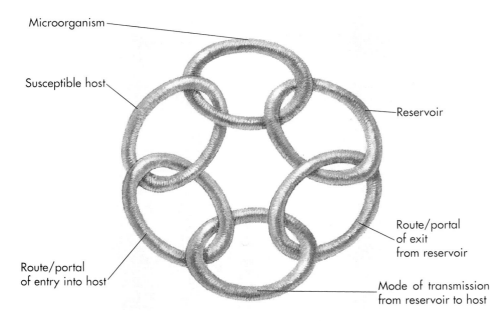

Fig. 7-1. The transmission of microorganisms from one person to another can be viewed as a chain with six links.

fection are called pathogenic, while those that do not are called nonpathogenic. Without a pathogenic organism, infection cannot occur.

The Reservoir

The second link is called the reservoir for organisms, where the organisms live. The human body is a reservoir for many different types of organisms, but organisms also live in animals, plants, soil, food, and water.

Portal of Exit from the Reservoir

The third link in the chain is the portal of exit from the reservoir. The organisms must exit from people, the reservoirs for organisms, to be transmitted to another. Portals or routes of exit include all natural body openings and openings made during medical procedures such as surgery. For example, organisms in the lungs exit the body when one coughs or sneezes. Organisms in the bladder exit in urine when voiding. Organisms in the intestinal tract exit in stool when defecating.

Modes of Transmission from the Reservoir

Organisms are transmitted from the route or portal of exit of one person (the reservoir) to the portal of entry of another person (the susceptible host) by several pathways or modes.

Direct Transmission (Person-to-Person)

Direct transfer of organisms from one person's portal of exit (such as the mouth or genitalia) to another person's portal of entry occurs during activities such as kissing and sexual intercourse. Direct transfer also occurs when droplets coughed by one person land in the eyes, nose, or mouth of another person, usually when they are within 3 feet of each other (Fig. 7-2). Direct transmission is an efficient way for organisms to be transmitted and is why droplet-transmitted diseases such as chicken pox and measles are transmitted quickly among children.

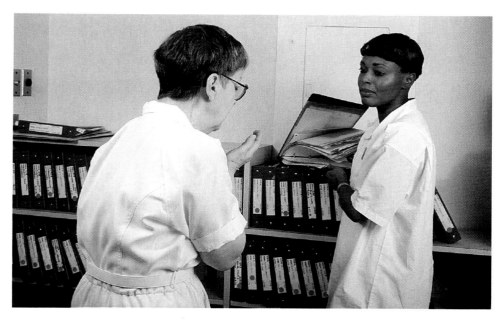

Fig. 7-2. Organisms can be transferred directly through droplets that may land in the eyes, nose, or mouth.

Indirect Transmission (Person-to-Intermediate Object-to-Person)

Indirect transmission is less efficient than direct transmission because there is an intermediate object between the portal of exit of the reservoir and the portal of entry of the susceptible host. Intermediate objects include hands, soiled linen or dressings, and contaminated water or food (Fig. 7-3).

In long term care facilities, hands are the most common intermediate objects in indirect transmission of organisms from one resident to another. Consider this example:

> You are taking care of Ms. Swenson and Ms. Ritter, who are bedridden and are roommates in a two-bed room. As you deliver lunch trays to both residents, you discover that Ms. Swenson has been incontinent of urine. You give Ms. Ritter her lunch tray but put Ms. Swenson's tray aside until you can clean her and her bed. Just as you finish cleaning Ms. Swenson, Ms. Ritter asks you to help her open a plastic wrapping on a cookie. You do not wash your hands, so your hands may have Ms. Swenson's urine organisms on them. Your contaminated hands touch the cookie and put some of these urine organisms on it. When Ms. Ritter eats the cookie, she eats some of Ms. Swenson's urine organisms. This is an example of indirect transmission.

Airborne Transmission

Airborne transmission of organisms occurs when the reservoir coughs microorganisms into the air and a susceptible host breathes them into the lungs. Only a few microorganisms are transmitted by this mode, including the bacteria that cause tuberculosis (TB). TB organisms will stay in the air until the ventilation system clears them out.

Portal of Entry into Susceptible Host

Most portals of entry are natural openings in the body. Microorganisms coughed from the lungs of a reservoir enter the lungs of a susceptible host when the person breathes them in through the nose and mouth. Microorganisms that can cause diarrhea enter when the susceptible host eats and swallows them. The portal of entry for sexually transmitted diseases is through the vagina or penis.

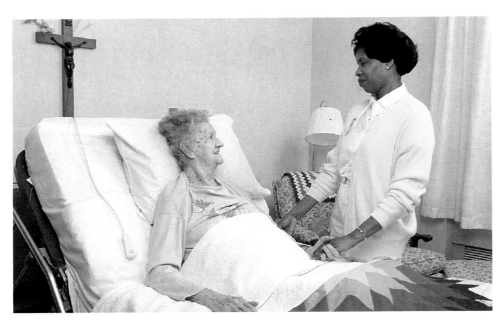

Fig. 7-3. Organisms can be transferred indirectly through intermediate objects such as hands, linens, dressings, or contaminated water or food.

Susceptible Host

All people are susceptible to infections caused by viruses, bacteria, and fungi. People are most susceptible when they are run down, after surgery, or in an acute phase of a disease. Many of these infections can be prevented by vaccines (such as for measles, mumps, rubella, hepatitis B, tetanus, diphtheria, whooping cough, polio, influenza). Chapter 23 describes your role in supporting a resident in infection control and prevention.

If only one link in the chain is broken, transmission will not occur. Many different infection prevention and control measures can be used to break different links in the chain.

STRATEGIES FOR BREAKING THE CHAIN OF INFECTION TRANSMISSION

The following sections describe how to break the chain at the different links by using infection prevention and control techniques. Remember, if only one link is broken, the chain of transmission of infection can easily be broken (Fig. 7-4). Consider the following strategies when you are providing care.

Breaking the Chain with Hand Washing and Other Strategies

Hand washing and the use of barriers breaks the chain at the portal of exit and at the mode of transmission. Many barriers also break the chain at the portal of entry. Environmental sanitation measures break the chain by eliminating environmental reservoirs. Many different patient care practices break the chain at the portal of entry link. Immunizations against many diseases break the chain for you and for residents at the susceptible host link.

Breaking the Chain at the Reservoir Link

When a person is diagnosed with an infection, treatment with antibiotics targets the reservoir link. Treatment will reduce the number of organisms and severity of the infection so that when the person gets well he or she is no longer a reservoir.

Procedures for food sanitation such as using clean equipment for preparation and adequate refrigeration for storage prevent food from being a reservoir for

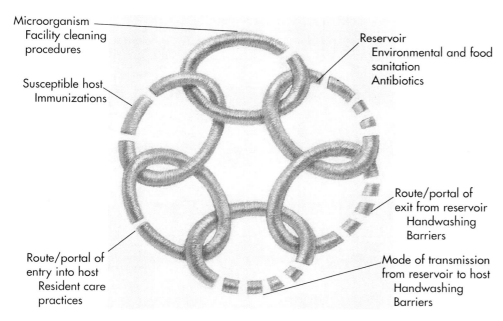

Fig. 7-4. The chain of transmission can be broken by many methods of infection prevention and control.

organisms that can make people sick. But if food sanitation is not maintained, large numbers of people can become ill from eating the contaminated food.

Breaking the Chain at the Mode of Transmission Link

Diseases such as gonorrhea, syphilis, and human immunodeficiency virus (HIV) infection are transmitted by direct contact during sexual intercourse, and there are no vaccines for these diseases. Ways to break the chain of transmission of sexually transmitted diseases include the use of barriers such as condoms.

Another organism transmitted by direct contact is the virus that causes fever blisters (*Herpes simplex* virus). For example, a resident has a fever blister on the lip. You have a cut in the skin of your index finger. You touch the fever blister with your finger during mouth care. The virus from a resident's fever blister can enter your body through the opening in your skin and cause you to develop a fever blister on your finger. Wearing gloves for mouth care is one way to break the chain. Another way is by using a mouth care cleaning sponge on a handle so you do not have to touch a resident's mouth with your fingers.

The chain can be broken at the airborne transmission route if the facility has adequate ventilation and staff identify residents with coughs at early stages. The use of masks can be effective if used properly—changed every 20 minutes.

Breaking the Chain at the Susceptible Host Link

People become immune to some microorganisms if they are infected only once. For example, the chicken pox virus and the hepatitis A (infectious hepatitis) virus confer lifetime immunity. Other microorganisms can cause infections again and again, because infection does not result in immunity. Many gastrointestinal diseases do not lead to immunity.

Breaking the chain at the susceptible host link depends on the microorganisms and the individuals involved. For example, the best way to protect susceptible hosts from vaccine-preventable diseases is to vaccinate them. The best way to protect susceptible hosts from becoming sick with organisms that are already in their bodies is to help them stay healthy.

TABLE 7-1.　Breaking links in the chain of infection

Link	How the Chain is Broken
The microorganism	Use of facility cleaning procedures
The Reservoir	Environmental sanitation
	Identify and treat infections with antibiotics
	Food sanitation procedures such as cleaning equipment and adequate refrigeration
The Portal of Exit	Use of hand washing
	Use of barriers like gloves and masks
The Mode of Transmission	Use of hand washing
	Use of barriers like gloves and masks
The Portal of Entry	Proper nursing care procedures
The Susceptible Host	Immunizations against disease

The best way to protect yourself from becoming ill with microorganisms from residents is for you to be immunized against those diseases that have vaccines, stay as healthy as you can, use barriers appropriately, and wash your hands often and well.

Table 7-1 summarizes the chain of transmission and the ways it can be broken. As you can see, simple common sense can break the chain of transmission.

Many of the procedures for breaking the chain are not just your responsibility. All departments must work together to control and prevent infection.

HAND WASHING

The facility has hand washing areas readily accessible to you. Wash your hands with soap and lukewarm running water as soon as possible before and after all care procedures to adequately wash contaminated material from the skin.

When soap and water are not available for washing your hands or other parts of the body, use an appropriate antiseptic hand cleanser along with clean cloth, paper towels, or antiseptic towelettes. When antiseptic hand cleansers or towelettes are used, wash the hands or other affected area with soap and running water as soon as possible.

You must wash your hands immediately or as soon as possible after removing gloves or other personal protective equipment. Wash your hands and any other skin with soap and water, and flush mucous membranes (eyes and inner surfaces of your nose or mouth) with water immediately or as soon as possible following contact with blood or other potentially infectious materials. This may happen if someone bumps you and a fluid splatters.

Almost any time is a good time to wash your hands at work. But at several specific times we must all wash our hands:

▶ Before and after each shift worked
▶ Before and after resident contact
▶ After using a restroom
▶ Before and after handling food
▶ After handling anything you think is contaminated (dirty), especially body fluids
▶ Before and after cleaning an area
▶ Before and after handling body fluids collected for testing
▶ After smoking cigarettes

Hand Washing

Follow these steps for proper hand washing procedure:

1. Remove your watch and roll up your sleeves. Note: you might consider keeping jewelry to a minimum to prevent the constant removal for hand washing.
2. Turn on the water to a comfortable temperature. Wet hands and wrists (Fig 7-5).
3. Apply soap to hands from the dispenser (Fig. 7-6).
4. Rub hands in circular motion causing friction for 10 seconds (Fig. 7-7). Lace your fingers together to wash in between them (Fig. 7-8). Clean under your nails.
5. Rinse hands with warm water, keeping them downward, allowing the water to run from the wrist to the fingers (Fig. 7-9).
6. Dry hands with paper towel. Start at the top of the fingers and work downward toward the wrists (Figs. 7-10 and 7-11).
7. Turn off faucets with paper towel (Fig. 7-12).
8. Discard paper towel in appropriate receptacle (Fig. 7-13). Note: You may want to use a lotion on your hands if they are dry. This will prevent them from cracking.

Remember, no procedure is more important than washing your hands to prevent the transmission of diseases and infection. Practice the procedure carefully and consistently.

USING BARRIERS

Barriers include gloves, gowns or plastic aprons, masks, and eye protection. ***Barriers do not replace hand washing but should be used along with hand washing.*** Barriers protect your hands, skin, clothing, eyes, and mucous membranes from organisms that may be in a resident's secretions or excretions. They also protect residents. Barriers protect residents from organisms that may be on your hands, skin, or clothing.

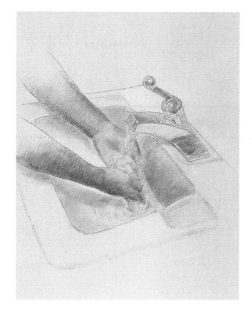

Fig. 7-5. Wet the hands and wrists.

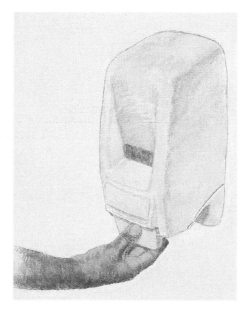

Fig. 7-6. Apply soap to the hands.

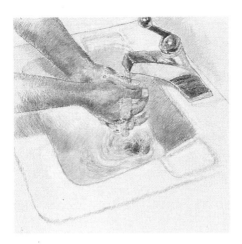

Fig. 7-7. Rub hands together in a circular motion.

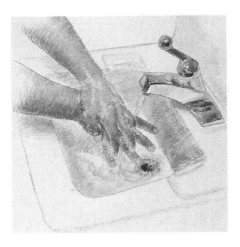

Fig. 7-8. Lace fingers together to wash in between them.

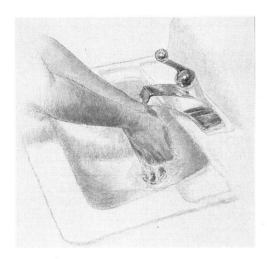

Fig. 7-9. Rinse the hands and keep them downward.

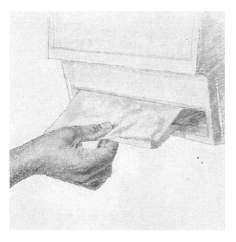

Fig. 7-10. Use a paper towel to dry hands.

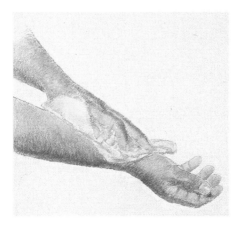

Fig. 7-11. Dry hands. Start at the tip of the fingers and work downward toward the wrist.

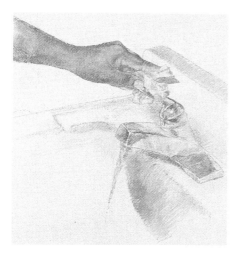

Fig. 7-12. Turn off water with paper towel.

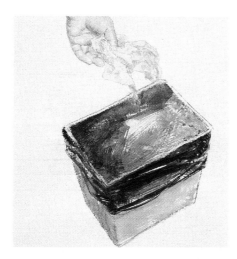

Fig. 7-13. Discard towel in appropriate receptacle.

Gloves

Gloves are made of a variety of materials. You usually use single-use clean disposable gloves made of latex, vinyl, or other synthetic materials. These gloves are packaged clean, not sterile. Some types of gloves fit better than others, and better-fitting gloves are needed for fine motor skills. Most of the tasks you do that require gloves will not require them to fit tightly or for the gloves to be sterile. Change gloves and wash your hands after completing care activities for one resident before caring for another. You don't want to carry organisms on your gloves from one resident to another.

If you are cleaning equipment or surfaces such as a bedside table, it is better to wear heavy utility gloves rather than single-use clean disposable gloves (Fig. 7-14). The chemicals in cleaning solutions are hard on the hands, and the heavy utility gloves provide better protection. These utility gloves can be reused for cleaning until they are cracked or worn out, just as you would use similar gloves many times at home.

Situations where you should wear gloves include cleaning a resident who is incontinent of stool and cleaning bedpans that have stool in them (Fig. 7-15). Organisms in stool easily get under the fingernails and are difficult to wash away, even with good hand washing.

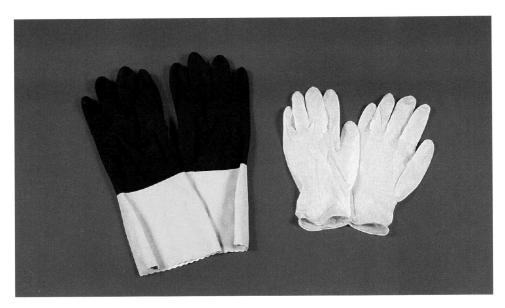

Fig. 7-14. When cleaning, heavy utility gloves are preferable to disposable latex gloves.

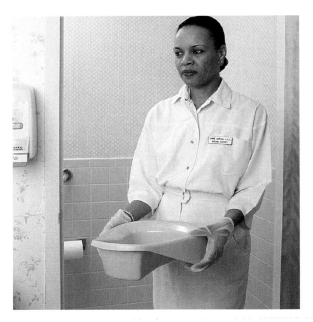

Fig. 7-15. Wear gloves when there is a possibility of coming in contact with stool.

Many tasks you perform do not require gloves if you can use another barrier between your hands and a resident's secretions or excretions. You usually do not need to wear gloves to handle a resident's urinary incontinence pad because the pad has a barrier backing made of plastic and you do not need to touch the wet surface. If you accidentally touch the wet surface, hand washing removes the urine from your hands quite well.

Some nurse assistants prefer to wear gloves to remove, handle, and clean a resident's dentures because of the oral secretions on them. Other nurse assistants handle dentures with a paper towel to provide a barrier between the nurse assistant's hands and a resident's oral secretions.

Whenever you are getting ready to do a task for a resident, ask yourself, "Will my hands touch something wet or moist?" If the answer is yes, ask, "Do I need to wear gloves or any other personal protection equipment, or can I use another, less expensive, barrier?" Wash your hands whenever you touch something moist and after your remove your gloves.

If gloves are being used alone, put them on immediately before your hands contact broken skin or mucous membranes. Put them on any time you need them as a barrier between you and a resident's secretions or excretions. Follow these steps for putting on gloves:

Putting On Gloves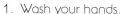

1. Wash your hands.
2. Slip gloves on, covering entire hand and wrist
   Note: If putting on gloves along with a gown and mask, put the gown on first, then the mask, and then the gloves. Be sure the gloves are pulled up over the gown cuffs.

Remove gloves when your task is completed. Remove them as described below if you are right handed. Reverse hands in each step if you are left handed.

Removing Gloves

1. Using your right hand, grasp the glove on the left hand at the inside of the wrist, turning it inside out as you pull it down over your left hand (Fig. 7-16)
2. Hold the used glove in a ball in your gloved right hand (Fig. 7-17).
3. Grasp the inside of the top of the right glove with the left hand (Fig. 7-18).
   Note: If you are wearing fitted, sterile gloves, you will not be able to grasp the inside of the top of the right glove—so, you must cuff the top of the right glove before you begin.
4. Pull the right glove down over the right hand and over the used glove you are holding. The right glove is now inside out and has the left glove enclosed in it (Fig. 7-19).
5. Discard the gloves in the trash can. Use your facility's infection control policies to guide your disposal of soiled waste (Fig. 7-20).
6. Wash your hands.

Gowns and Plastic Aprons

Gowns are a barrier used to cover the skin and clothing. Gowns may be made of cloth, paper, or plastic. You are the best judge of whether you need to wear a gown to protect your skin and clothing from a resident's secretions or excretions.

Plastic aprons are a barrier used to cover the front of your clothing and are particularly useful if your clothing may get wet, such as when assisting a resident with bathing. Plastic aprons are also useful for changing soiled linen that cannot easily be folded on itself to contain the soilage (Fig. 7-21).

Microorganisms are not transmitted efficiently by clothing, and there is no convincing evidence that care providers "carry germs home" to their children from the facility. However, nobody likes to wear soiled or dirty clothing, and gowns and aprons help keep clothing clean.

Gowns

If you are using gloves and a gown, apply the gown first, then apply gloves as described above. If the gown is for one-time-use only, follow these steps:

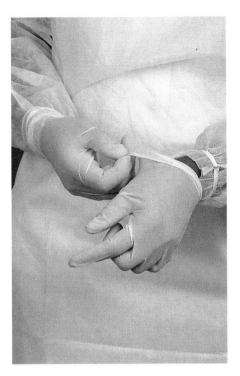

Fig. 7-16. With the right hand, grasp glove on left hand. Turn it inside out as you pull it off.

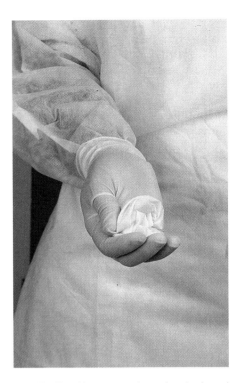

Fig. 7-17. Use your gloved right hand to hold the used glove in a ball.

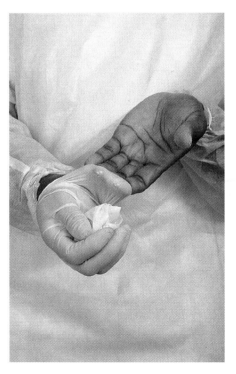

Fig. 7-18. Grasp inside of top of right glove with left hand.

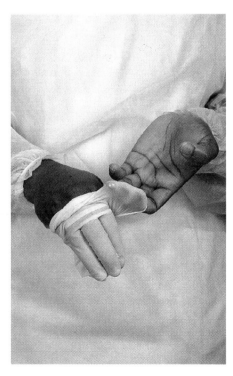

Fig. 7-19. Pull right glove down over used glove.

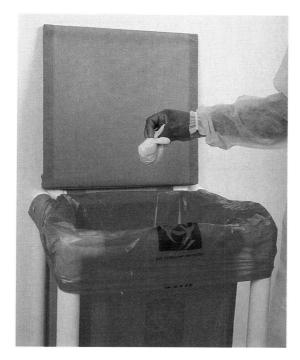

Fig. 7-20. Discard the gloves. (see Step 5).

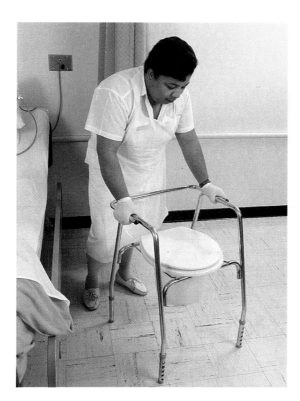

Fig. 7-21. A plastic apron helps protect the front of your clothing from contamination.

1. Open the gown (Fig. 7-22).
2. Put each arm in the gown's sleeves, with the opening in the back (Fig. 7-23).
3. Tie the gown at the neck and waist (Fig. 7-24)
   Note: Apply gloves afterwards and pull the gloves up over the gown's cuffs.

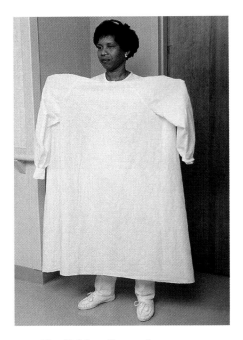

Fig. 7-22. Open the gown.

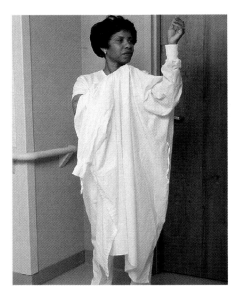

Fig. 7-23. Put each arm in the gown sleeves.

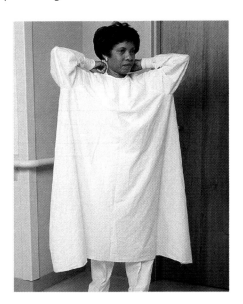

Fig. 7-24. Tie the gown.

Removing the Gown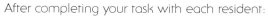

After completing your task with each resident:
1. Remove the gloves first, and discard them.
2. Remove the gown by untying the waist and neck (Fig. 7-25).
3. Grasp the cuff of one of the sleeves and pull the arm down over that hand (Fig. 7-26).
4. Pull the other arm off with the covered hand (Fig. 7-27).
5. Carefully roll the gown up, keeping the soiled surface inside (Fig. 7-28).
   Note: If the gown is made of cloth and needs to be laundered, discard it in the appropriate linen hamper. If the gown is made of paper and is disposable, discard it in the trash can according to your facility's policy. In most states, gowns can be discarded as regular waste.
6. Wash your hands.

In some facilities you may use the same gown again when caring for the same resident. Be careful not to contaminate the inside of the gown that will touch your clean clothes and skin.

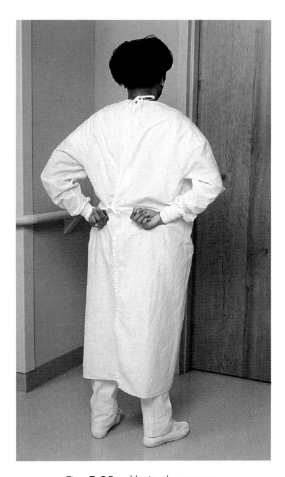

Fig. 7-25. Untie the gown.

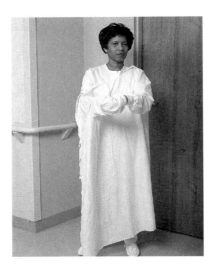

Fig. 7-26.   Pull the gown down off the arm.

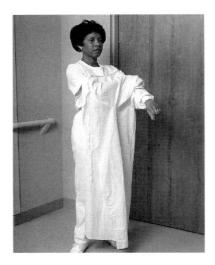

Fig. 7-27.   Pull the other arm off.

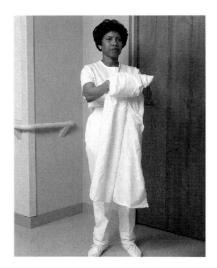

Fig. 7-28.   Roll the gown with the soiled surface inside.

Plastic Aprons

Plastic aprons usually have a strap around the neck and ties at the waist. They do not protect the arms. To put on a plastic apron, slip the strap over your head and tie it at the waist. The apron keeps the front of your clothes clean and dry.

Remove the plastic apron by untying the ties at the waist, pulling the neck strap over your head, and rolling the apron into a ball with the contaminated surface on the inside. This is similar to removing a gown except there are no sleeves. Discard the apron in the regular trash. Wash your hands.

If you are using gloves and a plastic apron, put on the apron, then the gloves. Remove the gloves, and then remove the apron. Wash your hands.

Masks

Masks protect the mucous membranes of the mouth and nose from splashes and may protect the wearer from inhaling airborne droplet nuclei from the air. Masks are an effective barrier to splashes or splatters (Fig. 7-29). However, few tasks are done by nurse assistants that result in splashing or splattering of your face, nose, and mouth.

The effectiveness of masks to protect the wearer from inhaling airborne droplets has not been proven. The mask must fit tightly enough for air not to be inhaled easily from around the sides of the mask.

Masks used in the operating room are intended to protect surgical patients from organisms in the care provider's respiratory secretions. Few situations in long term care facilities involve protecting residents from you with a mask. Although some believe you should wear a mask if you have an upper respiratory infection such as a cold, cold viruses are transmitted more easily from your hands. Hand washing is the best way to prevent transmission of the common cold.

Masks vary somewhat but all have a metal bar on the bridge of the nose and ties or straps to secure the mask. Follow these steps for putting on the mask:

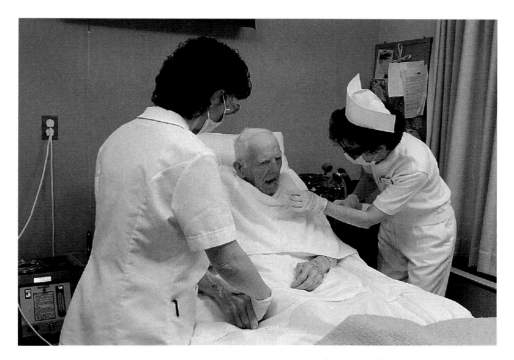

Fig. 7-29. Masks protect the mouth and nose from splashes.

1. Put the mask over your nose and mouth (Fig. 7-30).
2. Tie or secure the straps around the ears or back of the head so that the mask fits tightly (Fig. 7-31).
3. Pinch the metal piece on the bridge of the nose to provide a tight seal (Fig. 7-32).

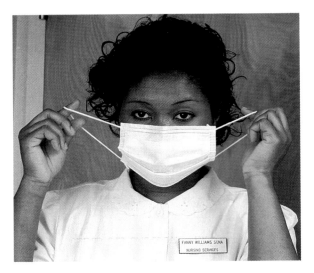

Fig. 7-30. Put the mask on.

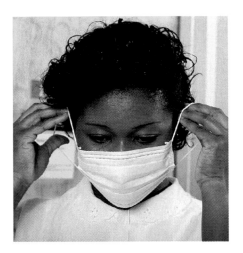

Fig. 7-31. Secure the straps.

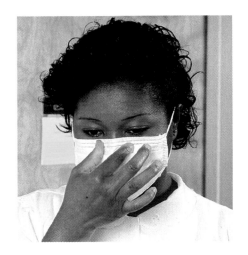

Fig. 7-32. Pinch the metal bridge.

Removing the Mask

1. Remove the mask by untying the ties or pulling the straps over the ears or head (Fig. 7-33).
2. Discard the mask in the regular trash, according to the facility's policy, and wash your hands (Fig. 7-34).

If you are using a mask, gloves, and a gown or apron, put on the gown or apron first, then put on the mask, then put on the gloves. Remove the gloves first, then the gown or apron, then the mask. Wash your hands when all barriers are removed.

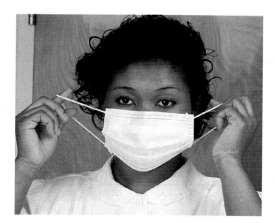

Fig. 7-33. Remove the mask.

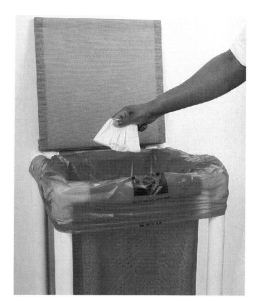

Fig. 7-34. Discard the mask and wash your hands.

Eye Protection

Eye protection provided by goggles or glasses with side shields protects the eyes from splashes or splatters. The OSHA Bloodborne Pathogens Standard requires that masks and eye protection be used together if splashing or splattering of the face is likely. Very rarely are nurse assistants in situations requiring this kind of protection (Fig. 7-35).

If you wear corrective lenses (glasses) and want to use them for splash protection, they must be equipped with side shields to protect you from splashing from the side. You may want to obtain side shields for splash protection so that you do not have to remove your glasses or use a pair of goggles on top of them if you are doing a task where you are likely to be splashed. The infection control practitioner for your facility can help you find appropriate side shields for your glasses.

If you do not wear glasses and need eye protection, you need to use goggles or a face shield. Goggles can be washed, dried, and reused many times. Most face shields can also be washed, dried, and reused many times. Some manufacturers make a combination mask and eye protection shield intended for single use only. These shields can be used with corrective lenses and provide adequate splash protection from the front and sides.

If you are using eye protection and a mask along with a gown or plastic apron and gloves, put on the eye protection when you put on the mask and remove it when you remove the mask. Wash your hands after you have removed all barriers.

CLEANING, DISINFECTION, AND STERILIZATION
Cleaning

Cleaning is the removal of soil from objects. Water, detergent, and scrubbing are used to clean things. Cleaning is done for infection control and prevention and to keep the environment pleasant and free of odors, dust, and dirt.

Housekeepers in facilities generally clean floors, carpets, walls, and large items regularly. They also clean drapes, curtain dividers, and furniture, as needed. When a resident is discharged, housekeepers may thoroughly clean the bed, chairs, overbed and bedside tables, and the entire area of the room so that the environment is clean and attractive for the next resident (Fig. 7-36).

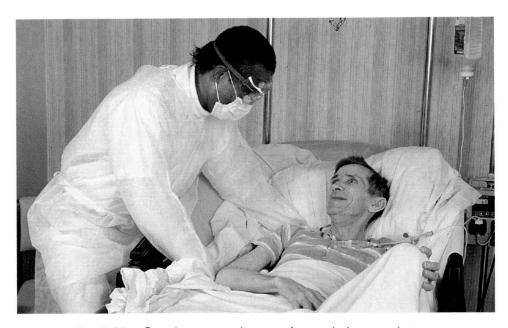

Fig. 7-35.   Goggles protect the eyes from splashes or splatters.

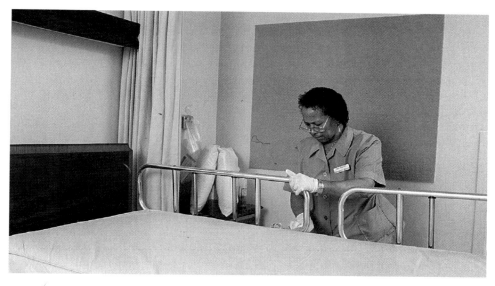

Fig. 7-36. After a resident is discharged, housekeepers thoroughly clean the room for the next resident.

In some facilities, nurse assistants may clean residents' immediate environment during daily care activities. Be sure you know who is responsible for cleaning what in residents' rooms so that tabletop items are cared for and discarded when needed.

Disinfection

Disinfection is a process that eliminates most but not all microorganisms on objects. This is usually done with special chemicals, sometimes combined with a detergent. This detergent/disinfectant is used for general cleaning of objects such as overbed tables, side rails, and plastic-covered mattresses. These items generally only need to be clean, but as an added measure of safety, some facilities like to clean them with a detergent that includes a disinfectant in the solution (Fig. 7-37). When you use these disinfectants, wear gloves to protect your hands from being burned or damaged, as you do at home when cleaning a bathroom or kitchen with chemical cleaners.

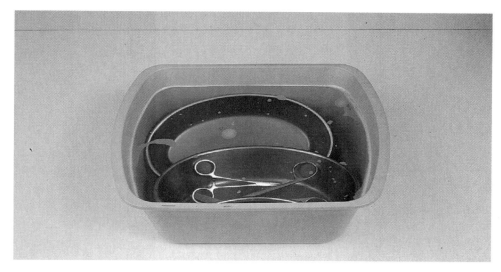

Fig. 7-37. A detergent/disinfectant can be used to clean and disinfect some things.

Sterilization

Sterilization is the complete elimination of all microorganisms. Many items used for resident care are purchased sterile, such as gauze pads, surgical supplies, urinary catheters, needles used to give injections, and bags of fluid used for intravascular (IV) therapy (Fig. 7-38).

An autoclave is a type of equipment that generates steam under pressure to sterilize things such as surgical instruments and operating room supplies. Objects that cannot stand the heat of steam are sterilized with ethylene oxide gas. Other chemicals also may be used to kill all organisms.

DESIGNATED CLEAN AND DIRTY AREAS OF THE FACILITY

Most facilities have designated clean and dirty utility rooms or areas to keep separate clean and dirty supplies, equipment, and functions. Clean utility rooms or areas are used to store supplies such as bandages and tape, dressings, urinary catheters and tubing, bed saver pads, bottles of irrigation fluid, irrigation sets, feeding tubes and supplies, bedside kits (with wash basin, water pitcher, cup, and emesis basin), and other clean supplies (Fig. 7-39). Some supplies for an individual resident may also be stored in that person's room if there is space.

Once a resident has used a supply or patient care item, it is considered dirty. Some used supplies such as soiled dressings or bed saver pads are disposable and are discarded into a waste can in that resident's room. Other supplies will be reused, but must be cleaned first. Follow your facility's policy for cleaning reusable supplies. When you take a piece of dirty equipment (such as a used bedpan) to the dirty side of the utility room to be cleaned, always wash your hands after you finish cleaning it. Then return the cleaned bedpan to the resident's bedside or bathroom. Wash your hands again before you take some clean supplies from the clean side of the utility room.

An alternative to using a dirty utility room or area for some cleaning functions is to use a resident's bathroom. The toilet there may be used to empty bedpans, urinals, and emesis basins. Bedpans can also be rinsed in a resident's bathroom if the toilet has a pull-down lever or spray cleaning device, but bedpans should not be washed out in the same sink that you or the resident will use for hand washing or brushing teeth. Stool in bedpans can contaminate sinks with microorganisms that

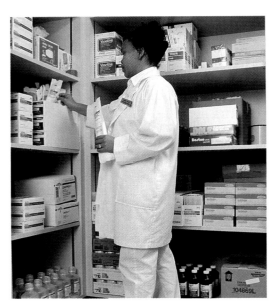

Fig. 7-38. Sterile items used for resident care are stored in special supply rooms.

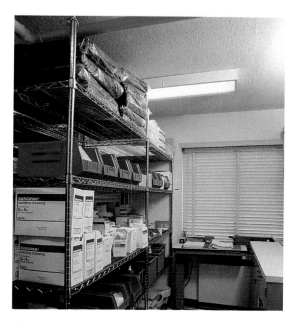

Fig. 7-39. Clean utility rooms are used to store clean supplies.

can then contaminate your hands later, or items used by other nurse assistants or others. If stool microorganisms from contaminated hands are ingested, they may cause gastrointestinal illness.

Dirty utility rooms or areas are also used for cleaning reusable equipment that may be used next with a different resident. For example, when a resident is discharged from the facility, reusable basins, bedpans, and urinals must be cleaned, dried well, and stored for another resident to use later. Dirty utility areas are also used to clean equipment such as wheelchairs when they are soiled by incontinent residents.

Most dirty utility rooms or areas have a deep flushing sink similar to a toilet so that liquid wastes can be poured into it and go directly into the sanitary sewerage system. Many dirty utility areas also contain waste receptacles for disposal of filled containers of sharps and other regulated waste ("red bagged trash"). Be sure you know the regulations for "red bagged trash" for your facility, as these regulations vary from county to county and from state to state.

PROTECTING YOURSELF FROM BLOODBORNE INFECTIONS

Several viruses can live in a person's blood without that person appearing sick right away. The viruses of special concern to nurse assistants and others in nursing facilities are the hepatitis B virus (HBV), the hepatitis C virus (HCV), and the human immunodeficiency virus (HIV).

Universal Precautions

To prevent transmission of these bloodborne viruses, the Centers for Disease Control (CDC) developed recommendations for facilities to use in handling the blood and certain body fluids of *all* patients. These recommendations are called universal blood and body fluid precautions (or universal precautions) (Fig. 7-40). Universal precautions are an approach to infection control and prevention. The basic concept is that all human beings, their blood, and certain body fluids are to be treated as if infected with HIV, HBV, and other bloodborne pathogens.

Because universal precautions are intended to prevent exposure to bloodborne pathogens, they apply only to blood and body fluids that transmit disease: semen, vaginal secretions, tissues, and joint and closed space fluids. They do not apply to

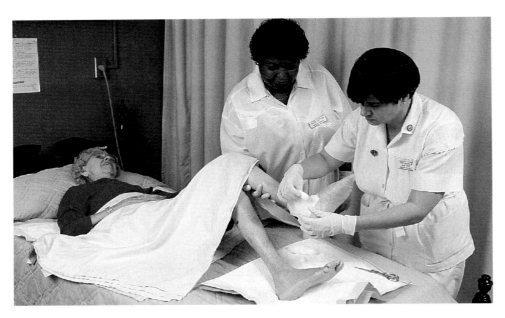

Fig. 7-40. Using gloves is a universal precaution used when changing the dressing of a resident's open wound.

feces, nasal secretions, sputum, saliva, sweat, tears, urine, and vomitus unless they contain visible blood.

In general, universal precautions involve *any* work practices that minimize or eliminate exposure to bloodborne pathogens. Information covered in the first section of this chapter on preventing the transmission of infection is considered part of universal precaution practices—the use of hand washing, barriers, and cleaning, disinfecting, and sterilizing.

The OSHA Bloodborne Pathogens Standard

The Occupational Safety and Health Administration (OSHA) Standard (1992) requires all health care agencies, including long term care facilities, to comply with the Center for Disease Control (CDC) recommendations for universal precautions. In addition, there are several other requirements of the Standard.

Preventing Needlesticks

Microorganisms in the blood of one person can enter the body of a susceptible host through accidental needlestick injuries. Consider the following example:

> The nurse has just given Ms. Anderson an insulin injection. Ms. Johnson, her roommate, faints out of bed just as the nurse removes the needle from Ms. Anderson's skin. The nurse quickly puts the needle and syringe down by Ms. Anderson's pillow as she rushes over to help Ms. Johnson.
>
> You are in the hallway and hear Ms. Johnson fall. You come in the room to see if the nurse needs help. You notice Ms. Anderson is very concerned about her roommate's fall. You go over to comfort her. You do not see the needle and syringe by the pillow until you feel a stick in your arm when you adjust Ms. Anderson's pillow.

In this case, the needle is an intermediate object that could transfer the blood from the patient to you through your skin. If Ms. Anderson had organisms in her blood, this needlestick could transfer those to you. In any case, you would need to participate in your facility's program for postexposure evaluation and follow-up of needlestick injuries.

Of course, you and the nurse know the nurse should have discarded the needle and syringe immediately after use in a needle disposal container (Fig. 7-41). However, Ms. Johnson's fall distracted her and Ms. Johnson needed immediate help. The nurse didn't take time to carry the needle to the disposal container outside the room before she helped Ms. Johnson. The nurse intended to return to Ms. Anderson's bed and discard the needle correctly as soon as she finished helping Ms. Johnson, but you came into the room while she was still helping her up from her fall. If you were the nurse, what would you have done?

Exposure Control Plan

All facilities are required by OSHA to have a written exposure control plan designed to eliminate or minimize employee exposure to blood and body fluids to which universal precautions apply. Every department in the facility is involved in the exposure control plan. Every employee should be aware of the plan and have access to it any time.

Engineering and Work Practice Controls. Engineering controls remove a hazard through devices. An example is a needle disposal container near the place needles and sharps are used, so that sharps can be discarded directly without need for recapping or transport to another location.

Work practice controls make job procedures safer. An unsafe practice is to recap a used needle with two hands because it is easy to slip and puncture the finger holding the cap (Fig. 7-42). An example of a work practice control is to use a one-handed scoop technique to recap a used needle if it must recapped to be transported elsewhere. In a later section you will learn more about special equipment used in infection prevention.

Personal Protective Equipment. Personal protective equipment includes barriers to prevent contact between the reservoir and the susceptible host. Gloves, masks and eye protection, and cover gowns or aprons prevent you from contacting

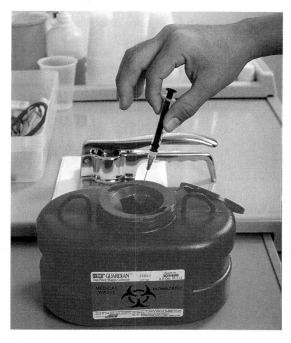

Fig. 7-41. Discard needles and syringes in the proper disposal container immediately after use.

blood or other body fluids from patients. The proper use of these barriers are described in Chapter 23 (Fig. 7-43).

Housekeeping. The facility's environment must be maintained in a clean and sanitary condition. A written schedule is required for cleaning the facility that includes methods for decontaminating surfaces or equipment soiled with blood or body fluids. If you have questions about how the OSHA Bloodborne Pathogens Standard is followed in your facility, the infection control practitioner can help you.

Hepatitis B Vaccination and Post-exposure Evaluation and Follow-up

OSHA requires all facilities to make the hepatitis B vaccine available to all employees who may have occupational exposure to blood or other infectious materials

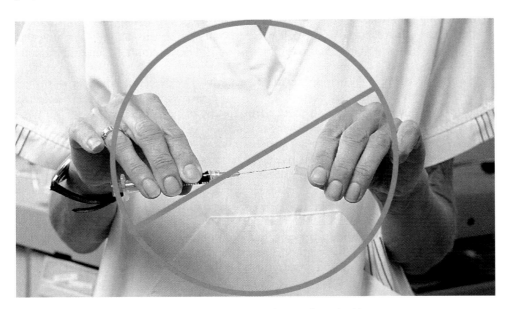

Fig. 7-42.   Never recap a needle with two hands. If you must recap a needle, scoop the cap onto the needle with the same hand that holds it.

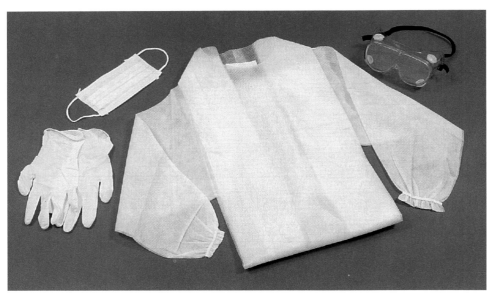

Fig. 7-43.   Personal protective equipment.

(Fig. 7-44). The facility cannot require the employee to take the vaccine or to pay for the vaccine. All facilities are required to provide postexposure evaluation and follow-up if an exposure incident occurs. This evaluation must be paid for by the employer, but it does not have to be done at the facility where the exposure occurred.

Information and Training Requirements

The OSHA Standard requires the employer to provide information and training to all employees during working hours. This training must include information about bloodborne pathogens, discussion of tasks that involve occupational exposure, and ways to reduce exposure risks.

Information About Bloodborne Pathogens. The OSHA Standard is intended to protect workers from all known and unknown diseases transmitted by blood. The viruses of greatest concern at present are hepatitis B virus (HBV) and the human immunodeficiency virus (HIV) that causes acquired immunodeficiency syndrome (AIDS).

HIV and AIDS. The signs and symptoms of HIV infection are extremely variable. HIV infection can be detected with an HIV-antibody test within a few weeks to several months after a person is infected, but HIV-infected persons may have no apparent signs or symptoms for an average of 10 years.

HIV is transmitted by contact with blood and other body fluids such as semen and vaginal secretions. Transmission occurs by sexual contact, sharing drug needles, receiving contaminated blood products, and being born to an HIV-infected mother.

Occupational transmission has occurred from puncture injuries with HIV-blood-contaminated needles and sharps, and from HIV-blood contact with broken skin or mucous membranes. The risk of infection from a puncture with an HIV-blood-contaminated sharp is about one chance in 300. That is, for every 300 health care workers who are punctured with needles contaminated with HIV-blood, only one would become infected with HIV. The other 299 or so do not become infected because their immune systems are strong enough to keep the virus from causing infection.

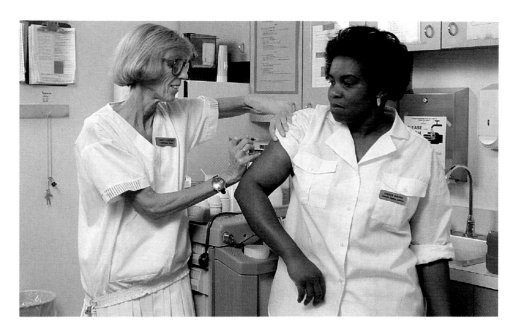

Fig. 7-44. OSHA requires that hepatitis B vaccine be available to employees who may be exposed to blood, or other infectious materials.

Tears, saliva, or other types of casual contact do not transmit HIV. Many studies have shown this. You do not have to worry about providing care for a resident with HIV as long as you follow the universal precautions.

Hepatitis B and Hepatitis C. Hepatitis B and hepatitis C are two viruses that cause inflammation of the liver. A vaccine to prevent hepatitis B is available, but there is not one for hepatitis C. Hepatitis C is transmitted in the same ways as hepatitis B and HIV infection. The good news is that hepatitis C is fairly rare, and few residents are likely to be infected with it.

Hepatitis B is far more common than HIV, and the hepatitis B virus (HBV) is present in high concentration in the blood of infected persons. This means HBV has a greater chance of infecting exposed persons. For example, if a person is stuck by a needle contaminated with HBV-infected blood, the risk for becoming infected ranges from 5% to 30%. Persons who have been immunized against hepatitis B will not become infected from sticks with needles contaminated with HBV-infected blood.

The most serious problem with hepatitis B and hepatitis C infections is that some people with these infections never get well. These are called chronic carriers. They have liver damage that may be so serious that they need liver transplants later in life. Preventing hepatitis B with vaccine will prevent this serious liver damage. Preventing hepatitis C with careful attention to sharps safety and barrier use when contact with blood is likely will help protect you from this infection.

Nurse Assistant Tasks Involving Exposure to Blood

Because nurse assistants do not administer medications to residents, they are not at direct risk for needle puncture injuries. However, nurse assistants may change sharps disposal containers and could be injured if needles are improperly disposed of, are sticking out the top, or have punctured the side of the container. **You must examine the sharps disposal container carefully *before* you handle it to prevent accidental injury.**

Because nurse assistants provide most of the care to residents, you may notice blood in drainage from a resident's wound or blood in a resident's stool, urine, or vomitus. Wear gloves in these clean-up activities to protect you from this blood of all residents (Fig. 7-45).

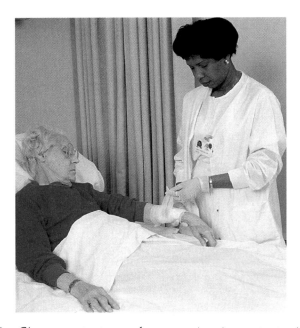

Fig. 7-45. Gloves protect you from coming in contact with blood when caring for a resident.

Situations are rare where you are likely to be splashed in the eyes, nose, or mouth with blood. These kinds of splashes are common in surgery and in critical care units but are very uncommon in long term care facilities, so you will rarely need to protect your eyes, nose, and mouth with barriers.

Nurse assistants sometimes clean up spills on the floor or in a resident's bathroom, and these spills can be bloody. The facility's procedure for cleaning up spills includes the use of an appropriate detergent/disinfectant, gloves, and a gown or plastic apron if the spill is large enough to soil your skin or clothing. The infection control practitioner or head housekeeper is your best resource for information about cleaning up spills.

SPECIAL EQUIPMENT AND SUPPLIES FOR INFECTION PREVENTION AND CONTROL
Sharps Safety Equipment

Punctures from sharps such as hypodermic needles and cuts from used scalpels put health care workers at risk for many infections, including HIV, HBV, and HCV. All facilities have policies and procedures for handling and disposing of used sharps. Sharps disposal containers should be located as close as possible to where they are used. In most facilities they are on medication carts and in medication rooms. Some facilities have sharps disposal containers on the walls of resident rooms, but other facilities do not because of concerns about resident safety if a resident were to tamper with the device.

Wastes Requiring Special Handling

The terms regulated waste, infectious waste, biohazardous waste, infective waste, and special waste are all used to designate wastes that require special handling. All states have regulations about management of wastes contaminated with blood or secretions and excretions.

Wastes that require special handling in most states include pathological wastes, lab cultures, liquid blood, and contaminated items that would release blood if compressed. The OSHA Bloodborne Pathogens Standard defines regulated wastes and sets requirements for handling, storage, or shipping. Regulated wastes are discarded in red bags or bags labeled with a special biohazard label (Fig. 7-46).

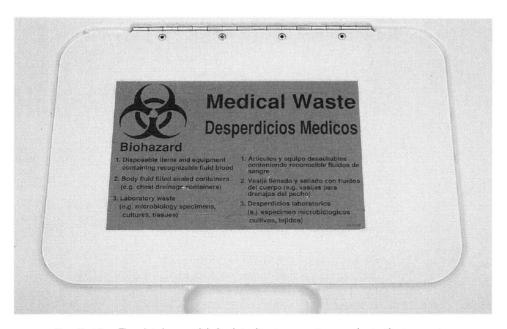

Fig. 7-46. The biohazard label indicates waste products that require special handling.

Check with your facility's infection control practitioner about regulations for waste because they differ from state to state and from facility to facility. If a resident is on isolation for a particular infection, then contaminated disposable supplies must be placed in a red bag (Fig. 7-47). Nondisposable items should be double-bagged. Chapter 23 discusses isolation procedures in more detail.

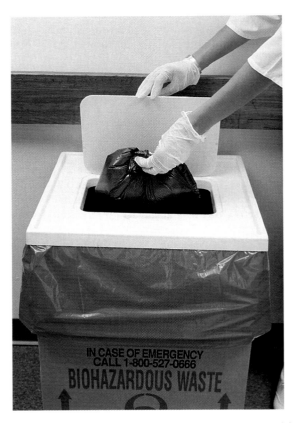

Fig. 7-47. Put disposable contaminated supplies in a red bag if the resident is on isolation for a particular infection.

INJURY PREVENTION

Just knowing something will not make a difference in your life if you do not do anything about it. We all know the importance of seat belts, for example. But have you ever been in a hurry to get to the store? Did you ever drive off not using your seat belt because the store was just a block away? Often people take shortcuts and skip important steps. But what if someone hits your car that one time you don't use your seat belt?

We all know that we should wear a seat belt, brush our teeth, look both ways before crossing the street, and limit fats and sugar. But do we always follow these common sense rules of healthy living? Sometimes we just think, "It won't happen to me." Ignoring common sense rules may not have immediate consequences. A second bowl of ice cream just once won't make you overweight. But other actions, like not wearing your seat belt, can mean pain, suffering, and injury to yourself or loved ones. Bad things won't happen every time, but once they do happen, all the wishing in the world cannot undo the bad results from an unwise or thoughtless choice.

No other nurse assistant role is more important than personal and resident safety. Yet as important as safety is, usually only a little extra effort is needed to prevent accidents and injuries. Most of the time you need only be mindful in your actions and use common sense to prevent injuries.

This chapter discusses common sense rules to prevent injury to you and residents. You will learn about good body mechanics to prevent injury to yourself when caring for residents. You will also learn how to prevent chemical and electrical hazards in the facility and your role in disaster preparedness.

ERGONOMICS

Ergonomics looks at the relationship between workers and their jobs. Studies have shown how job injuries can occur from repetitive body movements, awkward posture, using the wrong equipment, or using equipment wrongly. Repetitive job motions include bending, lifting, turning, and reaching. When you move in these ways, think about what muscles you are using and what kinds of injuries can occur. If you don't use the right equipment correctly or misuse your body when trying to perform your duties, you can seriously injure yourself.

Injuries result from not knowing how to do something safely or acting with bad habits. Sooner or later, an injury will happen if you are not careful to prevent it. As a beginning nurse assistant, you have the perfect opportunity to develop safe habits to prevent injury. You may even have some bad habits already. For example, unless you have been trained in body mechanics for moving and lifting, you might be bending over with your back when you lift something heavy. This habit can lead to serious injury. To break the habit you need to learn the correct way to lift something heavy without bending your back. Developing good work habits such as this lowers your risk of being injured. Other safety habits prevent other kinds of injury to both you and residents you work with.

Throughout this book, you will learn a variety of skills for caring for residents. Using mindful decision making and common sense safety principles applies to everything you learn to do as a nurse assistant. You also benefit from these good habits in your personal life and at home.

MINDFUL DECISION MAKING: INJURY PREVENTION

Consider injury prevention, or safety, one of the most important parts of your job. Being mindful about safety means paying attention to details, always assessing the situation, and being observant. It also means a willingness to ask questions and to change. Ask the charge nurse about any procedure or equipment or anything else you are not completely sure about (Fig. 8-1). Never put yourself or your resident at risk. Ask the charge nurse to help you to learn to evaluate situations. Remember, every resident and situation is different, and your actions have to change with each resident's unique needs.

Common Sense Rules

Following are common sense rules for the safety of all residents as well as your own. They include environmental concerns affecting both you and residents. The safety rules are grouped by how they concern residents, you, and the environment. Some of the safety rules involve all three. Consider each resident's own safety needs. For example, needs of residents with visual impairments may be different from those with hearing impairments. The key is to know your residents and their special needs. With this knowledge you will be able to adjust your common sense safety rules.

Resident

▷ Check each resident's path before walking for potential trip hazards such as a bed crank.
▷ Encourage residents to use handrails and grip rails.
▷ When bathing residents, test the water temperature carefully to be sure it is not too hot.
▷ Always turn the hot water off first and then the cold just in case hot water drips on a resident's skin or yours.
▷ Encourage residents to always use their assistive and prosthetic devices. For example, put on glasses when getting up at night to use the bathroom.
▷ Always respond to call lights immediately. Be sure the call bell is close by and that residents know exactly how to use it.

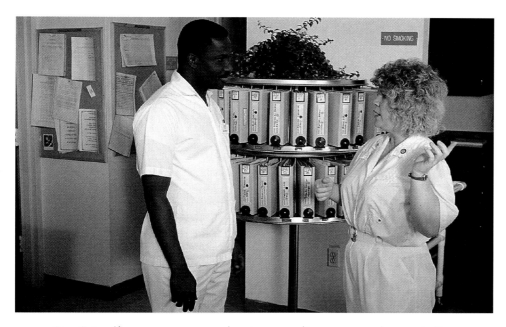

Fig. 8-1. If you are unsure about any policy or procedure, ask the charge nurse.

▷ Familiarize residents with all aspects of their surroundings.
▷ Always keep each resident's bed in its lowest position when a resident is resting or not in bed.
▷ Inspect assistive devices residents use, such as walkers and canes. Be sure that rubber tips are on and fit correctly.
▷ When moving a resident, always lock any moveable equipment, such as wheelchairs, shower chairs, beds, etc.

Nurse Assistant

▷ Wear nonskid shoes.
▷ Avoid jerky movements, such as fast, awkward turns. When you turn, move your feet so that your body can follow smoothly. Avoid twisting motions.
▷ Never reach high overhead for something; use a stool (Fig. 8-2).
▷ Always use proper body mechanics.
▷ Never run down a hallway; use caution when turning corners, because someone may be there.
▷ Never use electrical equipment near water.

Environment

▷ Always clean up spills immediately.
▷ Keep residents' rooms and hallways free of clutter.
▷ Make sure hallways are well lit.
▷ Use night lights.
▷ Always store chemicals like cleaning solutions and medicines in their proper place.

By following these common sense rules, you can know you have done everything to protect residents and yourself from injury.

BODY MECHANICS

Being able to lift safely is an important part of your job. When assisting a resident with many kinds of care, pushing an equipment cart, or lifting a box of supplies, always take care to ensure good body positioning. This is called good "body

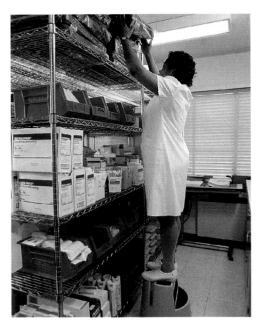

Fig. 8-2. Use a stool to get items that are out of reach.

mechanics" and helps to prevent injury to you and residents. Body mechanics are the way you use your body to do something.

Proper body mechanics maximize the body's efficiency by using the body efficiently and minimizing stress. With good body mechanics the body has to do less work in any particular task. Poor body mechanics can injure the back or other areas. Even though injuries like strains and sprains may not seem too serious, over time smaller injuries accumulate to cause a more serious injury. Not using good body mechanics every time you do something puts you at risk for injury. Remember your back all day long. Before you lift something, take a minute to assess the situation. If you are lifting a resident, find out first if he or she can help you. If you have any doubts about your ability to lift someone or something, get help.

Principles of Body Mechanics

Think of the principles of body mechanics in terms of three steps. Step 1 is what to consider before lifting, moving, or positioning. Step 2 is preparing yourself, and Step 3 is how to do the lifting, moving, or positioning.

Things to Consider

▶ Adjust the height of the bed. Move it up when providing care, such as when giving a complete bed bath, and down when moving someone out of the bed. Adjusting the height will reduce the amount of bending you will have to do (Fig. 8-3).

▶ Never reach over things, like bed rails, tables, or people. Bring what you need close to you to avoid reaching injuries.

▶ If you are moving a resident in bed, consider putting your knee up on the bed. This lets you to get closer to residents without reaching. Note: If you are concerned about infection control, place a barrier (such as a sheet or towel) between your knee and the bed sheets (Fig. 8-4).

Preparing Yourself

▶ Separate your feet about shoulder width apart to widen your base of support for better support and strength.

▶ Put one foot slightly in front of the other, giving you a stronger base of support.

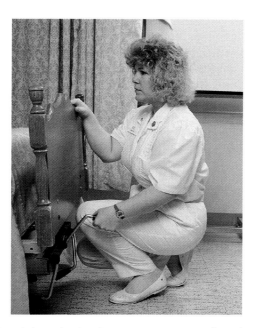

Fig. 8-3. Adjust the bed as necessary to reduce bending.

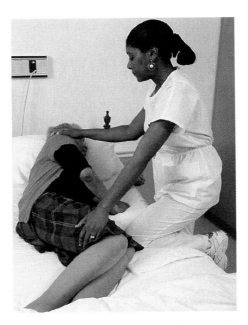

Fig. 8-4. Put your knee on the bed to get closer to the resident without reaching.

- Tighten your abdominal muscles by pulling in your stomach to support your spine.
- Concentrate on keeping your back straight when lifting. Keeping your back straight will prevent injury.
- Bend your knees and lift using your leg and arm muscles. Leg and arm muscles have the greatest strength (Fig. 8-5).

How to Move

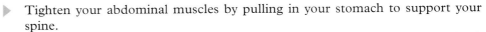

- Get as close as possible to what you are lifting or moving. "Hugs" are very supportive: bring a resident or the item you are moving as close to you as possible. Getting close gives you more strength (Fig. 8-6). Try carrying something with your arms stretched out versus close to you.
- Keep your palms up when lifting: get under what you are lifting. This uses the biceps, the strongest arm muscles.

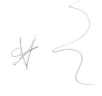

- Breathe in deeply before you begin to lift and breathe out while you lift. This helps pump blood and oxygen to muscles.
- Always rock to gain momentum for a lift or move. Rocking consists of moving slightly back and forth or side to side. It shifts your weight to and from the object you are moving. This motion increases your strength in the move. But always be careful not to move a resident too fast, which could potentially cause injury.

Apply these principles as you learn the procedures of resident care. In Chapter 13, " Moving and Positioning," you will learn many different skills for helping a resident move in bed and between bed and chair. You can injure your back in any procedure if you are careless about body mechanics. Be mindful about doing it the right way and your body will thank you for it.

Body mechanics help prevent injury. It is like deciding to wear your seat belt: no one but you can make the decision, but the decision can prevent injury.

ENVIRONMENTAL AWARENESS

In addition to being safe in your actions, you need to be aware of the environment in the long term care facility and control it to prevent injuries.

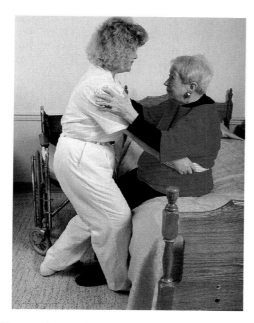

Fig. 8-5. With your knees bent, lift using your arm and leg muscles.

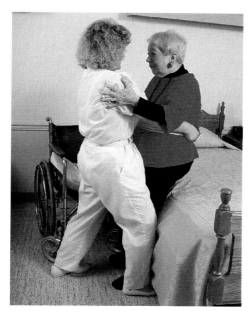

Fig. 8-6. While moving the resident, bring her or him as close to you as possible.

Wet Floor

Everyone is responsible for cleaning up spills. Whether you make or find a spill, you must ensure it is cleaned up immediately. Even if you are responding to a medical emergency, think to call out and get someone else to take care of the clean-up before someone slips and is seriously injured.

The clean-up is simple. First make sure that everyone is alerted to danger. Mark the location with an easily seen "Wet Floor" sign (Fig. 8-7). If the wet area is large, use additional signs. Don't leave to get the sign, but request another staff member to bring you the sign and clean-up equipment.

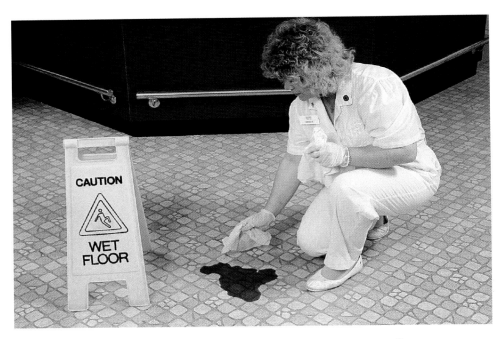

Fig. 8-7. A "Wet Floor" sign will alert others of a spill.

Dry the floor as much as possible. If a high traffic location or a very large area is involved, ask the housekeeping department to dry the floor immediately. Remove warning signs afterwards or others may get in the habit of ignoring them.

When working with water, such as when giving showers, be extra careful. Don't assume that everyone is on the lookout. You know of the increased chance for a slip or fall, but not everyone will be as aware as you. Keep your eyes open and your work area clean and dry. Watch out for your co-workers.

Remember: It is everyone's job to clean up spills. The guidelines above apply not only to wet areas but also to any kind of slipping or tripping hazard on the floor, such as urine, broken floor tiles, soap, paper clips, bed cranks, food, etc.

Electrical Safety

Electrical safety also is everyone's concern. While working with and around electricity, follow these guidelines:

▷ Never use electrical devices around water.
▷ Always dry hands before using electrical equipment.
▷ Never use extension cords or outlet expanders. These are prohibited by law in facilities.
▷ If you're not currently using the device, then turn it off.
▷ Report any electrical shock to your supervisor. The device should be removed from use until it is repaired.
▷ Never attempt to repair an electrical device yourself.

Also pay attention to electrical items family members bring in. Things like electrical razors, televisions, fans, radios, and lamps should be examined by maintenance staff for potential electrical problems. In some facilities this inspection is a set policy before the item can be used (Fig. 8-8). Supervise any residents' use of equipment.

With any electrical device, always watch to be sure the device is in working order. Watch for frayed cords, sparks, excessive heat, missing guards, exposed wires, or any cracks that may indicate the device may not be in proper working order. Report any such conditions immediately to your supervisor.

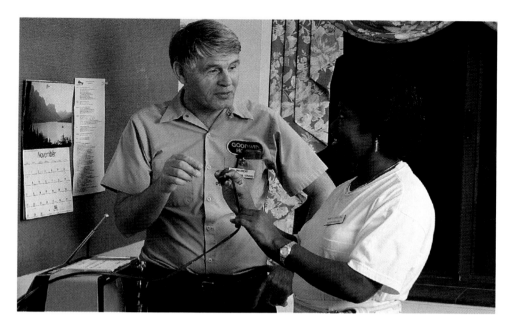

Fig. 8-8. The maintenance staff should inspect electrical items before use.

Chemical Training

By law, all employers must educate employees about chemicals used in the work place. In care facilities, these chemicals usually mean disinfectants and cleaners. Follow their directions for use, and you and your residents will be completely safe.

If you will use any hazardous chemicals, you will receive specialized training about them. This training is called hazard communication training or "Haz Com" and is required by Occupational Safety and Health Administration (OSHA) standards. This training includes any information you need to know to ensure safety.

Material Safety Data Sheets (MSDS)

As part of your training about chemicals, you will learn about Material Safety Data Sheets (MSDS), which describe chemicals you will use. Each sheet has a complete listing of the chemical contents, a physical description, fire and health hazards, precautions and clean up procedures, disposal requirements, needed personal protective equipment, and first aid procedures. Your facility keeps these sheets in an accessible location like the nurses station (Fig. 8-9).

Container Labeling

You will also be trained about container labeling. You must get in the habit of reading and following labels because they contain most of the information you need to protect both you and your residents (Fig. 8-10). If you find a container that isn't labeled, do not smell it to guess what it is or use it in any way. Take it to the charge nurse immediately.

Emergency First Aid for Chemical Exposures

How you act in the event of a chemical exposure depends on what kind of chemical you are using. Following is the general emergency first aid related to chemicals:

▶ Follow the guidelines in the material safety data sheet for the chemical.
▶ See your supervisor immediately, who will contact the local Poison Control Center if needed for what actions to take.
▶ If you or a resident inhales the chemical, get to fresh air.

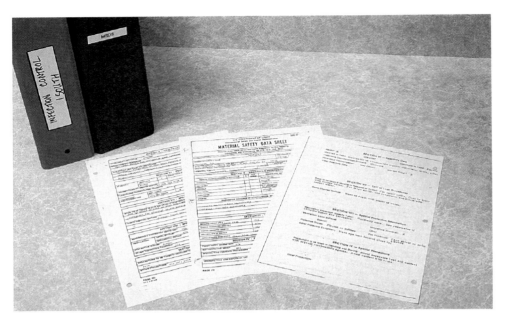

Fig. 8-9. Material Safety Data Sheets describe the chemicals you will use.

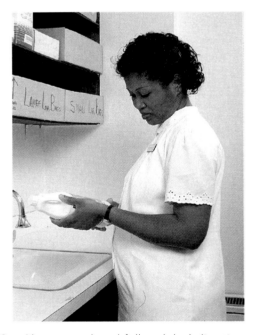

Fig. 8-10. Always read and follow label directions carefully.

▷ If you or a resident gets it on your skin, rinse it off with lots of running water.
▷ If you or a resident swallows it, do not induce vomiting. Rinse out your mouth. Wait for instructions from the Poison Control Center (Fig. 8-11).
Spills or Splashes to Your Eyes
▷ Immediately flush your eyes with cool running water for at least 5 minutes.
▷ Remove contact lenses.
▷ Continue flushing for at least 15 minutes, holding eyelids apart to ensure rinsing of the entire eye.

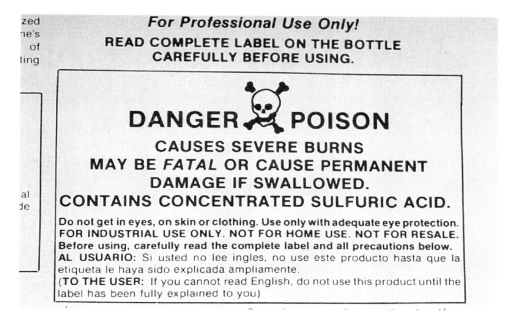

For Professional Use Only!
READ COMPLETE LABEL ON THE BOTTLE
CAREFULLY BEFORE USING.

DANGER ☠ POISON

CAUSES SEVERE BURNS
MAY BE *FATAL* OR CAUSE PERMANENT
DAMAGE IF SWALLOWED.
CONTAINS CONCENTRATED SULFURIC ACID.

Do not get in eyes, on skin or clothing. Use only with adequate eye protection.
FOR INDUSTRIAL USE ONLY. NOT FOR HOME USE. NOT FOR RESALE.
Before using, carefully read the complete label and all precautions below.
AL USUARIO: Si usted no lee ingles, no use este producto hasta que la etiqueta le haya sido explicada ampliamente.
(**TO THE USER:** If you cannot read English, do not use this product until the label has been fully explained to you)

Fig. 8-11. The Poison Control Center gives specific instructions on what to do if poison is ingested.

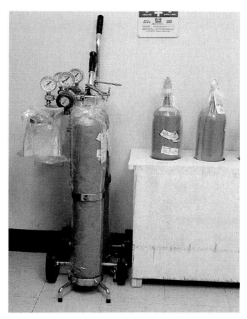

Fig. 8-12. Oxygen may be administered from green tank bottles of compressed gas.

Safety Around Oxygen Use

Oxygen (O_2) is an important gas in your facility. Because of the risk of explosion, you must remember certain important facts and follow certain precautions around oxygen.

Oxygen is administered in several different ways: from a valve in the wall, from green tank bottles (of various sizes) of compressed gas (8-12), or from the little machine called an oxygen concentrator. Regardless of the source of the oxygen, certain precautions always apply:

▸ Oxygen is not flammable itself but supports fire explosively, so eliminate all flame and spark sources. This includes smoking when oxygen is in use.

▸ Always put "No Smoking —- Oxygen" signs on doors where oxygen is in use (Fig. 8-13).

▸ NEVER apply any kind of lubricant to hoses or fittings used with oxygen, as this can conduct a spark. If the pieces don't go together smoothly, inform the charge nurse.

In addition, follow these guidelines when using compressed oxygen cylinders:

▸ Be sure the cylinders are chained to the wall. Even if they are in a two-wheeled hand truck, they must be chained to ensure that they cannot be knocked over (Fig. 8-14).

▸ Keep the outlet valve protection caps in place.

▸ ALWAYS use a hand cart to transfer large cylinders.

▸ NEVER drop cylinders or let them hit each other violently.

▸ Report empty cylinders to the charge nurse.

For information about oxygen use with residents, see Chapter 24, Management of Common Chronic Illness and Problems.

DISASTER PREPAREDNESS

All facilities have written disaster plans to follow in case of an emergency. These plans usually say that employees must first remove residents to safety and then give care to those residents. Regardless of problems caused by the disaster, you must still meet the needs of your residents.

Disaster plans cannot assign tasks to specific people because of staffing differences day to day. Emergency tasks are assigned by job description. Therefore you need to be familiar with your facility's disaster plan and know what role the nurse assistants have in case a disaster strikes. Disasters may include natural disasters such as unsafe weather conditions and fires, discussed in the following sections.

Weather

The weather conditions you need to prepare for depend on your local weather. Emergencies can occur suddenly or with advance warning, such as a hurricane

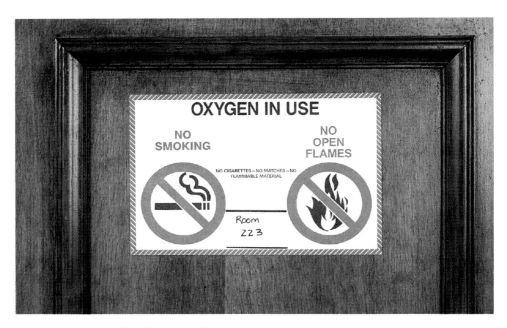

Fig. 8-13. "No Smoking-Oxygen" signs should be in plain view where oxygen is in use.

coming. The charge nurse will inform you when you need to evacuate residents. This may be done in an internal evacuation, in which residents are moved to another section within the facility, or an external evacuation, in which residents are transported to another site.

Evacuations follow a principle called "priority of movement." This is the order in which residents are taken out of the facility. The order starts with residents who require the least amount of assistance. This frees staff members to assist those who are more dependent and less able to move themselves to the new location. Usually the order occurs in this manner:

1. Ambulatory residents
2. Residents who require wheelchairs and walkers
3. Bed-ridden residents

To evacuate bedridden residents, you use emergency transfer methods that are quick, efficient, and safe. These are different from the transfer techniques you use normally. These emergency methods are described in Appendix D.

Fire

Fire preparedness is a major responsibility for all employees. As a new employee you will learn the facility plan as part of your orientation. Fire procedures are displayed in each department and at each nursing station near the phone. Local emergency phone numbers (for fire, police or sheriff, ambulance, poison control, etc.) should also be posted.

Fire drills on each shift are held at least once a quarter. Your full participation in the drills is essential to ensure that you and the rest of the staff are as prepared as possible.

To prevent fires, follow these guidelines:
▷ Report any unsafe condition so that corrective measures can be taken promptly.
▷ Enforce smoking regulations. Safety ash trays should be used. Cigarettes must always be out when discarded.
▷ Never store anything within 18 inches of a sprinkler head. Be sure that linen and food carts are not parked in front of or hide manual fire alarm "pulls."

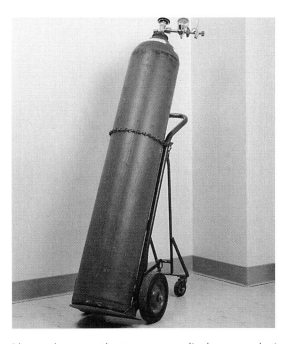

Fig. 8-14. Always be sure that oxygen cylinders are chained so that they cannot be knocked over.

> Make sure that corridors and exits are kept free of nonwheeled obstructions. Exit doors should never be locked or blocked (Fig. 8-15). Never block smoke or fire doors. Doors to maintenance areas, elevators, equipment rooms, and boiler rooms should always be kept closed.

Your role in emergency preparedness is so important that you must always be alert for problems. Stay involved in prevention activities, and everyone around you will be safer.

If You Are the First to Notice a Fire

If you walk in on a fire or are first to see it, do this:

1. Stop and quickly assess the situation.
2. Yell for help and/or sound the alarm.
3. Immediately remove all residents from the area. Do this quickly because smoke inhalation causes most deaths in fires. If possible, discontinue oxygen treatments.
4. Do not open the windows.
5. Close the door to the room. Most doors in health care facilities are called fire doors. They help contain a fire for at least 1-2 hours.
6. Evacuate residents in rooms on both sides of the affected room.
7. Never open a closed door during a fire unless you have no option. If you must open a door, put your hand on it first to check if it is warm and look for smoke coming from underneath. If so, do not open the door because the oxygen that would enter the room will cause the fire to explode, which would seriously injure you and expand the fire.
8. Move residents at immediate risk to the end of the wing farthest from the fire or off the wing or unit entirely if instructed to do so.
9. Fight the fire with a fire extinguisher only if it is very small and contained, such as in a waste basket. Do not attempt to fight any larger fire because it can expand out of control very quickly.

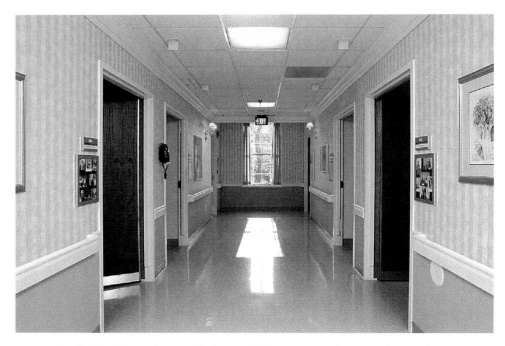

Fig. 8-15. Fire safety guidelines include ensuring that corridors and exit doors are never blocked or locked.

If a Fire Alarm Sounds on Another Wing or Unit

1. Clear residents out of the halls into their rooms and close the doors. Remember the rooms have fire doors on them.
2. If several residents are in a gathering area, close the doors to that large room rather than going through fire doors to return them to their rooms, unless the fire is in the immediate area. Act calmly and reassure residents.
3. Make sure the halls are free from obstructions.
4. Wait for further instructions.

If an Evacuation Is Ordered

Evacuate residents in this order:
1. Those nearest the fire
2. Ambulatory residents
3. Ambulatory residents who need assistance
4. Residents who use wheelchairs
5. Residents with severe medical complications
6. All charts and medication carts

The reason for this order is that if evacuation begins with residents with severe medical complications, the process will take longer and more residents likely will be caught in the burning area. If ambulatory residents are removed first, more residents will be saved (Fig. 8-16).

THE "RIGHT TO KNOW" LAW

As an employee, you have a right to access to certain kinds of personal records. In addition to your employment and medical histories and job description, you have the right to see other documents affecting safety in the facility. Two specific documents you can request are:

▶ Your departmental chemical inventory list and Material Safety Data Sheets
▶ A copy of the OSHA "Access to Employee Exposure and Medical Records Standard"

You may want to see these if you have questions about what chemicals you may be exposed to on the job or what to do in an emergency. Submit a written request

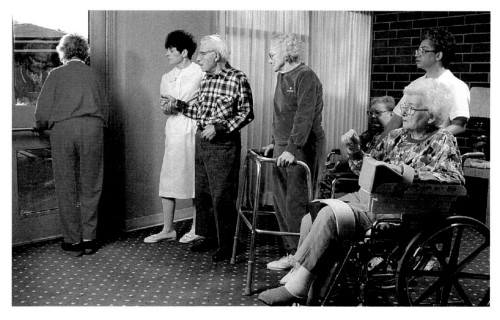

Fig. 8-16. Residents must be evacuated in a specific order.

through your supervisor. Include your full name, the date of your request, a general description of the information desired, and your signature.

INCIDENT REPORTING

Sometimes, no matter how careful and mindful one is to prevent injuries, an accident does happen. As human beings, we're not perfect. Even if you follow the rules, a problem can occur. In such cases you may need to make an incident report.

This is called an incident report rather than an "injury report" because you should report not only injuries but any "incident." An incident is anything that goes wrong that should be fixed. If you see a problem, never wait until someone gets hurt to make a change. Regardless of whether the incident involves equipment, staff, or a procedure failure, tell your supervisor immediately. The sooner it's reported, the sooner it can get corrected. Chapter 12, "Communication on the Job," discusses in more detail how to complete an incident report.

9

HEALTH PROMOTION: A WAY OF LIFE

What does health really mean to you? Take a minute to visualize a healthy person. What images come to mind? A person involved in a physical activity such as walking or jogging? Can you imagine the person's facial expression: is he or she smiling?

Health is more than just the absence of disease. Good health involves a number of factors and life-style choices. These all contribute to your physical, mental, and social well-being:

- Nutrition
- Exercise
- Staying drug free
- Avoiding alcohol and tobacco
- Managing stress
- Maintaining a positive attitude

In this chapter you will learn the benefits of good health. People in good health enjoy their job much more than someone who is often tired or sick. The quality of care you provide is enhanced if you feel healthy and have a positive attitude. Other staff can count on you not to call in sick. All this is health promotion, which depends on good nutrition, exercise, and a positive attitude. These concepts are important for you and residents you work with. Understanding how you can improve the quality of your life will help you improve the quality of life for others (Fig. 9-1).

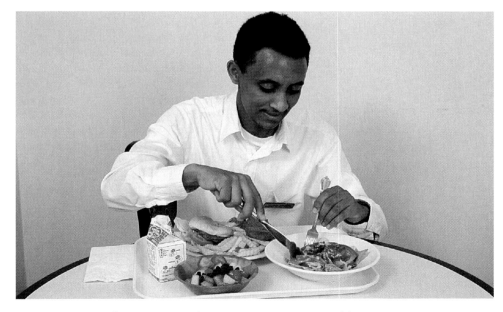

Fig. 9-1. Practicing good nutrition, exercising, and keeping a positive attitude will help you to enhance the quality of care you provide.

WHAT IS HEALTH PROMOTION?

Health promotion is working to achieve a state of health and well-being. Factors that influence health in a positive way affect the mind as well as the body.

FACTORS THAT INFLUENCE A HEALTHY LIFE-STYLE

We all benefit from good health. Good health allows us to lead a full, active life and to achieve our maximum potential. This is true for residents as well. Consider the following examples of two nurse assistants. As you read the descriptions think about which you would like to be most like. Maria is a 38-year-old mother of two. She is full of energy, always smiling and offering assistance to her co-workers. She has formed a walking group at lunch and organizes a pot luck dinner for others once a month. Nancy is also a 38-year-old mother of two. She is always late for work, and she never smiles and complains constantly about work. If you ask her to help, she does, but you never hear the end of it. She is overweight and eats junk food for lunch. She never participates in social functions. What is the difference between these nurse assistants? Do you think it has to do with good health? Good health comes from a combination of factors:

▶ Good nutrition
▶ Exercise
▶ A healthy attitude

In addition, a healthy life-style also involves certain life-style choices we make. Staying drug free, avoiding the use of tobacco, and using alcohol in moderation or not at all can help us reach a higher level of health. These substances can negatively affect our lives and job performance. Drugs can impair our mental and physical functioning. Tobacco use is linked with many diseases such as lung cancer, heart disease, and emphysema. Alcohol abuse can lead to malnutrition, impaired mental and physical ability, and cirrhosis of the liver and is linked to certain cancers such as breast and esophageal cancer.

Managing stress is also an important part of health. Stress affects health in many ways. Not being able to cope with stress in daily situations may predispose us to illness. We all have stress in our lives. To develop a more positive attitude and live the healthiest life possible, we must learn to manage stress in a way that allows us to keep functioning at our best both personally and professionally.

DEVELOPING A POSITIVE ATTITUDE

A healthy attitude begins with a positive outlook. If a group of people look at a glass half filled with water, some will say it is half empty and some will say it is half full. People have different attitudes and often see things differently. People who describe the glass as half full may have a more positive attitude than those who describe it as half empty. A positive attitude influences how you live your life, how you view your job, and how you treat residents.

It is easier to have a positive outlook when you feel good about yourself. And a good attitude is easier to maintain when you are well rested. Get plenty of sleep: 7-9 hours per night. A positive attitude can brighten your day as well as the residents'. Try to follow these principles:

▶ Every day think how important you are to yourself and others.
▶ Maintain a cheerful attitude, which can be contagious!
▶ Be mindful of and open to others' point of view.
▶ Stay calm when things get hectic or a crisis occurs.
▶ Try to think through difficult situations before responding.
▶ Maintain a compassionate, caring attitude.
▶ Emphasize the positive. See the glass as half full, not half empty.
▶ Accept yourself without judgment. Be the best you can be.
▶ Take charge of your life. Visualize what you want for yourself and your family and work to achieve it.

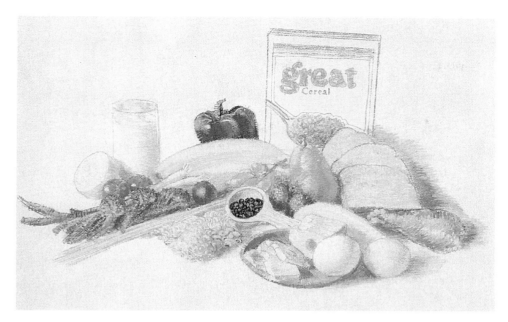

Fig. 9-2. Healthy food choices.

A positive attitude improves one's self-image and leads to a sense of happiness and well-being. This in turn helps us cope with stress and sadness. When you have a healthy attitude, you can better nurture this attitude in others. As a nurse assistant, your day-to-day attitude will have a direct impact on residents' attitude and quality of life.

GOOD NUTRITION

Nutrition affects quality of life for young and old alike. Guidelines help us understand what we should eat to maintain good health. Nutrition is even more important for a frail elderly person. As a nurse assistant, one of your most important roles is assisting residents with meals and monitoring their intake (described in Chapter 16). Understanding what foods people need and what amounts helps you encourage residents to make healthy food choices and to make healthy choices for yourself (Fig. 9-2).

What is good nutrition? Good nutrition depends on eating a variety of foods and maintaining an appropriate body weight. Variety helps ensure you get all the nutrients your body needs to be as healthy as possible. Some people can get by with poor nutrition but do not feel as good or function as well. The United States Department of Agriculture and Department of Health and Human Services have issued guidelines for good nutrition:

1. Eat a variety of foods in a balanced diet that includes a daily intake of:
   - 3-5 servings of vegetables
   - 2-4 servings of fruit
   - 6-11 servings of grains (breads, cereals, rice, and pasta)
   - 2-3 servings of milk, yogurt, and cheese
   - 2-3 servings of meat, fish, poultry, dry beans and peas, eggs, and nuts
   More servings of fruits and vegetables are now being recommended. Eating more servings from these groups may reduce the risk of heart disease and cancer in some people.
2. Maintain healthy weight. To lose weight, lose one half to one pound per week. Exercise regularly (Fig. 9-3).
3. Choose a diet low in fat, saturated fat, and cholesterol (Fig. 9-4).

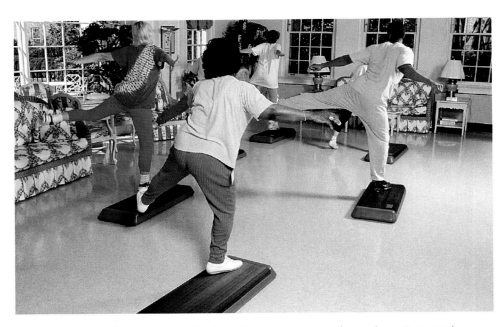

Fig. 9-3. Regular exercise is an important part of good nutrition and maintaining a healthy weight.

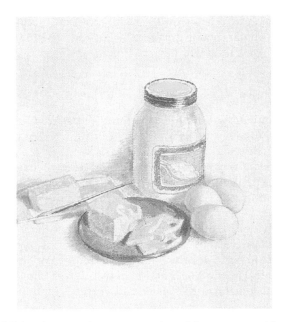

Fig. 9-4. While dieting, decrease intake of fat, saturated fat, and cholesterol.

▷ Limit fat in the diet to 30% or less of total calories
▷ Limit saturated fats to less than 10% of total calories
▷ Eat less fat from animal sources such as beef, pork, and organ meats
▷ Use fats and oils sparingly in cooking
▷ Use small amounts of salad dressings and spreads, such as butter, margarine, and mayonnaise
▷ Choose liquid vegetable oils more often because they are lower in saturated fat

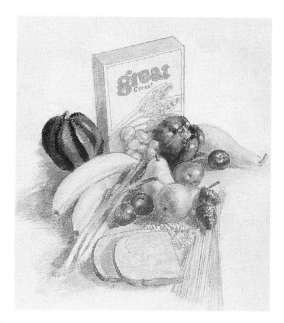

Fig. 9-5.   Always eat plenty of vegetables, fruits, and grain products.

▷ Trim fat off meat, take skin off poultry
▷ Eat cooked dry beans and peas sometimes instead of meat
▷ Use egg yolks and organ meats in moderation
▷ Use skim or low-fat milk and milk products

4. Choose a diet with plenty of vegetables, fruits, and grain products (Fig. 9-5).
   ▷ Have dark-green leafy and deep-yellow vegetables often
   ▷ Eat dry beans and peas often
   ▷ Eat some starchy vegetables, such as potatoes and corn
   ▷ Eat citrus fruits or juices, melons, or berries
   ▷ Choose fruits as desserts and fruit juices as beverages
   ▷ Eat products from a variety of grains, such as wheat, rice, oats, and corn
   ▷ Eat several servings of whole-grain breads and cereals

5. Use sugars only in moderation.
   ▷ Sugars and sugar-laden foods are high in calories and low in nutrients
   ▷ Sugar on food labels may appear as fructose, glucose, maltose, lactose, molasses, high-fructose corn syrup, honey, and fruit juice concentrate
   ▷ Sugar contributes to tooth decay—to keep teeth and gums healthy, brush and floss regularly, and use a fluoride toothpaste

6. Use salt and sodium only in moderation.
   ▷ Use little or no salt in cooking and at the table
   ▷ Eat little of salted snacks, such as chips, crackers, pretzels, and nuts
   ▷ When planning meals, consider that:
      ▷ fresh and plain frozen vegetables prepared without salt are lower in sodium than canned ones
      ▷ cereals, pasta, and rice cooked without salt are lower in sodium than ready-to-eat cereals
      ▷ milk and yogurt have less sodium than most cheese
      ▷ fresh meat, poultry, and fish have less sodium than most canned processed ones
      ▷ most frozen dinners and combination dishes, packaged mixes, canned soups, and salad dressings contain much sodium, as do condiments such as soy and other sauces, pickles, olives, catsup, and mustard

7. If you drink alcoholic beverages, do so in moderation.
   - ▶ Moderation is defined as no more than two drinks a day for men and no more than one drink a day for women; one drink is considered to be:
     - ▶ 12 oz of regular beer
     - ▶ 5 oz wine
     - ▶ 1 oz of distilled spirits (80 proof)
   - ▶ Women who are pregnant or trying to become pregnant should not drink at all because alcohol may harm the fetus
8. If you never smoked, don't start. If you do smoke, consider the well-being of others and smoke outdoors. Avoid the smoke of others (secondhand smoke).

What Is a Serving?

In the guidelines above, a serving may not be a typical "helping" of what you eat. Here are some examples of servings:
- ▶ For bread, cereal, rice and pasta, one serving means:
  - ▶ 1 slice of bread
  - ▶ 1 oz of ready-to-eat cereal
  - ▶ cup of cooked cereal, rice, or pasta
  - ▶ 3 or 4 small plain crackers
- ▶ For vegetables, one serving means:
  - ▶ 1 cup of raw leafy vegetables
  - ▶ cup of other vegetables, cooked or chopped raw
  - ▶ 3/4 cup of vegetable juice
- ▶ For fruits, one serving means:
  - ▶ 1 medium apple, banana, or orange
  - ▶ cup of chopped, cooked, or canned fruit
  - ▶ 3/4 cup of fruit juice
- ▶ For milk, yogurt, and cheese, one serving means:
  - ▶ 1 cup of milk or yogurt
  - ▶ 1 oz of natural cheese
  - ▶ 2 oz of processed cheese
- ▶ For meat, poultry, fish, dry beans, eggs, and nuts, one serving means:
  - ▶ 2-3 oz of cooked lean meat, poultry, or fish
  - ▶ cup of cooked dry beans, 1 egg, or 2 tablespoons of peanut butter equals 1 oz of lean meat

How much is an ounce of meat? Here's a guide to determining what a portion of meat, chicken, fish, or cheese weighs:
- ▶ 1 ounce is the size of a match box
- ▶ 3 ounces are the size of a deck of cards
- ▶ 8 ounces are the size of a paperback book

The Food Pyramid

Nutritional information is summarized in the food pyramid (Fig. 9-6). The pyramid's pieces represent the basic five food groups (levels 1-3) and the fats, oils, and sweets commonly found in our diets (level 4). The size of the food-group piece represents the recommended number of daily servings from that food group. For example, the grain group is the largest because it includes most recommended servings.

The triangle and circle shapes scattered throughout the pyramid's pieces represent added and naturally occurring fats and oils in some foods, as well as added sugars. Many triangles and/or circles in a food group piece mean that many of the foods in that category contain a large amount of natural or added fat, oil, and/or sugars.

If you start at the bottom of the pyramid and work your way up, you can see how selections from the food groups can be put together for a healthful diet. When you are familiar with the food pyramid, try some menu planning for a few days; write

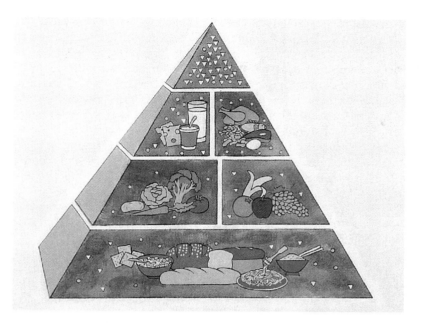

Fig. 9-6.   FDA Food Pyramid.

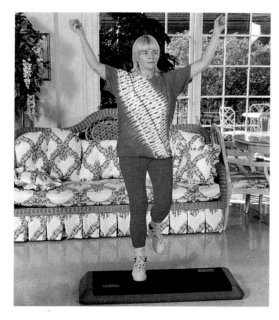

Fig. 9-7.   Step aerobics is one form of aerobic exercise.

down specific foods you to eat for each meal. You will find that this planning helps you make sense of the number of servings for each food group. This planning then becomes a natural part of your diet.

EXERCISE AND HEALTH

Exercise and movement is a vital part of life. Exercise can help you stay healthy and independent. Exercise can also help bring people back to health.

There are two basic types of exercise. One is aerobic, meaning "with oxygen." Aerobic exercise is a low-grade steady activity that increases your heart rate and the amount of oxygen delivered to body tissue (Fig. 9-7). Walking, jogging, swimming, and cycling are examples of this type of exercise.

The other form of exercise is anaerobic, meaning "without oxygen." This form of exercise does not increase the supply of oxygen to body tissues. This is an activity of high intensity and short duration, such as weight lifting or sprinting.

It is best to combine both types of exercise. Your doctor can help you determine how hard and how much exercise is best for you. Exercising for 30 minutes three to four times a week can help you become more physically fit. One is never too young or old to benefit from exercise! Exercise improves the health of a 19-year-old or a 90-year-old. It benefits both you and residents.

Remember the healthy person you visualized at the beginning of this chapter. Most people visualize an active person with a strong body and good muscles. Exercise is necessary for anyone to build and maintain a healthy body, as shown in Table 9-1.

TABLE 9-1. Health Benefits of Exercise

Exercises helps:	Which helps to prevent:
Increase muscle strength	Muscle weakness
Maintain joint mobility/flexibility	Contractures, osteoporosis
Improve coordination	Falls
Improve self-image	Anxiety and depression
Maintain or reduce weight	Obesity
Improve circulation	Prevent vascular disease and leg ulcers caused by poor circulation
Reduce many factors that contribute to heart disease	Heart disease
Reduce tension	Stress

LIFE-STYLE CHANGES

Just as good nutrition and exercise affect health, so do other life-style choices. Follow these guidelines to make positive changes in your own life-style:

▶ Drink lots of water (about 2 quarts) every day.

▶ Snack on popcorn (without butter or salt), pretzels, fruit, or raw vegetables instead of candy and sweets.

▶ Take your lunch instead of ordering fast food. Include foods from the major food groups.

▶ Begin an exercise routine.

▶ Go for a walk at lunchtime or after work.

▶ Take the stairs instead of the elevator.

10

INTRODUCTION TO THE APPLICATION

Do you know the saying, "It's not what you do, but how you do it"? Think of a simple task, such as opening and closing a door. The actual opening and closing is always the same, but how it is done can send different messages. The door can be pushed open hard so it bangs the wall, or it can be opened so quietly that no one hears you come in. The door can be closed softly or slammed shut. How you do even a simple thing can show your anger, frustration, or distraction—or it can show you are considerate and caring. This is why it is important to pay attention to how you do even the simplest tasks.

This chapter focuses on how to provide the best care. The themes of care described here create a framework for how to give care. You will learn what each theme means and how to use it when performing any skill as a nurse assistant.

WHAT IS A THEME?

A theme is something repeated over and over to send a message. It's that part of a song you cannot get out of your head. The words may change from verse to verse, but the tune or melody, the musical theme, never changes. The tasks you perform every day are like the words of the song. The specifics may change throughout the day, or be different for different residents because of their preferences, but the themes of care should always stay the same and send the same message. In every interaction with a resident, these themes must be part of what you do. Weave them into every daily task. Themes of care help you balance the art of caregiving with the science of nursing.

If you incorporate the themes of care into every service you provide, you will provide quality care in a timely, efficient manner. The next section describes the seven themes of care. Many of these will be familiar to you already from earlier chapters. Now, however, you will learn to apply this knowledge in specific areas of your work.

THEMES OF CARE

The seven themes of care involve both the art of caregiving and the science of nursing. Caregiving themes include communication, autonomy, and respect. Nursing themes include safety, infection control, and observation. Time management is a general theme of care for performing in an efficient manner.

▸ **Communication:** In Chapter 6 you learned how we send and receive messages. You communicate with residents throughout the day. If you did not communicate with a resident or notice nonverbal messages, how would you know if a resident was unhappy or in pain? How would a resident know that you were about to help him or her to bathe, when you start to remove his or her clothes? Residents have the right to know what is happening to and around them (Fig. 10-1). Communication is crucial for developing a trusting relationship with each resident and other staff.

▸ **Autonomy:** Autonomy means deciding for oneself how to live one's life. Being autonomous is being independent and making your own decisions. You must help each resident be as independent as possible. Encourage residents to take responsibility for their care through choices. If you become too protective or do

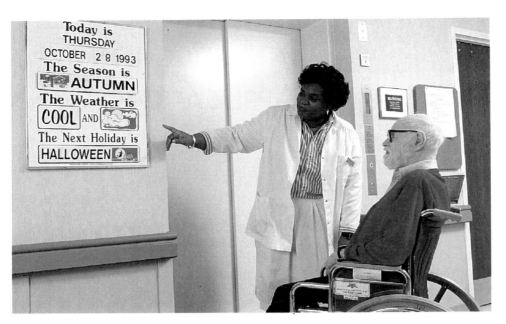

Fig. 10-1. Communication with residents helps develop trusting relationships.

something for a resident instead of letting him or her do it, the person's autonomy is undermined (Fig. 10-2).

▷ **Respect:** Everyone deserves to be treated with respect. Simple courtesies, such as knocking on doors, saying please, and asking permission, are ways you can be respectful. Ask yourself, "If I was this resident, how would I like to be treated?" Treating each resident with respect must be part of everything you do (Fig. 10-3).

▷ **Safety:** Safety means being free from harm or risk, secure from threat or danger. The facility's environment is structured to be a safe place where everyone can focus on giving care in a home-like setting. However, if care becomes a quick and careless routine, injuries and accidents are likely. Residents' safety and yours depend on planning your actions thoughtfully in every situation (Fig. 10-4).

▷ **Infection Control:** Prevent the transmission of infection by using the infection control procedures described in Chapter 7. The transmission of microorganisms can be kept to a minimum if everyone practices these principles (Fig. 10-5). Incorporate this theme in all your caregiving actions.

▷ **Observation:** You have already learned that observation means to watch and pay attention to details. You must pay close attention to any changes in a resident and report them immediatley. Remember, since you spend the most time with residents, you will see changes first (Fig. 10-6).

▷ **Time Management:** The ability to organize your activities and perform them efficiently is *time managment*. Take control and prioritize your tasks by deciding

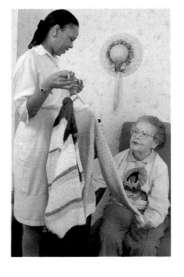

Fig. 10-2. Encouraging residents to make choices promotes autonomy.

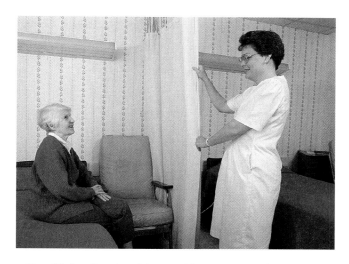

Fig. 10-3. Treat residents with respect and courtesy.

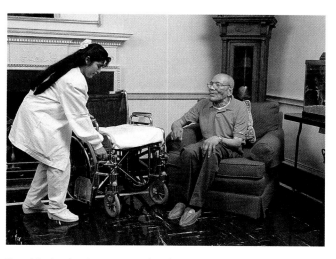

Fig. 10-4. Locking a resident's wheelchair helps ensure his or her safety.

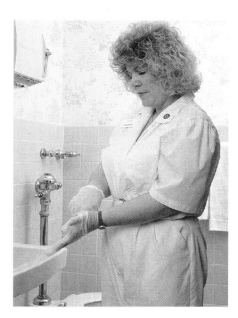

Fig. 10-5. Wearing gloves is one way to prevent the transmission of infection.

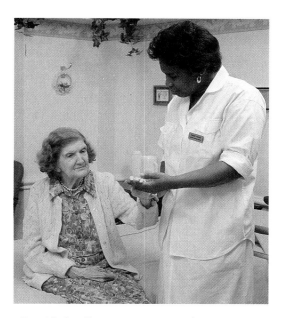

Fig. 10-6. If you notice any changes in a resident, report them immediately.

what is most important, and you will become more efficient (Fig. 10-7).

Each of these themes is important, and you should work to incorporate them all into your everyday caregiving.

HOW TO USE THEMES IN YOUR WORK

You can incorporate the themes of care into your daily work if you think of each task as consisting of three parts:

1. You prepare and get ready to do a task.
2. You do the task or procedure.

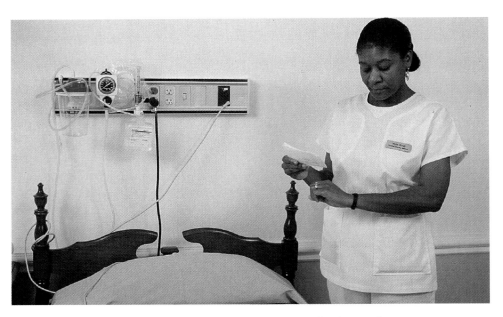

Fig. 10-7.   Learn to organize by prioritizing on the basis of importance.

3. You complete or finish the job.

Remember, think about the themes of care as you carry out the steps of each task. How you perform the process is as important as finishing the task. Ask yourself the following questions every time you begin:

1. What do I need to do before I begin?
2. How should I do this task?
3. What do I need to do to complete the task?
4 How can I incorporate the themes of care in this task?

Let's look at an example. Assisting with a shower is a common task for nurse assistants. If you consider the questions above, your preparation for the shower will include the following steps:

1. Schedule shower room. Be sure it is clean. Hang an "Occupied" sign.
2. Gather all supplies needed for a shower, such as a washcloth, towels, and bath blanket. Having things ready before you start is good **time management**.
3. Knock on the door, and wait for the resident's permission before entering. Knocking shows you have **respect** for the person's privacy.
4. Introduce yourself, and identify the person. Introducing yourself is also **respectful**. Identifying a resident ensures you are helping the correct person, a **safety** issue.
5. Explain what you would like to do, and ask a resident how much assistance he or she needs and what his or her preferences are. By doing this, you are **communicating,** showing **respect,** and encouraging **autonomy**.
6. As needed, prepare each resident's own supplies, such as soap, deodorant, and lotions. This step is also good **time management**. Using a resident's personal supplies promotes **autonomy**.
7. Assist the resident to the shower. This ensures the resident's **safety**.
8. Help the resident get ready. Encourage each resident to do whatever part of the shower he or she is able to do. This encourages residents to continue to be independent and **autonomous,** and you are also observing a resident's capabilities. This **observation** can help you encourage residents to maintain or improve that level.
9. Turn on the water and check the temperature. This **safety** measure ensures the resident does not get burned.

Because you are prepared, you can complete the shower without stopping to get other supplies or wasting time. Nurse assistants who plan each task also enjoy their work much more. Residents are happier, and the whole experience is more enjoyable for both of you. You can thus balance the skills and art of caregiving.

Now, let's look at another example. Suppose you are to give Mrs. Jones a shower. Without thinking, you follow these steps:

1. You walk into Mrs. Jones's room.
2. You say hello to her.
3. You tell her what is going to happen.
4. You assist her out of bed and to the shower.
5. You open the shower room door and find a mess. Another resident's towels and supplies are there.

Now you have to stop, tell Mrs. Jones you forgot the supplies, and leave to get them. You leave Mrs. Jones sitting on a chair in the shower room. While you are gone, she needs to go to the bathroom. She gets up and slips on a wet spot on the floor. You come back and find her on the cold, wet floor. How could you have prevented this situation? If you had considered the question above and planned the shower carefully and mindfully, you could have prevented this situation.

As you can see, much of your job involves preparation. Being prepared for a specific task reduces your workload and gets the job done efficiently. All nurse assistant skills, like bathing residents, bed making, or moving residents from bed to chair, involve preparation. Often, you will use the same preparation steps over and over again for each procedure. However, because resident needs and preferences change and the environment or setting changes, small variations in preparation may be necessary.

The example above shows the importance of mindful preparation. Mindfulness and the seven themes are important throughout the task, as well. The chapters in this section of the book describe the specific steps for doing the actual tasks. How you end these tasks, similar to how you prepare for them, is also similar for most daily tasks. The completion steps let a resident know you are done, help him or her to get comfortable, and give the person a chance to ask questions.

Tables 10-1 and 10-2 list the common steps of preparation and completion. Each step includes a rationale, the reason for performing the step. The third column gives the themes of care incorporated in the steps.

TABLE 10-1. Common Preparation Steps

Step	Rationale	Theme(s)
Knock on the door and wait for permission before entering.	Lets a resident know you are requesting permission to enter the room.	Respect, Autonomy, Communication
Introduce yourself.	Residents must know who is entering the room.	Respect, Autonomy, Communication
Tell what you would like to do and check if this time if OK.	Residents have a right to know what kind of care is being provided.	Respect, Autonomy, Communication
Check the resident's identification.	You must be sure you are providing care to the right resident.	Safety
Provide privacy by closing doors or pulling the curtain completely around the bed.	You must always consider each resident's right to privacy.	Respect
Gather supplies located outside a resident's room.	This will save you time, help you to plan, and prevent injuries that could occur if you leave a resident unattended.	Safety, Time Management
Gather supplies that belong to the resident.	This will save you time, help you to plan, and prevent injuries that could occur if you leave a resident unattended.	Safety, Autonomy, Time Management

Continued.

TABLE 10-1. Common Preparation Steps—cont'd

Step	Rationale	Theme(s)
Prepare the equipment and environment. Lock wheelchair or bed wheels, adjust the height of the bed, lower side rails if used, move things around for adequate space to work. Make sure equipment and rooms needed are reserved and clean.	This will save you time, help you to plan, and prevent injuries to both you and the resident	Safety, Time Management
Offer assistance: Encourage each resident to do the task. Offer (if needed) to get supplies from the bedside table or other storage area. Offer (if needed) to get supplies ready: remove the toothpaste cap, open containers. Offer (if needed) to do the task. Note: Encourage residents to do as much as possible for themselves.	Giving residents choices helps them feel in control and independent.	Respect, Autonomy, Communication
Wash your hands.	Prevents the transmission of infection.	Infection Control
Wear gloves, goggles, mask, gown when needed.	When needed, these items protect residents and staff from the transmission of infection.	Infection Control
Bring proper container to dispose of dirty items, such as plastic trash bag.	Using the proper container reduces the transmission of infection and helps identify how the dirty items are thrown away.	Infection Control
Raise or lower bed to proper working height.	Reduces injury to your back, makes your work more comfortable.	Safety
Lower side rails.	Reduces injury to your back.	Safety
Lock bed or wheelchair wheels.	Prevents injury while transferring residents.	Safety
Ask yourself questions such as the following:		
Is this normal for the person?	Helps you determine changes in the resident.	Observation
Is this part of a resident's routine?	Helps you ensure you are meeting a resident's needs.	Autonomy
Is all the equipment available and working?	Helps prevent any problem while performing the skill	Safety, Time Management
Are there any changes a resident would like?	Encourages a resident to choose to change the routine at any time.	Autonomy
Explain what you are about to do.	Gains cooperation and makes a resident feel involved and in charge of his or her plan of care.	Communication, Autonomy, Respect
Discuss plans for the day or evening.	Courtesy, politeness.	Communication, Respect, Autonomy
Discuss any needs or wants with each resident.	Makes each resident feel involved and in charge of his or her plan of care.	Communication, Respect, Autonomy

The steps you incorporate into your plan of care may change from task to task and even movement to movement, because caregiving is not exact. Quality care means meeting individual needs. This means you must be flexible and adapt care to meet each resident's preferences. Different equipment and environments may also lead to adjusting the preparation steps.

The most common preparation steps you will use are:

1. Ask the question. "What do I need to do before I begin the skill?"
2. Get supplies from outside the resident's room (Fig. 10-8).
3. Knock on the door and wait for permission before entering (Fig. 10-9).
4. Introduce yourself (Fig. 10-10).
5. Identify the resident (Fig. 10-11).
6. Explain what you would like to do (Fig. 10-12A).
7. Get all supplies ready (Fig. 10-12B).
8. Wash your hands (Fig. 10-13).
9. Prepare the environment by locking the wheelchair or bed wheels, moving things out of the way, raising or lowering the bed, and lowering side rails if used. Provide for privacy (Fig. 10-14).
10. Prepare a resident by asking what the person can do and what he or she would like you to do, and assist with clothing removal, and so on (Fig. 10-15).

Always perform these steps before you begin. Add any others from Table 10-1 based on the resident's preferences and needs.

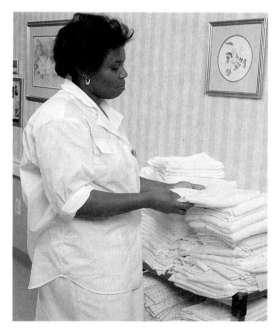

Fig. 10-8. Prepare yourself for the resident's plan of care by getting supplies ready before the skill.

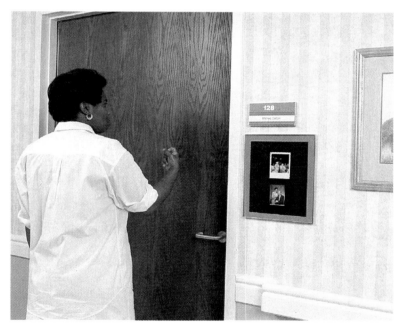

Fig. 10-9. Knock on the door and wait for permission before entering.

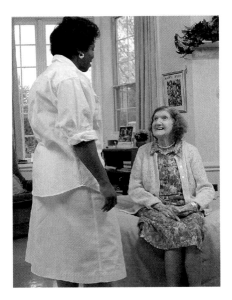

Fig. 10-10. Introduce yourself to the resident.

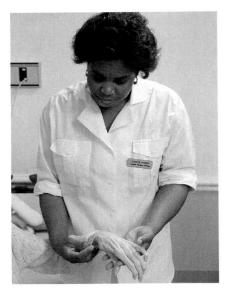

Fig. 10-11. Identify the resident.

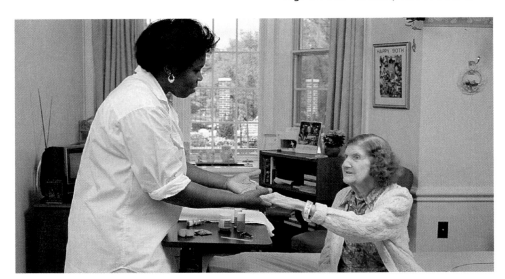

Fig. 10-12. A, Explain what you want to do.

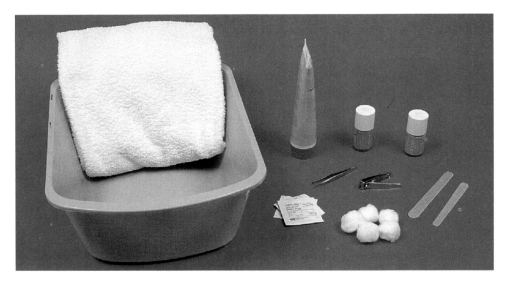

Fig. 10-12. B, Get supplies ready.

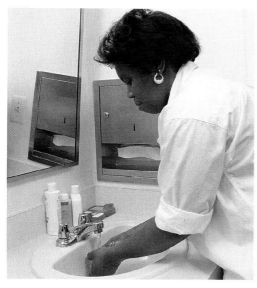

Fig. 10-13. Wash your hands.

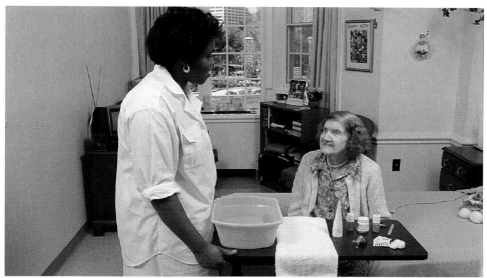

Fig. 10-14. Positioning and lowering the bedside table is an example of preparing the environment.

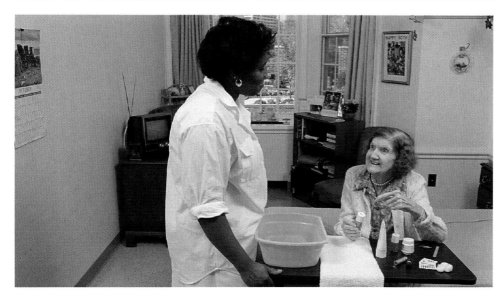

Fig. 10-15. Always ask the resident what he or she can do and assist where he or she needs help.

Like the preparation steps, the exact completion steps used may vary. The most common completion steps you will use are the following:

1. Ask yourself, "What do I need to do to complete the skill?" (Fig. 10-16).
2. Make each resident comfortable with proper positioning, placing pillows correctly, making personal items available, and providing proper lighting for reading (Fig. 10-17).
3. Check a resident's environment: clean supplies and put them away, throw away disposable items, raise side rail if ordered, place bed in lowest position, position the call bell or device within reach (Fig. 10-18).
4. Ask resident if he or she needs anything else (Fig. 10-19).
5. If necessary, record and report that you have completed the procedure and any unusual observations (Fig. 10-20).

TABLE 10-2.   Common Completion Steps

Step	Rationale	Theme(s)
Put call bell or the facility's call device close to a resident.	Residents must be able to reach you throughout your shift.	Safety
Lower bed.	Bed should always be in its lowest position so residents can move in and out.	Safety
Raise side rail if ordered.	Remind residents to use the call bell for assistance.	Safety
Make sure resident is in proper body alignment.	Proper positioning of all body parts prevents injury to resident's joints and skin.	Safety, Respect
Use proper body mechanics.	Prevents injury to yourself and residents.	Safety
Dispose of all items in their proper containers.	All facilities have separate containers for items like linens and contaminated disposable and reusable supplies. Prevents the transmission of infection to residents and other staff members.	Infection Control
Remove gloves and dispose of them in the proper container.	Prevents the transmission of infection to residents and other staff members.	Infection Control
Wash hands	Prevents the transmission of infection.	Infection Control
Check with the resident to be sure everything is satisfactory.	Gives resident the opportunity to ask for something else or request a change. Gives you feedback on what you have done.	Observation, Communication
Provide comfort: Fluff pillows. Position small pillows behind a resident's lower back and under the feet. Get a foot stool. Put a blanket on his or her lap. Put sweater on the shoulders. Put personal items close to a resident. Provide adequate lighting. Note: You must ask each resident if he or she wants the above comfort measures.	Making residents comfortable is part of your responsibility.	Autonomy, Respect
Record the completed procedures on facility records.	This helps staff identify what is a resident's normal pattern.	Observation, Communication
Report any changes in a resident or in a resident's environment to the charge nurse. Note: Often you are the first person to notice when something is wrong with a resident.	This helps the charge nurse take action to identify potential problems with a resident.	Observation, Communication
Complete the skill without any distractions or interruptions.	Residents have the right to be cared for in a focused, directed way.	Time Management, Communication, Respect

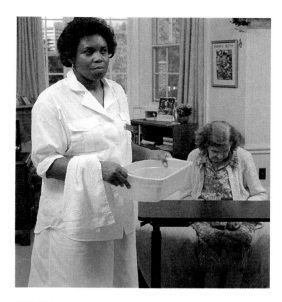

Fig. 10-16. When you have completed your skill, always question what else you need to do to finish up.

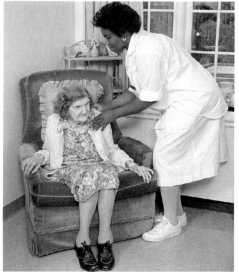

Fig. 10-17. After the skill is completed, make sure the resident is comfortable.

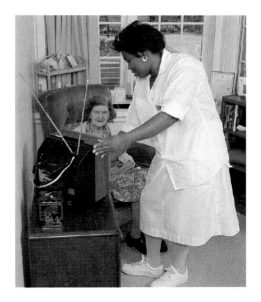

Fig. 10-18. Check the resident's environment.

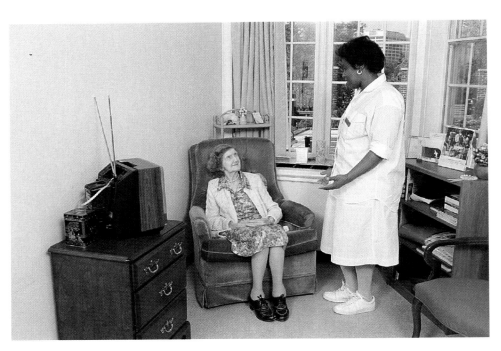

Fig. 10-19. Ask a resident if she or he needs anything else.

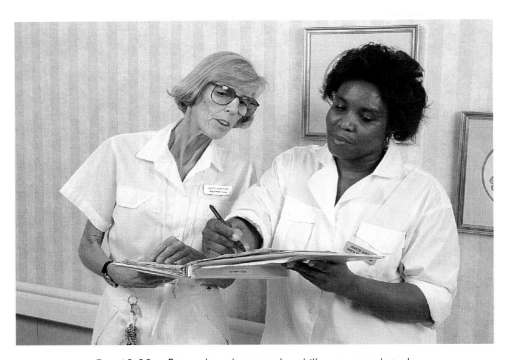

Fig. 10-20. Record and report the skill you completed.

Become familiar with these preparation and completion steps and use them with all skills you perform. You can change the order of some steps for a resident's needs, but always prepare for and finish the skill. These steps help you incorporate the themes of care: communication, autonomy, respect, safety, infection control, observation, and time management.

THE FORMAT OF SKILL DESCRIPTIONS

In the following chapters you will learn many skills. The steps in these skills are numbered to help you learn what to do first, second, third, etc. At the beginning of each skill is a reminder that looks like this:

This is to remind you of what you need to do before beginning and to prepare for the procedure.

The skill is then described, step by step

Learn the procedures in the order outlined, but remember that you need to be flexible in some steps based on a resident's preferences.

At the end of each skill you will see a reminder that looks like this.

This is to remind you of what to do to complete the skill and to follow the standard completion steps like putting away all items used, washing your hands, throwing away dirty items, making each resident comfortable, checking if anything else is needed, and reporting and recording when necessary.

Remember:

▶ Resident preference
▶ Common preparation steps
▶ Equipment and supplies needed
▶ Environment preparation
▶ Resident preparation

Remember:

▶ Meet resident needs
▶ Common completion steps
▶ Clean and put away equipment and supplies
▶ Environment completion (Is it safe? Is it clean?)

IN THIS CHAPTER YOU LEARNED TO:

▶ define the themes of care
▶ list general questions to be considered when beginning a skill
▶ list the commonly used preparation and completion steps

11

WORKING WITH NURSING STAFF

IN THIS CHAPTER YOU WILL LEARN TO:

▶ describe the nursing team

▶ explain the importance of developing a trusting relationship with the charge nurse and co-workers

▶ list four questions to ask when receiving an assignment

▶ describe the approach to care used in your facility

▶ list at least three factors that influence care

We all have relationships with many other people. Some relationships are casual and passing, and others are involved and complicated. Developing positive relationships takes hard work. You must be open, honest, and reliable. You must be willing and able to communicate your needs, to listen well, and most of all, to change your behavior if necessary.

As a nurse assistant, you will be forming relationships every day. You will work closely with many people from different departments. You will work with many residents and their families.

This chapter is about the nursing team. You will learn who is on the team, what everyone does, and what their responsibilities are. Your role on the nursing team is discussed, along with how to develop relationships with the charge nurse and your co-workers. In addition, you will learn about factors that can influence care.

THE NURSING TEAM

In Chapter 1 you learned many different people provide services for residents in long term care. The largest department is the Nursing Department, led by the Director of Nursing. Nursing departments are typically organized as shown in Table 11-1. You will spend more time with members of the nursing team than with anyone else on the interdisciplinary team.

Table 11-1 depicts an organizational chart. Solid lines show a reporting relationshp. Dotted lines imply a relationship but not a direct reporting one. All team members working together to provide the service.

▶ The Director of Nursing develops the philosophy—a belief about quality care—and approach of care for the nursing staff to follow as well as determine the staff requirements.

TABLE 11-1. Organizational Chart

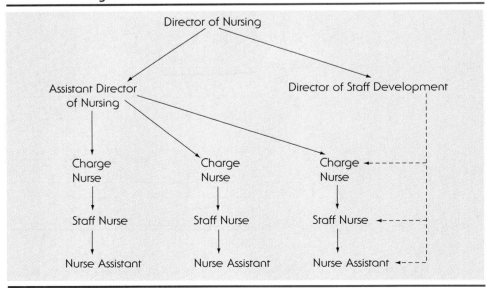

2 ▶ The Assistant Director of Nursing helps the Director of Nursing put into use in care this philosophy and approach.

3 ▶ The Director of Staff Development usually reports directly to the Director of Nursing. This person oversees staff education in the philosophy and approach to nursing care.

4 ▶ The Charge Nurse reports directly to either the Assistant Director or the Director of Nursing, depending on the facility. She or he has the day-to-day responsibility for supervising resident care. The charge nurse gives the specific care assignments. The charge nurse may also have some responsibility in staff education.

5 ▶ Staff Nurses. The number of staff nurses depends on the staffing requirements of the facility. The staff nurse is responsible for special treatments and medications. A staff nurse may be the charge nurse on some shifts.

6 ▶ Nurse Assistants report directly to charge nurses or staff nurses. Nurse Assistants give 80% of all resident care.

Developing a Relationship with the Charge Nurse

Your relationship with the charge nurse is important for quality care. You need to feel you are partners to reach the caregiving goals for each resident in your care. The charge nurse can also help you understand how best to provide care. She or he is a resource for problem solving and teaching and can help you direct your inservice education (Fig. 11-1). To develop an effective relationship with the charge nurse, you need to demonstrate reliability, trustworthiness, and open communication. Follow these guidelines to develop a good relationship with him or her:

1. Be on time for work every day (Fig. 11-2).
2. Be open and flexible in accepting your assignment.
3. Ask questions about things you do not understand. Make sure you understand what the charge nurse expects of you.
4. Be patient when you need the charge nurse's help. (Remember, the charge nurse has other responsibilities too.)
5. Report any resident changes immediately to the charge nurse.
6. Communicate any problems or concerns you may have.
7. Be accountable and honest.

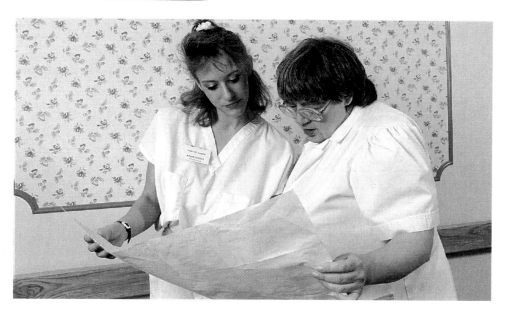

Fig. 11-1. It is essential to have a good relationship with the charge nurse.

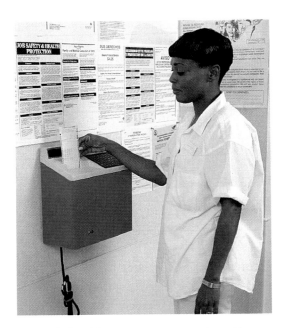

Fig. 11-2. Always come to work on time.

Developing Relationships with Co-workers

A positive relationship with your co-workers is also important. Although every nurse assistant has his or her own assignment, you should help each other and work together. For example, sometimes residents will ask you for assistance even though you are not assigned to them. Residents expect their needs met when they ask. You must never say, "I can't do that. I'm not your nurse assistant."

You should assist this resident with his or her request and then report this information to the nurse assistant assigned to the resident. If the request is something you cannot do, simply tell the person, "I cannot do that. Let me get the nurse assistant caring for you. You then can offer the assigned nurse assistant your help. With some tasks, such as moving a very weak resident, you need another's help to prevent injury for both of you. You can do some nurse assistant skills on your own, but with many others you will need help from your co-workers.

Developing an effective working relationship with your co-workers is very important. Following are some things you can do to help develop positive relationships:

1. Offer your help to co-workers.
2. Go to lunch together (if staffing allows).
3. Share ideas about caregiving (but remember, respect residents' rights to confidentiality).
4. Be available to help co-workers when needed.
5. Call in sick only when you are ill.
6. Attend continuing education classes together.
7. Be honest and reliable.
8. Be open to learn about and accept cultural differences.
9. Be supportive and helpful to others as long as it doesn't interfere with your care.
10. Respect others' opinions and beliefs.

Remember, although the charge nurse guides your activities, your co-workers are the ones who assist you when needed. You must work to get along with them. A supportive work environment is also more pleasant (Fig. 11-3). When everyone co-operates and works together, residents receive quality care.

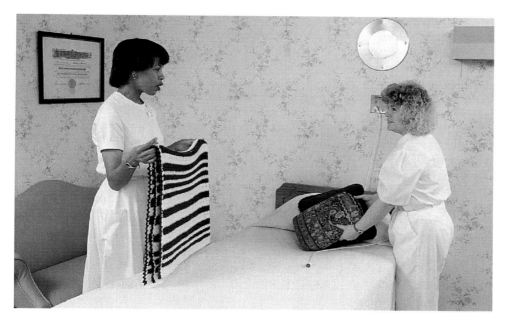

Fig. 11-3.   A supportive relationship with co-workers creates a pleasant and cooperative work environment.

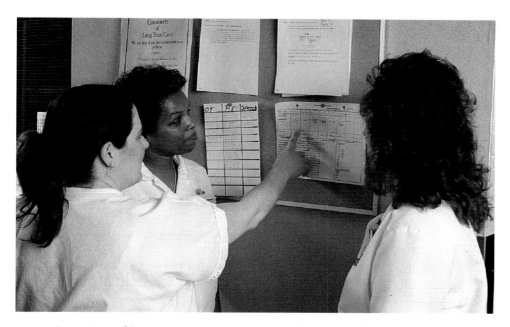

Fig. 11-4.   Obtain your assignment on a daily basis from the charge nurse.

Daily Assignments

At the beginning of your shift every day, you receive your assignment from the charge nurse. This assignment includes the residents you will care for that day (Fig. 11-4). In some facilities you may meet with staff on the previous shift to hear their report on residents. Sometimes you get all the information from the charge nurse, such as information about what occurred on the previous shift. For example, a resident who usually sleeps all night was up pacing. Treatments and medication status

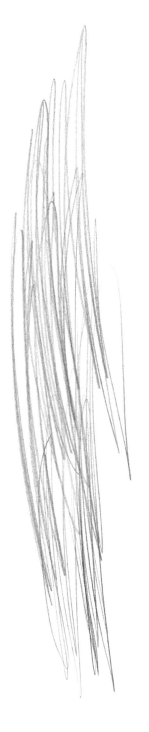

would be included. Carefully review your assignment and ask the charge nurse any questions. Never begin giving care without having all the information you need, including the following:

▶ Do any residents have special needs today?
▶ Do I need the charge nurse at any time for a treatment?
▶ Are there any activities the charge nurse wants done first?
▶ Do any residents have any specific appointments to keep?

Review your assignment with the charge nurse and talk about anything you feel uncomfortable doing. For example, a resident needs to go to the hospital for an X-ray and you have never done this. Discuss the procedure with the charge nurse. The charge nurse can teach you more about the tasks you will be doing. Openly discussing your assignment lets the charge nurse know when you need help and when you can be independent. Remember, be honest with the charge nurse about things you do not feel comfortable doing. Never try to do anything you have not learned to do. For example, if you did not discuss how to send a resident for an X-ray, you may have forgotten to send the resident's chart and perhaps the X-ray would not have been done. By communicating openly with the charge nurse, you will find her or him to be a great resource and educator.

APPROACHES TO CARE

Different approaches to nursing care are used in different facilities. The director of nursing usually sets the facility's approach based on a philosophy of caring, residents' needs, available staff, and costs. An approach called team nursing is common in long term care. The charge nurse is the team leader and makes assignments based on the needs for the shift. The charge nurse assigns team members to specific residents, but nurse assistants work together as a team to deliver care. For example, nurse assistants may discuss how to accomplish feeding a large number of residents. They may decide to change their own lunch breaks so everyone can help with feeding, regardless of who is assigned. They report back to the team leader with any problems or concerns they may have about residents.

With team nursing, a group of nursing team members is assigned to care for a group of residents, and together all the care is provided.

Two other nursing approaches are called functional and primary nursing. With the functional nursing approach, nurse assistants have specific tasks rather than specific residents as the focus of care. For example, you might have the responsibility of giving all the showers for the day, while another nurse assistant makes all the beds. Sometimes this approach is used at times of staffing shortages. If a nurse assistant calls in sick, the charge nurse may assign tasks to other nurse assistants so that all care activities are done.

In the primary nursing approach, a registered nurse or licensed practical nurse has the primary responsibility for residents' needs. You work with the nurse and care for the same residents each day. Together, you are responsible for residents' care 24 hours a day. On other shifts other staff members carry out the plan of care you, the nurse, and each resident set. This approach is more common in hospitals and facilities where residents are assigned to nurse assistants for a long time.

In all approaches the focus is always on giving quality care to residents. You will learn which approach is used in your facility when you begin to work. You will also learn that many factors influence the approach and quality of care. Be open to all approaches, be aware of what influences care, and remember always to keep residents' needs your primary concern.

FACTORS THAT INFLUENCE CARE

A facility's approach to care influences how care is provided. Besides the overall approach, other factors influence care:

1. *Resident's Needs:* A resident's needs must always be the primary focus of care. You should always ask yourself, "Is this what this resident wants or needs?"
2. *Philosophy of Caring:* The direction for care activities is set by the director of nursing. Different directors have different ideas about how things should be done. You will learn your director of nursing's emphasis for care in the facility where you work (Fig. 11-5).
3. *New Treatments or Equipment:* Facilities are always looking for better ways to deliver care. Your facility may try new things such as products for treatment of skin breakdowns or new back protection devices.
4. *Federal and State Regulations:* The framework for delivery of care is federal and state regulations, such as the Federal Rules and Regulations and Occupational Safety and Health Administration (OSHA) standards. These rules and regulations influence how much, and how often, care is provided to ensure quality caregiving.
5. *Staffing:* The reliability of staff has a major influence on care. If staff members often call in sick or if there is much turnover, continuity in team building and resident care will be compromised. All the factors above are also greatly influenced by the attitude of the nursing staff.

These influences sometimes lead to changes in how the nursing department delivers care. You may not always know the reason for a change. But if you keep an open mind, ask questions, and keep residents' well-being the highest priority, you will be more comfortable with changes.

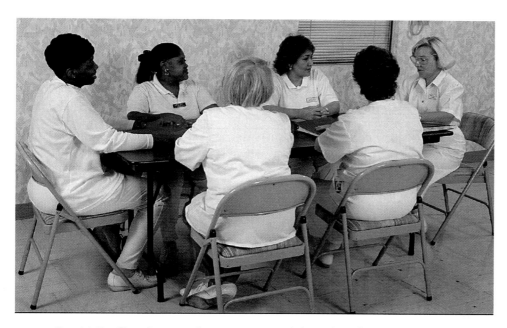

Fig. 11-5. The director of nursing sets a philosophy of caring.

IN THIS CHAPTER YOU LEARNED TO:

▶ describe the nursing team.

▶ explain the importance of developing a trusting relationship with the charge nurse and co-workers.

▶ list four questions to ask when receiving an assignment.

▶ describe the approach to care used in your facility.

▶ list at least three factors that influence care.

12

COMMUNICATION ON THE JOB

Think back to a special event months ago, like a birthday or holiday. Try to remember the event in detail: what people there were wearing, what they said, what they ate and how much, what their mood was, what time each person came and went, and similar details. Notice how you have forgotten many facts? It's only human to forget specifics like these.

Because of our memory limits, insurance companies ask us to write down the facts and details after a car accident. We can then remember these specifics by reading the notes months or even years later if necessary. If we didn't write down the details, the "facts" of the case would be only the events that we remembered, and much would be lost. We might not know at the time how important some of these details are and therefore might not pay enough attention to them to remember them, but later it could turn out that the forgotten specifics were very important.

Your documentation on the job has the same purpose. Most of what you write down is used by members of the health care team in the care of a resident, but some facts that you write down may be used months or years later. You and your facility can accurately state the facts with certainty because you wrote them down.

From your first minute on the job as a nurse assistant, you are flooded with information. People talk to you, give you things to read, show you things, and encourage you to ask questions. This is two-way communication: you are not only listening, observing, and reading, but also talking, being observed, and documenting (writing things down). Providing the best care for residents depends on clear, thorough, and accurate information. Other health care team members, including residents, depend on information you communicate.

This chapter focuses on the skills you will use to communicate clearly on the job as you observe, report, and document activities and participate in assessing each resident and developing the care plan.

GETTING INFORMATION ABOUT RESIDENTS AND CARE ACTIVITIES

As you care for residents, you will receive much information from residents themselves and others through a variety of means.

Residents

Each resident is the main source of information. As the key person on the health care team, a resident can give you valuable information about his or her care preferences and needs. Be sure to verify this information with the charge nurse. In some cases, residents might be confused or "wish" that something that they tell you were true. For example, a resident may tell you that she or he is going home tomorrow. You must verify this with the charge nurse before starting to prepare for discharge. Residents' feelings and preferences are especially important to listen to and to report or document. This way, other members of the health care team can understand a resident better and give more personalized care.

A Resident's Chart

A resident's health record, also called the medical record or the chart, is the main communication tool used by the health care team (Fig. 12-1). It belongs to the facility and is a legal record of a resident's stay in the facility. As the basic tool for

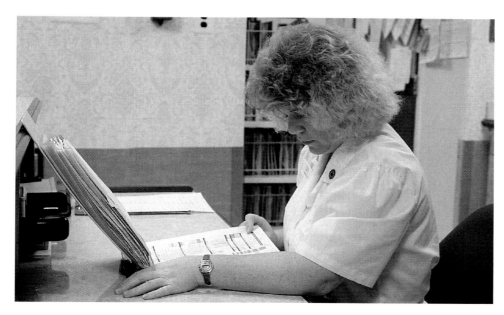

Fig. 12-1. A resident's chart must be complete, accurate, and confidential.

planning, recording, and evaluating a resident and the care provided, the chart also helps organize all information you and others gather about a resident. The chart is confidential. Because it is a record of each resident's condition and care at the facility, it must be complete and accurate.

There is a common saying: "If it isn't charted, it didn't happen!" This means that information not on the chart is not communicated for other members of the health care team to act on. Weeks or years later, no one will remember all the facts clearly, so it's as if it never happened. We generally remember what occurred but forget specific details. The purpose of the chart is to provide information about each resident that is permanently accessible to the facility, the staff, and that resident.

A typical chart includes history (past conditions and events), current records, and proposed (future) plans for that resident on many different pieces of paper (Fig. 12-2). All health care team professionals record information in the chart, such as the following:

▶ Identifying information (name, medical record number, birth date, etc.) is often on a form called the face sheet.

▶ A resident's admission papers that outline the reason for admission are part of the record.

▶ Each resident or representative signs permission forms (called "Consent for Treatment") and instruction forms (for example, "No cardiopulmonary resuscitation"), which become part of the chart.

▶ Some parts of the chart include documentation from just one discipline. The physician's orders, for example, are written by a resident's doctor.

▶ Other parts of the chart include documentation from many disciplines in progress notes written in paragraph form. Examples are notes from the dietician, the respiratory therapist, and the physical therapist.

▶ Test results such as lab tests, X-rays, and hearing tests are also collected in the chart.

▶ Any graph or flow sheets used for recording nursing activity such as vital signs, weights, bowel movements, ADL (activities of daily living) Sheets and I & O (intake and output) are added to the record as completed.

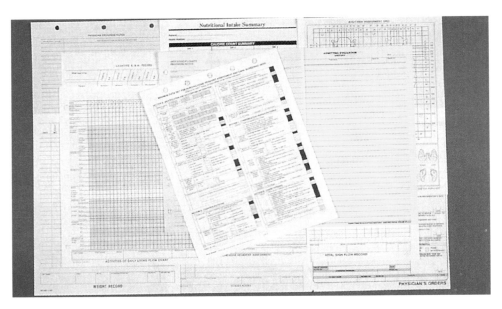

Fig. 12-2.   A chart is composed of the resident's history, current records, and proposed plans for the future.

Nurse assistants often document information on flow sheets. A flow sheet is a list of objective facts: information you see, hear, smell, and touch. The facts on the flow sheet all concern the same subject over time. Examples of flow sheets are the vital sign record, the intake and output record, and the weight chart. Collecting information on a flow sheet makes it easier to see how facts change over time. You can evaluate your observations by comparing them with other findings. For example, it may not seem important that a resident did not have a bowel movement today until you discover this is the fourth day in a row that he or she has not had a bowel movement. By recording facts about residents, you can monitor their progress (Fig. 12-3).

Additional information from each department is documented in the medical record. For example, if you care for a resident whose speech is unclear, you need to know if there are other ways to communicate with him or her. You can read the speech therapist's notes to find out that the person can use an alphabet board to spell out words. You can also look at the care plan. This part of the chart describes how the team is working together to help a resident achieve his or her goals. You can look at the care plan to see what the speech pathologist is doing and recommending.

Sometimes, the chart is kept all together in one place in a holder like a notebook or covered clipboard. In other facilities, sections of the chart are kept in different places. For example, the weight chart for all residents may be stored in one notebook near the scales to make it easier to record weights. The weight sheet is still a part of the health record even if it is kept in a different place. It is still a legal record.

Sometimes, you will document information on worksheet forms. A worksheet is a temporary form where you write down information, but it is not a part of the chart. For example, a resident whose intake and output are being recorded might have a worksheet where staff can record amounts throughout the day. At the end of the day, these numbers are added together and the total intake and output are recorded in the chart. The worksheet is then discarded. You need to know which forms are worksheets and which are a permanent part of the chart since the documentation rules for worksheets are not as strict.

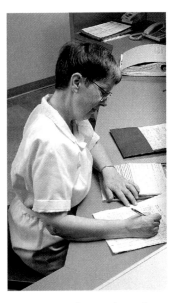

Fig. 12-3. Recording facts about residents on flow sheets is used to monitor the progress of a resident over a period of time.

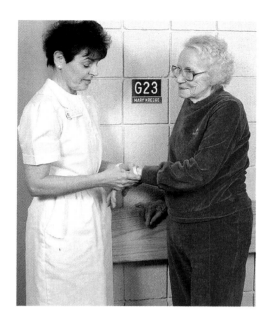

Fig. 12-4. Door cards are used to communicate information about a resident.

Other Communication Devices

Other communication devices give you additional information about a resident. These can be different in each facility, so you must ask questions about the information in your own facility. A resident's wristband always has his or her name on it and may include other information as well. For example, some facilities identify residents who have diabetes or other diseases or conditions by using different colored wristbands. The only true way to identify a resident is with the wrist band or by asking a resident his or her name. If you do not know a resident who cannot state his or her name, always check the wristband. If a resident is not wearing one, talk to the charge nurse.

Words and symbols on residents' door cards may communicate other information. The door card is the sign on or beside the door of a resident's room with his or her name on it (Fig. 12-4). For example, some facilities use colored dots on the door card to identify blind or deaf residents who need special help in case of emergency. Signs with words or symbols by a resident's bed provide more information. You must be aware of and understand all this information so that you can provide safe and thorough care for each resident.

Other People

Others with whom you work also tell you about each resident. Staff in all departments who have worked with a resident have gathered much information. Other nurse assistants often have personalized information you can use to provide individualized care. Families and visitors can also communicate much about residents. Of course, be careful to verify any information that you get from families and visitors because they may not always know the full situation. For example, a family member may tell you that a resident always took a nap after breakfast at home. When you check with the charge nurse, you learn he or she has a physical therapy appointment after breakfast. This information allows talking with the person to see if he or she would prefer changing the appointment time to take a nap at the usual time. You shared the information that a resident usually napped after breakfast and perhaps saved him or her from going to bed and having to get up again immediately.

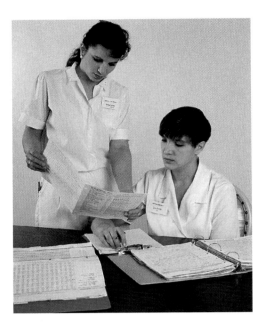

Fig. 12-5. Each resident, staff member, and family member becomes valuable asset for clarifying information.

Facility Policies and Procedures

Facility policies and procedures are the rules for how to do things in the facility. The information in policies and procedures tells you how and why things are done. For example, you may consult a procedure called "Completing the Personal Possession Record" when you are listing the items that a resident brings from home. Policies and procedures provide general information about residents to help you care for specific residents. For instance, if the "Policy and Procedure for Residents Leaving the Facility" states that residents are to sign out in the Leave Notebook, this may remind you to ask a resident if he or she will be returning for the next meal. You must follow facility policies and procedures so that your actions are consistent and correct.

There is so much information on the chart, in other places in the facility, in facility policies and procedures, and from staff, each resident, and the visitors that you are challenged to keep it all straight. Once you are familiar with all these sources, gathering information will become second nature to you. When communicating with members of the team, resident, or family, if you are unsure of anything—ask! Don't assume anything you're not sure of. Asking questions and clarifying information are useful and necessary aspects of communication for the whole health care team (Fig. 12-5). You receive information and share information with others, adding your own observations and ideas to the chart and other records.

THE DIFFERENCE BETWEEN OBJECTIVE AND SUBJECTIVE INFORMATION

Your observations of a resident are an excellent source of information. Objective information is factual information—that everyone will agree with. You make observations by looking, listening, feeling, and touching. For example, "this resident weighs 127 pounds" and "that resident's skin is warm and dry" are observations of objective data.

Subjective information is your guess or "hunch" about what you observe. If you see that a resident did not drink any milk at lunch, you might interpret that fact by guessing that he or she does not like milk. Your guess is subjective; it might be right or wrong because it is not a fact. Perhaps this resident likes milk but did not drink it this time for another reason. The subjective information you provide from your hunches can be very helpful as long as you identify it as subjective information.

Imagine a situation where you hear a loud crash and then a resident yelling, "Help me! I fell." When you run into the room, you see the person lying on the floor with the tray table tipped over. You guess that he or she fell down. You report to the nurse, "I heard a loud crash, then I heard him call, 'Help me! I fell.' When I walked into the room, I saw him lying on the floor with his tray table on the floor beside him. I think that he fell." By clearly identifying which information is objective facts (in this case, what you heard and what you saw) and which information is your subjective guess ("I think that he fell"), you have made a clear and accurate report of the situation.

Now imagine that actually something else happened. The resident carefully got down on the floor, pushed his tray table over, and then started calling, "Help me! I fell." He wants his family to think that he fell because he thinks they may come to visit him when the nurse calls them to report the "fall." The objective data that you reported is still correct, but your guess was wrong. Fortunately, you identified it as a guess (as subjective information) and not as a fact (objective information). The report would be inaccurate if the subjective information ("I think the resident fell") was given as though it were an objective fact ("The resident fell"). Accurate observations and reporting combine subjective and objective information with clear identification of facts and guesses.

Good observations include detailed information. You will know more about the situation if you use all of your senses. For example, danger signs in a resident with diabetes are heavy sweating, a red face, "fruity" smelling breath, and the person saying, "I don't feel right." You want to gather as much information as you can (in this case, quickly) to make a thorough report. For example, is the room very warm or is the person too heavily covered with blankets, which might account for the sweating and red face? Do you notice a particular odor in the room? Asking a resident for more detail ("What do you mean, you don't feel right?") will also give you more objective information. You then report the information to the charge nurse so that appropriate actions can be taken. Your accurate observations and reports increase the quality of care.

HOW TO REPORT INFORMATION

You report information in a variety of ways. Usually you report it to the charge nurse, but sometimes you may need to report to other facility staff. Since all staff maintain the confidentiality of resident information, you can safely report information to other health care professionals in the facility. Use a private place to report where others will not overhear.

Because information about a resident is confidential, be careful with information given to families and visitors. Even fairly routine information may not seem that way to others. For example, tell a resident's husband that his wife slept that afternoon for 2 hours. He becomes alarmed and says, "She never sleeps that long. She must be sick!" Always talk with the charge nurse first before making reports to residents or families.

Routine Reporting

At the end of your shift always report to the charge nurse about residents you have been caring for. This is routine reporting and includes objective and subjective information not immediately important. With routine reporting, you provide information about the care you gave during your shift. Before you give your report, ask yourself, What did I see, hear, smell, or touch when caring for each resident? Was there anything new or changed? Did I meet each resident's needs? Much general information does not need to be reported before the end of the shift. For example, "Mrs. Jones is continuing to walk without limping" and "Mr. Smith wants us to tell the night shift to wake him up at 7 in the morning because his son is telephoning him at 7:15" are examples of general reporting. You can make general reports any time convenient for you and the person you are reporting to.

Immediate Reporting

Some observations must be reported immediately. Dangerous situations (frayed electrical cord, for example), unusual incidents (such as a resident falls or you suspect resident abuse), resident complaints of ill health (such as a resident complains of pain or dizziness), and unusual observations (like a temperature of 103° F or a normally alert resident who is confused and agitated) must be reported right away.

"By a Certain Time" Reporting

A third type of reporting falls between immediate and general. This is "by a certain time" reporting and includes information needed by a set time. For example, the nurse may need a resident's temperature before the doctor calls. If you are unsure when to report something, talk to the charge nurse.

Usually, you make your reports directly to another person, speaking information face to face. Sometimes you report things with a written note or a form. A written request to the maintenance department to tighten a faucet handle is an example of a report that can be written for later action.

INCIDENT REPORTS

In Chapter 8 you learned an incident report is needed to protect residents, yourself, the facility, and the people involved in the incident. An incident report documents the incident and the facts surrounding it (Fig. 12-6). Some incidents involve later legal action, so the incident report is an important document. You may provide objective information (what you heard, saw, smelled, and touched) to someone else who fills out the report, or you complete it yourself. The guidelines for documenting an incident are the same as for documenting in the chart (described in the next section).

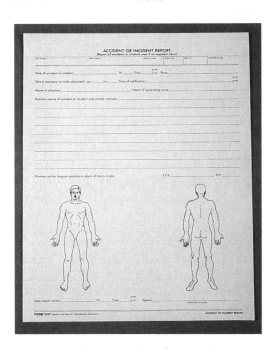

Fig. 12-6.   An example of an incident report.

YOUR ROLE IN DOCUMENTATION

Documentation is the term used for written reports the facility maintains. To document something means that you write it down. In addition to residents' charts, you also document on worksheets and facility records such as incident reports. The written record usually communicates to other staff, but your documentation may be used in other ways, perhaps by an insurance company or even in a legal case in court. Therefore all health professionals follow the same guidelines for documentation.

Even documentation that seems routine is important. Imagine this situation. You take a resident's blood pressure and write it on the vital sign sheet. It is 150/86, not an especially high reading for an elderly woman, but compared with her usual blood pressures around 100/60, it is quite high. You can report this possibly serious change only because you had compared it to previously recorded blood pressures in the resident's record.

When you are documenting, you may discover important information that needs to be reported. For example, as you record a resident's weight, you discover that he or she has lost weight since the last recorded weight. You report this information to the nurse in addition to documenting it. Documentation involves watching for trends. When completing the tray monitor record, you discover a resident often leaves the vegetable uneaten. Since the dietician can use this information to better plan meals, you report it to the dietician in addition to writing it down.

Before you document anything, be sure to know your facility's policies and procedures for your documentation. Each facility is different. In some, nurse assistants write progress notes. Progress notes are phrases and sentences written down about a resident and the care provided. This information is listed by date. It may include the following:

1. General statement on care provided
2. Appointments and activities attended
3. Any complaints voiced
4. General statement on psychological well-being
5. Visitors noted, including doctor's visits

Some facilities use flow sheets in the form of check-off sheets that require only your initials and simple documentation (for example, an "L" for large if a resident had a large bowel movement). You may record intake and output numbers on worksheets, which someone else such as the unit clerk or charge nurse later totals and writes in the chart, or you may record them directly in the chart yourself.

Your facility may use a combination of charting methods. For example, an assignment sheet may need your initials on one side but have a few lines on the other side for progress notes. Regardless of the formats used, follow the guidelines for documentation in the next section.

Guidelines for Documentation → P 174

The guidelines for documentation are common sense rules that keep the documentation in the chart clear and easy to read and prevent misunderstandings. The box at the top of page 174 lists guidelines for documentation. They also help prevent altering of the record. These guidelines maintain the chart as a legal record. If entries in the chart cannot be read or seem wrong or changed, it will be very difficult to know the facts for certain.

You must use neat handwriting or printing when making entries into the record since an entry that cannot be read is like an entry that isn't there at all. Health professionals are not allowed to skip lines or leave open spaces because someone could at a later time or date write something in that space. If there is a space in your charting that you initial after doing a task, for example, use your facility's system for recording in that space when you do not complete the task. Leaving the space empty would allow someone to change the record later. Chart only your own ac-

Guidelines for Documentation

1. The resident's name should be on every page of the chart and is written on each new page before anything else is written.
2. Write all entries in permanent blue or black ink, not pencil or felt tip markers that may smear when wet.
3. Print each entry or write legibly so that it is easy to read. Pay attention to your penmanship. You can use neat, orderly printing instead if it is easier to read.
4. Charting is continuous. Do not leave spaces or skipped lines between entries.
5. Document only your own actions and observations.
6. Do not tamper with or change entries made into the chart unless you make an error. If you make an error, correct it immediately and properly (as described below).
7. Use standard medical terminology and standard abbreviations. (See Appendixes A and B.)
8. As required, write down the date and the time of each entry.
9. Sign each entry and include your title after your name (or in some cases, initial the entry when your signature is somewhere else on the form).

tions and observations. Charting for someone else is illegal. All staff are responsible for their own work.

How Do I Correct a Mistake in Documentation?

The health record and most forms on which you document are legal records. People who look at records for legal purposes examine alterations closely. Lawyers, state surveyors, other inspectors, and insurance company officials are some of the people who might scrutinize residents' records. Therefore all health professionals use a standard method for correcting mistakes in documentation. If you make a mistake you must correct it so that other members of the health care team are reading accurate information. Imagine that you are writing a sentence in the health record and misspell a word. To correct it, draw a single line through the word, print "error," add your initials and the date above the misspelled word, and then write the correctly spelled word and continue on (Fig. 12-7A and 12-7B). If you obliterate the word with X's or scribble over the word, the reader cannot tell what was written under the scribble or X's. A person could claim that you had originally written something else, and you would not be able to prove that wrong.

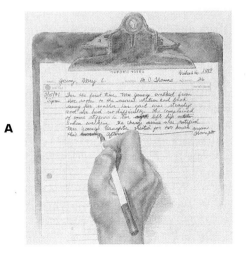
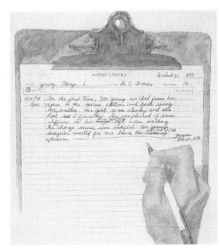

A　　**B**

Fig. 12-7. **A,** The wrong way to correct a documentation error. **B,** The right way to correct a documentation error.

If you have to correct a large area of writing, indicate the reason why you are making the correction. Many health professionals have written a detailed progress note only to discover it is written on the wrong resident's chart! If that happens to you, draw one large X or single lines through each line of charting, and write "wrong resident" in the margin with your initials or signature (Fig. 12-8).

Sometimes it is difficult to correct a mistake in your documentation. When your charting requires that you write your initials or numbers in a little box, there may not be enough room to correct the mistake in that place. Draw a circle around the entry and write on the reverse side of the sheet (or in the margin if there is not room on the reverse) to describe what happened, including the date, your initials, and the correct information (Fig. 12-9). Some mistakes are difficult to correct. Perhaps you cannot find enough room on the form to correct an error, or you realize days or weeks later that you made a mistake. In these unusual cases, talk with the charge nurse or the medical records department for correction guidelines. Your responsible attitude and desire to have only accurate information in the record is a sign of a good health care professional. The box at the bottom of this page lists guidelines on how to correct errors.

RESIDENT ASSESSMENTS

An assessment is an evaluation of a condition. If your television won't turn on, you assess the problem (maybe it isn't plugged in, maybe the batteries in the remote control are dead. . .). You evaluate the condition by looking at all the related factors. Health care includes many assessments of a resident and his or her condition. The first step in assessment is gathering data, and as you know, that includes collecting objective information. As nurse assistant, you are vital in the assessment process, especially in gathering data, because you spend so much time observing residents. All other departments use and depend on your observations and assessments of residents.

The most important assessment for every resident in a Medicaid/Medicare facility is the Resident Assessment Instrument (RAI). The RAI has two parts, the Minimum Data Set (MDS) and the Resident Assessment Protocols (RAPs) (Fig. 12-10). An RAI must be completed within 14 days of a resident's admission to the facility. Then a new RAI is done at least yearly and each time a resident has a major change in condition. A partial assessment (called a Quarterly Review) is completed every 90 days. You may be asked for information for the RAI or MDS.

Guidelines for Correcting Documentation Errors

▶ Draw a single line through the error. Do not completely cover the error with X's, scribbles, or "whte out." Do not erase entries. What you wrote should rremain readable.

▶ Print the word "error," your initials, and the date beside the error.

▶ If you are correcting a charting mistake in a small box, circle the mistake and write the correction, the date, and your initials on the reverse side of the sheet.

▶ If you are correcting a large amount of charting, indicate the reason why in the margin. (For example, "wrong resident" or "charted entry twice.") This is not necessary for correcting short entries.

▶ Ask for help from the nurse or the medical records department if you cannot figure out how to correct a documentation mistake clearly.

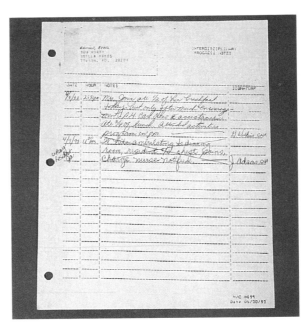

Fig. 12-8. Correct a mistake on a large area of documentation by drawing a large X or single lines through each line and note the reason for the correction.

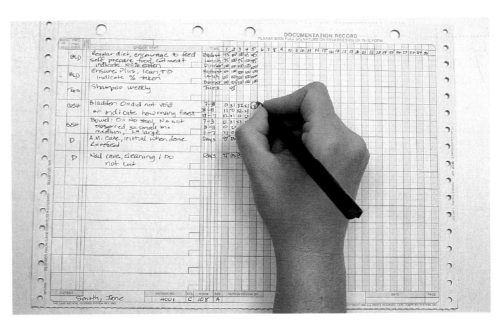

Fig. 12-9. To correct a mistake in a box or small area, draw a circle around the entry and make notes regarding the correction on the reverse side.

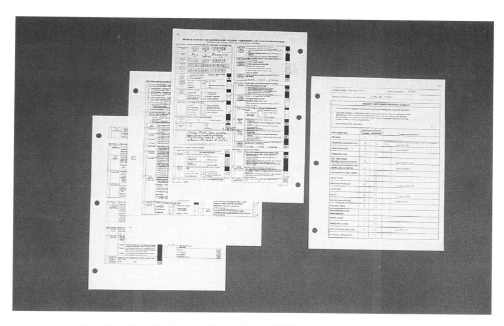

Fig. 12-10. The Minimum Data Set (MDS) and the Resident Assessment Protocols (RAPs).

The RAI has several different sections, usually completed by staff in the different departments, such as dietary and social services. Each section includes items observed by many different staff members, including you. Memory, communication and hearing, vision, emotional and social behavior, activity patterns, nutrition, and dental status are all assessed on the MDS. Two areas on the RAI are especially important to the nursing department. One involves the activities of daily living (for example, dressing, hygiene, mobility, eating, and bathing), and the other assesses bowel and bladder continence. Although you do not write in the form yourself, the nurse asks for your information to complete them. As with all of reporting, you clearly identify objective information ("Mr. Brown puts on his own shirt but he doesn't button the buttons himself") and subjective information ("I think that he could button his shirt himself if he had bigger buttons").

Some items on the RAI may have different definitions from what your facility usually uses. For example, "bed mobility" on the MDS includes not only how a resident turns from side to side in the bed but also how he or she sits up and lies back down. Be certain that you understand the item you are observing and reporting so that you give accurate and thorough information.

As the health professional who spends the most time with residents, you are often the person who first observes a change in condition. A big change caused by a serious illness will be apparent to everyone, but small, gradual changes are often identified first by nurse assistants. Imagine a resident who has been able to do his own dressing and hygiene with set-up help from you. Over the last few days, you observe and report that he is needing a little more help. You and other staff start observing him more closely and assess these changes. A new RAI is done when a resident has a significant change to try to determine why the change is occurring and what the staff can do to slow down deterioration and help the person improve. Without your observations and report, this subtle change might be missed. Individualized resident care starts with a thorough and accurate assessment from nurse assistants and other staff who know a resident well and who can communicate their observations clearly.

After the MDS is completed, a resident is assessed in more detail in possible problem areas. For example, a resident may have a problem with mobility. You provide information once again to assist the staff in this RAI process. Then the total information is used to develop the person's care plan.

RESIDENT CARE PLAN

A resident care plan is a written, interdisciplinary document that lists a resident's needs and goals as well as the actions and approaches the facility will take to assist a resident to meet his or her goals. Many health professionals in the facility have input into the plan. The care plan is a tool for all staff to use to ensure continuity in care. The care plan is usually located at the nurse's station so all staff have access. It may be in a looseleaf notebook or a kardex. A kardex is a file system for information about each resident.

The care plan is based on assessments on admission and is fully developed within 7 days of RAI completion. The care plan is never considered "done" because it changes to reflect changes in a resident, including both progress and decline, and other information that you and other staff gather about a resident's needs, preferences, strengths, weaknesses, and goals.

The care plan lists each resident's medical, nursing, and psychosocial needs. These are often called problems. For each problem, an objective or goal is written. An example of a problem is "Resident cannot walk," and a possible goal for that problem would be "Resident will be able to walk 10 feet within 90 day." The care plan also lists what staff will do, called approaches, to help a resident meet the goal. For example, "Take to physical therapy every morning at 9 A.M." (nurse assistant), "Stand resident at parallel bars for 2 minutes three times a day" (physical therapy), "Encourage resident to use his legs to move his wheelchair" (all), and "Range of motion exercises to both legs 5 times per leg at bedtime" (nurse assistant). To assist the care plan team in evaluating a resident's progress, a time frame (sometimes called a goal date) is set. Table 12-1 gives an example that identifies the problem, goal, time frame, approaches, and responsible department.

Your observations and experience with a resident are especially important in both developing the care plan and in keeping it up to date by observing and re-

TABLE 12-1. Section of a Resident's Care Plan

Problem	Goal	Approaches	Discipline
Poor appetite and weight loss	Gains 2 pounds within 3 weeks	Weigh every Friday A.M.	Nurse assistant
		Monitor tray and record intake	Nurse assistant
		High protein and drink at 10 A.M. and at bedtime	Nurse assistant and dietary
		Resident likes ice cream Offer ice cream if he refuses to drink high-protein drink	Nurse assistant
		Offer snacks at BINGO	Activity department
		Son will eat with resident at noon. Serve tray in A wing lounge.	Nurse assistant

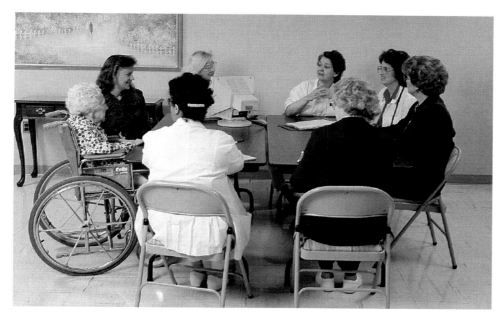

Fig. 12-11.   A care conference includes the health care team, the resident, and family and is held to help evaluate the resident's current plan of care.

porting whether it is working. In the example above, you might discover that this resident also likes peanut butter sandwiches at bedtime. If you suggest this addition to the care plan, the staff who work with this resident will know that even when he is refusing the protein drink and ice cream, another alternative might appeal to him.

Management information system (MIS) computer programs are becoming popular in long term care facilities. Computers allow staff to document, retrieve, track, and save information like never before. The risk of losing paper is completely eliminated. If you are working in a facility that uses computers, you will learn this method on the job.

Your Role in the Care Plan Meeting

The interdisciplinary team, including a resident and family, reviews and as needed revises the care plan at least every 90 days. Some disciplines write their information for this review. Most, however, sit down with a resident and family to discuss the care plan and his or her progress toward meeting the goals. This is sometimes called a care conference (Fig. 12-11). Problem solving is an important part of this meeting, with everyone sharing ideas, observations, and information. A care plan meeting requires good communication skills because many people are sharing a lot of information and struggling with sometimes difficult situations. Your role is to come well-prepared, knowledgeable about a resident, open to new ideas and approaches, and ready to share information. Since some areas of any resident's care and progress may be sensitive, your tact is especially important. It can be exciting for a resident to participate in this meeting, but it also might be stressful, so your professional and caring support of every resident is needed.

TELEPHONE COURTESY

Being courteous is very important in your job. You have a great opportunity to give good impressions of your facility to others. Telephone courtesy is as important as the courtesy given in person. Always think of how you would feel if you were treated rudely on the phone. It is easy to be rushed in your work and to find the telephone an irritation, but remember that rudeness or curtness is never appropriate. You are a representative of the facility you work for.

When you answer the phone you should:

▶ State the facility's name, the unit, and your name.

▶ Find out why the caller is phoning by asking how you can help.

▶ Assist the caller with a request. This might involve bringing a resident to the phone or finding the appropriate staff person to answer a question. Never yell or call out for the person requested but go and get him or her.

▶ Never put a caller on hold for more than 2-3 minutes. Never leave the telephone receiver unattended.

▶ If you cannot answer a caller's request, take the caller's telephone number and say you will give the message to the right person who can call back.

▶ Thank the caller for calling.

▶ Be sure you follow through on anything you say you will do.

COMMON MEDICAL TERMS AND ABBREVIATIONS

Imagine meeting with a banker to discuss a loan. You are already a little nervous, and then the banker starts to use financial and banking terms you never heard before. You feel lost, and understandably so, because it's like the banker is speaking a foreign language! This is a common feeling for many people. Medical terms like "perineum" replace words the general public uses (such as "crotch" or "privates"). Medical terms and abbreviations are used throughout the medical record.

As you gain more experience in health care, the terminology will become more familiar to you. Remember, however, that the medical terms that you use with ease may not be understandable to everyone, especially residents, visitors, new staff, or staff in other departments. Medical terminology is quite confusing to people new to health care, and may even cause funny situations. A new resident in a facility was asked by the nurse assistant if he needed to urinate. He replied, "No, I don't have to do that—I've just got to pee." This example may be humorous, but misunderstandings can also cause dangerous situations. Generally, you should communicate with residents with simple terms ("I'm going to wash between your legs now" instead of "I'm going to wash your perineum now"). Define words a resident might not understand ("I'm going to take an axillary temperature now. That means I'm going to put the thermometer in your armpit.")

Because so much documentation must be done, you generally use standard medical terminology and abbreviations. Most facilities have established standard terms and abbreviations. Sometimes facilities use different terms. Some facilities have their own abbreviations as well, so don't be embarrassed to ask what something means. It is much worse not to ask and to make a wrong guess. Think of the doctor who was confused because he read that a resident was walking with SBA (stand-by assistance) and thought that SBA was some new kind of leg brace.

Appendices A and B include common medical terms and abbreviations for your reference. You generally use standard medical terms when documenting, but even more important than using a complicated term is to document clearly. Sometimes health professionals think that they must use "official" medical terms and discover that they could have used a simpler term and communicated the information more clearly.

Next chapter 15 page 237

IN THIS CHAPTER YOU LEARNED TO:

- name all the locations in which resident information can be found.
- explain the difference between objective and subjective information.
- explain when and how to report and document information.
- explain the role of the nurse assistant in the care planning process.
- identify medical terminology and abbreviations.
- be courteous on the telephone.

13

MOVING AND POSITIONING

Did you ever fall asleep in one position, such as on your back with your arms at your sides and your legs straight, and wake up in a totally different position, such as on your stomach with your arms across the bed, and wonder how you got there?

Our bodies are in constant movement to stay comfortable. Sometimes we move consciously, such as when we shift our weight to feel more comfortable when sitting on a park bench. Sometimes movement is unconscious when the body changes positions to keep the blood flowing freely to all parts to prevent stiffness.

Movement of our limbs and our bodies is extremely important. Although residents you work with will have varying physical needs and abilities, moving is important for all. Moving and positioning our bodies also has psychological importance. Without the freedom that comes from mobility, one has difficulty meeting basic needs. Often a resident's self-esteem depends on at least some independence in mobility. Regardless of residents' individual needs for assistance, your goal is to help them optimize their mobility. With residents who have difficulty assisting in their care because of limited ability to move, you need to find ways for them to participate and become as independent as possible.

In this chapter you will learn why movement and positioning are so important. You will learn how to assess residents' mobility in different situations and how to help them move safely and efficiently. You will also learn how to position residents in various body positions for comfort and safety when they cannot independently change positions through the day.

MOVING AND POSITIONING

The human body is designed for continual movement. Each system in the body is in a constant state of change. When a person stops moving or has restricted movement, the body adapts and slows down to accommodate. Because the body systems are interconnected, a small change in movement can affect all body systems. In addition, because aging generally slows down the functioning of body systems, long term care residents are affected even more by such movement changes. Someone who has been confined to bed for even a short time may experience stiffness or general weakness (the muscular system), decreased appetite or constipation (the digestive system), shortness of breath or dizziness when moving (the circulatory and respiratory systems), skin redness (the integumentary system), and slowed movement (the nervous system). Movement is essential for keeping all of the body's systems functioning well.

"Positioning" is the term for how you help residents sit, lie down, or change position when they have trouble moving themselves or forget to change positions. Even residents who can move by themselves may need help positioning themselves if they are having trouble getting comfortable or are having skin problems from not changing positions often enough. The positions best for the individual resident depend on his or her body type, medical needs, equipment needs, skin condition, and comfort.

Certain areas of the body are prone to pressure sores caused by the weight of the body or pressure from the mattress or linens (Fig. 13-1). Usually pressure sores can be prevented by proper moving and positioning. Moving and positioning also helps

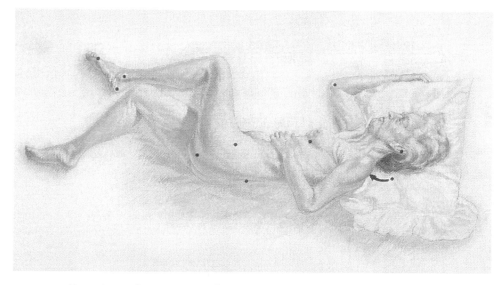

Fig. 13-1. Some areas of the body are prone to pressure sores.

reduce swelling in an arm or leg, prevents stiffness in a limb, and keeps tubes or needed equipment lines from being pulled.

Moving and positioning are important for many reasons in addition to helping a resident stay mobile and preventing skin problems. Moving and positioning also helps residents be as comfortable as possible by preventing pain and discomfort that result from stiffness, pressure, and poor circulation.

As with all other care, you must first assess and observe residents before choosing the best way to move or reposition them. For example, when positioning a resident, look for and consider the following factors that influence positioning:

▶ Spinal deformities (such as rounded back, forward head, leaning to one side)
▶ Areas of redness
▶ Bandaged areas, casts, or splints
▶ Arms, legs, hands, or feet in a stiff position or swollen
▶ Intravenous tubes or other medical lines
▶ Oxygen being administered
▶ Recent surgical sites

Be sure to keep these factors in mind when positioning a resident. Chapter 20 on "Restorative Activities" discusses in detail how to position a resident with these specific factors.

Preparing to Move or Position a Resident

Before you begin to help move or position a resident, you must know what the doctor and charge nurse expect. Ask yourself key questions to assess this resident and situation. Think about yourself, the resident, and the environment and ask yourself these questions:

1. Think about your own capabilities and limitations:
   ▶ Can you do what's needed? Do you need help?
   ▶ Do you understand the doctor's orders and the charge nurse's expectations?
2. Think about the resident:
   ▶ How much help does this resident need to move? How large is this resident?
   ▶ Does this resident have any special needs or behaviors to consider before you start the move?
   ▶ Does this resident have any physical condition that affects moving him or her, such as fragile skin or bones? How much weight is allowed to be placed on the limb? How much limb motion is allowed?

▷ Does this resident use an assistive device (such as walker or cane) or brace?

▷ Observe the resident's ability and function, and ask the charge nurse and co-workers about his or her needs.

▷ Does this resident understand what you are asking him or her to do? Can he or she see and hear you or need glasses or a hearing aid to see or hear better?

▷ What equipment is needed to most easily move this resident?

▷ Where are the resident's shoes and socks?

▷ What tubes and equipment surround the resident? IV tube, oxygen line?

▷ Does this resident have any dressings or open wounds?

▷ Can this resident tolerate all positions?

3. Think about the environment:

▷ How is the lighting in the room? Noise level? Commotion in the room?

▷ Are obstacles (medical equipment, appliances, extra linens, personal possessions, furniture) in the way?

▷ Is the bed at the proper height? Is everything close?

▷ Can you maneuver around the tubes or equipment surrounding this resident?

▷ Are there distractions in the room, such as television, radio, family members, or ongoing nursing care of another resident in the room?

▷ What chair and seating device does this resident use?

These questions are an important part of your assessment before beginning to help move or position a resident. Continually evaluate for changes throughout moving and transferring procedures.

When to Get Help

Based on your assessment of a resident and situation, decide whether you need help to move or position him or her. Always get help if you are at all unsure. You may need help for many reasons. If you are unsure how a resident will respond, are unfamiliar with him or her, or are uncomfortable lifting him or her by yourself, be safe and get help!

Communicating with Residents

Communicating with residents and your co-workers is important for moving and positioning. Serious injury can occur if someone does not understand how the move is to be done. Giving clear directions is important. Everyone must know what to do and when to start to do it. Be sure to communicate clearly with residents about their role. Ask them to do things on the "count of three" or push off the bed to help you raise them to a standing position. Or you might ask them to grasp the siderail while you are turning them toward you. Remember, residents need to help and be a vital part of the move. You must never do for residents what they can do for themselves.

Moving

The move will be successful if you assess each resident and situation and consider the questions listed earlier for preparing to move a resident. Also apply what you learned in Chapter 8, Injury Prevention, about using proper body mechanics to prevent injury to residents and yourself. Consider each situation individually and adapt your approach to meet each resident's needs. Work closely with the charge nurse and the physical therapy departments to adapt for each resident's own needs. *Note:* Never move a resident by pulling on or under his or her arm. Many arteries, nerves, and veins run under the pit of the arm. Pulling applies pressure that can damage blood vessels or nerves. As well, many older residents have osteoporosis or fragile bone structures that can be easily dislocated or broken. Take care to

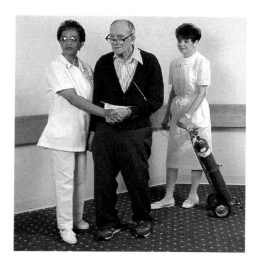

Fig. 13-2. When walking with or moving a resident, never lift him or her under the arms.

avoid lifting a resident under his or her arm when moving or walking him or her (Fig. 13-2).

If a resident is supine (lying on the back) and needs help moving up, down, or to the side of bed for personal care or repositioning, use the following procedures. Remember, first place the bed in the best position for the move. For example, put the bed in a flat position to move the resident up in bed, and raise the head of the bed when helping a resident out of bed. Be sure to ask him or her and the charge nurse which is best.

Moving Up in Bed When a Resident Can Help

1. Move the pillows against the headboard. Put the head of the bed flat if this resident can tolerate it.
2. Assist the resident to bend his or her knees up and place his or her feet flat on the bed. Place one arm under his or her shoulders and the other under the upper thighs.
3. On the count of three, have him or her push down with the feet and lift up the buttocks (This is called bridging) while you help move him or her toward the head of the bed.
   Note: You may also try having the resident help pull up in bed using the bedrails (Fig 13-3).

Remember:

▶ Resident preference
▶ Common preparation steps
▶ Equipment and supplies needed
▶ Environment preparation
▶ Resident preparation

Remember:

▶ Meet resident needs
▶ Common completion steps
▶ Clean and put away equipment and supplies
▶ Environment completion (Is it safe? Is it clean?)

Moving Up in Bed When a Resident is Unable to Help

1. Call another staff person to assist you.
2. Remove the pillow and place it against the headboard. Put the head of the bed flat if this resident can tolerate it.
3. Help the resident to cross his or her hands over the body.
4. Roll the draw sheet up from the side toward the resident until you and your helper

Remember:

▶ Resident preference
▶ Common preparation steps
▶ Equipment and supplies needed
▶ Environment preparation
▶ Resident preparation

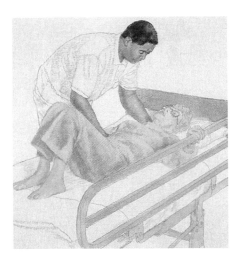

Fig. 13-3. The resident may use the bedrails to move up in bed.

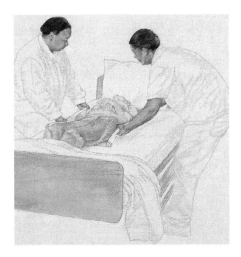

Fig. 13-4. Move the resident who is unable to help.

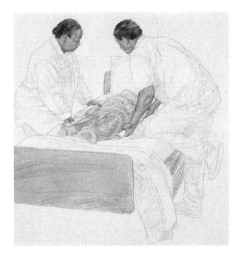

Fig. 13-5. To get as close to the resident as possible, put one knee on the bed.

both have a tight grip with both hands. Keep your palms up if that gives you more strength for moving him or her (Fig. 13-4).

Note: You can put one knee on the bed to get as close to the resident as possible (Fig. 13-5).

5. Count aloud to 3, and you and your helper lift the resident up to the head of the bed while you use good body mechanics. You can do this in stages until he or she is in position.
6. Unroll the drawsheet and tuck it in.

Moving to the Side of the Bed When a Resident Can Help

1. Stand on the side to which you plan to move this resident.
2. Assist him or her to bend the knees up and place his or her feet on the bed.
3. Help him or her to bridge (lift up the buttocks) and move his or her buttocks over to the side of the bed (Fig. 13-6).
4. Help the resident move his or her legs over, and then the head and upper body by sliding your arms under him or her and gliding them toward you if the resident needs help.
5. You can do this in stages to reach the desired position.

Remember:
▶ Meet resident needs
▶ Common completion steps
▶ Clean and put away equipment and supplies
▶ Environment completion (Is it safe? Is it clean?)

Remember:
▶ Resident preference
▶ Common preparation steps
▶ Equipment and supplies needed
▶ Environment preparation
▶ Resident preparation

Remember:
▶ Meet resident needs
▶ Common completion steps
▶ Clean and put away equipment and supplies
▶ Environment completion (Is it safe? Is it clean?)

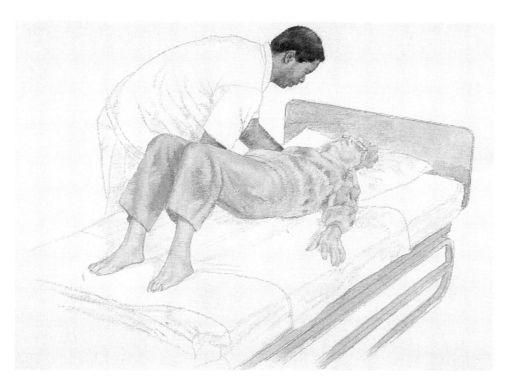

Fig. 13-6. Help the resident move to the side of the bed.

Remember:

▶ Resident preference
▶ Common preparation steps
▶ Equipment and supplies
  needed
▶ Environment preparation
▶ Resident preparation

Remember:

▶ Meet resident needs
▶ Common completion steps
▶ Clean and put away
  equipment and supplies
▶ Environment completion
  (Is it safe? Is it clean?)

Moving to the Side of the Bed When a Resident Is Unable to Help

1. Stand on the side to which you plan to move the resident.
2. Ask the resident to fold his or her arms across the chest, or do this for him or her if necessary.
3. Slide both your hands under the resident's head, neck, and shoulders and glide him or her toward you on your arms (Fig. 13-7).
4. Slide your arms under the resident's hips and glide them toward you (Fig. 13-8).
5. Slide your arms under his or her legs and pull them toward you (Fig. 13-9).
   Note: Keep the resident in proper body alignment.

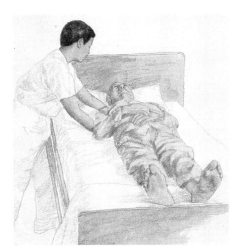

Fig. 13-7. Glide the resident's head, neck, and shoulders toward you on your arms.

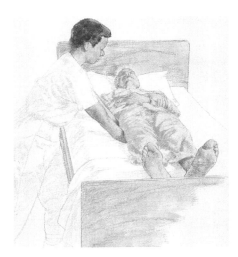

Fig. 13-8. Glide the resident's hips toward you.

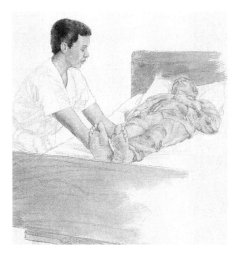

Fig. 13-9. Glide the resident's legs toward you.

Moving a Resident to the Side of the Bed Using a Drawsheet

1. Call another staff person to help you.
2. Help the resident place his or her arms across the chest.
3. Both you and your helper (on other side of bed) roll up the drawsheet from the sides toward the resident until you both have a good tight grip with both hands. *Note:* The staff person who is moving the resident away may want to put one knee on the edge of the bed to prevent injury caused by reaching too far (Fig. 13-10).
4. Count aloud to 3, and on 3 both of you lift the resident to the side of the bed. You can do this in stages until the desired position is reached.
5. Unroll the drawsheet and tuck it in.

Remember:

▶ Resident preference
▶ Common preparation steps
▶ Equipment and supplies needed
▶ Environment preparation
▶ Resident preparation

Remember:

▶ Meet resident needs
▶ Common completion steps
▶ Clean and put away equipment and supplies
▶ Environment completion (Is it safe? Is it clean?)

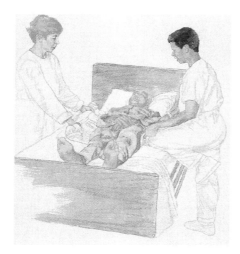

Fig. 13-10. Putting one knee on the edge of the bed prevents having to reach too far.

Turning a Resident from Supine to Side Lying for Personal Care

1. Help the resident bend his or her knees up one at a time and place his or her feet flat on the bed (Fig. 13-11).
2. Then place one hand on his or her shoulder farthest away from you and the other hand on the hip farthest from you (Fig. 13-12).
3. On the count of 3, help the resident roll toward you (Fig. 13-13). Raise the side rail (if used). Continue personal care. *Note:* Some residents may be more comfortable guiding the turn by holding onto the side rails.

Remember:

▶ Resident preference
▶ Common preparation steps
▶ Equipment and supplies needed
▶ Environment preparation
▶ Resident preparation

Remember:

▶ Meet resident needs
▶ Common completion steps
▶ Clean and put away equipment and supplies
▶ Environment completion (Is it safe? Is it clean?)

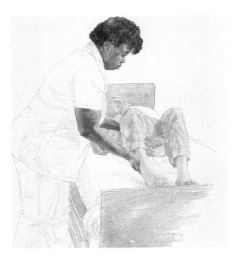

Fig. 13-11. After helping bend the resident's knees, place the feet flat on the bed.

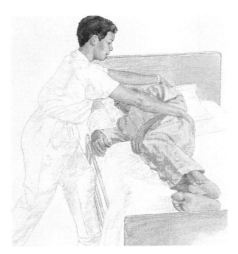

Fig. 13-12. Place your hands on the resident's farthest shoulder and hip.

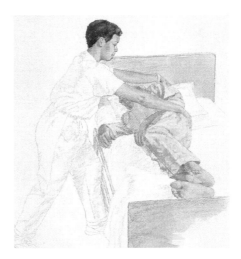

Fig. 13-13. Gently help the resident roll toward you.

Moving the <u>Resident from Supine Position to Sitting</u>

Note: Before you can transfer a resident from bed to a chair, the resident first needs to sit up on the side of the bed. The resident sits by rolling onto the side and then sitting up.

1. <u>Help the resident roll onto his or her side facing you or elevate the head of the bed and lower the side rails, if used</u> (Fig. 13-14).
2. <u>Reach under the resident's head and put your hand under the shoulder</u> (using your arm closer to the head of the bed). His or her <u>head should be supported by and resting on your forearm.</u> (Fig. 13-15).
3. <u>With your other hand, reach over and behind the resident's farthest knee</u> (Fig. 13-16).
4. <u>Using your legs and arms to do the lifting, bring the resident's head and trunk up as you swing his or her legs down to the sitting position. Hold his or her legs, letting the knees rest in the crook of your elbow</u> (Fig. 13-17).

   Note: Your arm behind the resident's head and trunk must stay in contact with the resident once he or she is sitting up, to prevent him or her from falling backward. Also remember to stay directly in front of the resident so you can block him or her with your body for safety (Fig. 13-18).

   If you need a second staff person to help you assist the resident to sit up, both of you stand on the same side:

   ▷ <u>One of you lifts the resident's head and trunk, while the other lifts his or her legs.</u> Or one does most of the lifting while the other stands on the opposite side of the bed behind the resident and assists as needed (Fig. 13-19).

Remember:

▷ Resident preference
▷ Common preparation steps
▷ Equipment and supplies needed
▷ Environment preparation
▷ Resident preparation

Remember:

▷ Meet resident needs
▷ Common completion steps
▷ Clean and put away equipment and supplies
▷ Environment completion (Is it safe? Is it clean?)

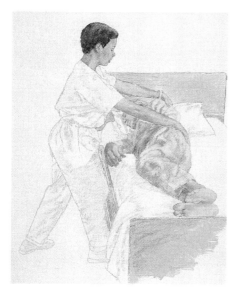

Fig. 13-14. Help the resident roll onto his or her side.

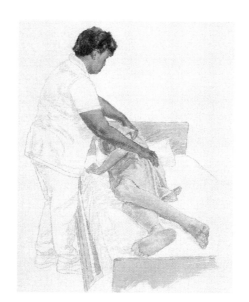

Fig. 13-15. Support the resident's head on your forearm.

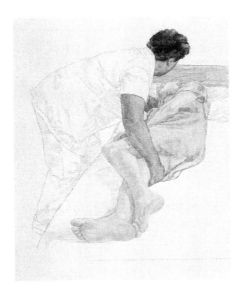

Fig. 13-16. Reach over and behind the farthest knee.

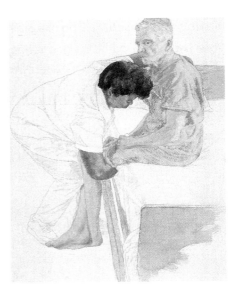

Fig. 13-17. Bring the resident's torso up and legs down simultaneously.

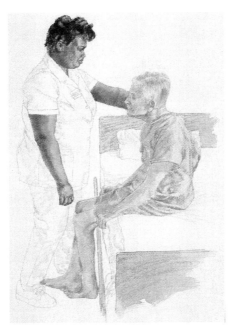

Fig. 13-18. Stand directly in front of the resident.

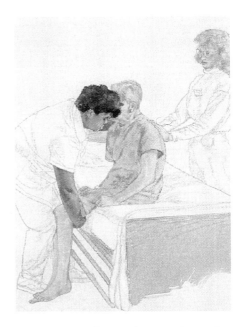

Fig. 13-19. One of you does the moving while the other stands on the opposite side to assist as needed.

Moving the Resident from Sitting to Supine Position

Note: Before moving a resident from sitting to the supine position, be sure he or she is sitting far enough back and up on the bed. He or she should be centered in the bed with the back of the knees against the mattress. Help him or her push down on the floor with the feet and down on the bed with the hands to move his or her body back onto the bed in the sitting position (Fig. 13-20).

1. Place one hand behind the resident's shoulder and let the head and neck rest on your forearm. Place your other hand under the knees and let his or her legs rest in the crook of your elbow. Position your arms as if you were carrying someone in front of you.
2. Use your legs to lift and breathe out as you help the resident lift his or her legs up onto the bed, and gently lower the trunk and head onto the bed (Fig. 13-21). *Note:* You might want to elevate the head of the bed before helping the resident into the supine position. Once he or she is in bed, you can lower the head of the bed.

Remember:

▶ Resident preference
▶ Common preparation steps
▶ Equipment and supplies needed
▶ Environment preparation
▶ Resident preparation

Remember:

▶ Meet resident needs
▶ Common completion steps
▶ Clean and put away equipment and supplies
▶ Environment completion (Is it safe? Is it clean?)

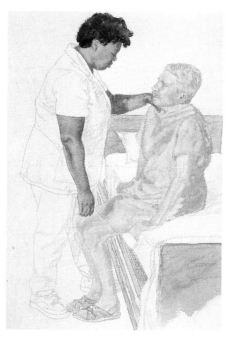

Fig. 13-20. Help the resident push down as his or her hands and feet move back on the bed.

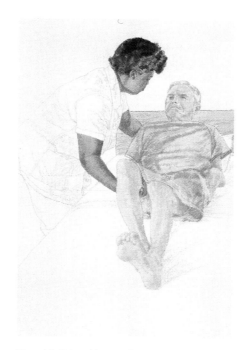

Fig. 13-21. Move the resident's torso and legs back onto the bed simultaneously.

TRANSFERRING

"Transfer" means moving a resident from one surface to another, such as from bed to chair, chair to toilet, bed to commode, and so on.

Using a Guard Belt

Place a guard belt (also called a transfer or gait belt) around a resident's waist to help you move him or her safely and without injury. It is safer for residents because it avoids straining or injuring their arm or leg. Residents often feel more secure when moving using a guard belt.

Note: Do not use a guard belt with residents who have a broken rib, abdominal wound, tubes such as a G-tube, or an opening such as a colostomy.

1. Turn the belt right-side-out. Most belts have a label on the outside to indicate which side is the outside.
2. Place the belt around the resident's waist (over clothes). You can do this with the resident either lying or sitting.
3. Once the belt is around the resident's waist, put the end through the teeth of the buckle and through the hoop, and tighten the belt firmly, but not so tightly that you cannot get your fingers under it to hold it when transferring the resident (Fig. 13-22). (If he or she is sitting, be sure to tighten it again when standing.)
4. Now you are ready to proceed with any of the following transferring procedures.

Transfer Considerations

When starting to transfer a resident from the bed to the chair, be alert for any of the following problems that may occur. If any of these occurs, let the resident back down onto the bed as described below. Then use a different action or get help.

▶   You lose your grip on a resident.
▶   A resident's legs give out.
▶   A resident gets dizzy. Sometimes a change in position can cause dizziness due to the pooling of blood in the extremities. If you wait a few minutes, the dizziness may go away. This is called postural hypotension.

The following problems may also occur:

▶   If you are helping a resident stand and you feel you do not have a good grip or enough leg support, help him or her sit down again and change your position to give more support.
▶   If a resident's legs start to give out or extend past your legs, block his or her legs with yours and help him or her sit again. You may need to get help (Fig. 13-23).
▶   If a resident becomes "floppy" or passes out, help him or her sit and then lower him or her to the supine position if needed and call the charge nurse. (See the later section in this chapter on stopping a fall.)

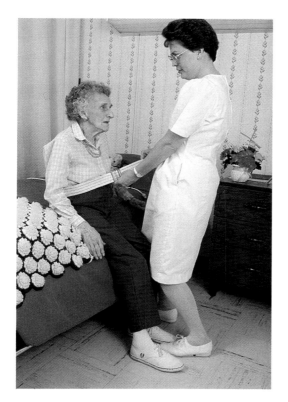

Fig. 13-22.   Apply the guard belt and tighten it so that it fits firmly.

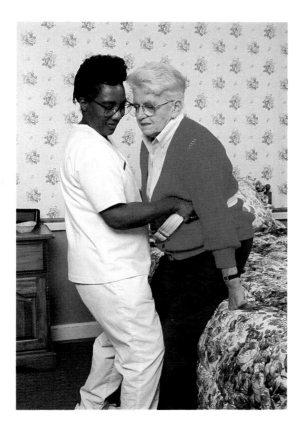

Fig. 13-23.   Block the resident's knees to prevent a fall.

Before transferring a resident, make these preparations:

▶ The resident's chair is locked and set up sideways to the bed with the arm of the chair next to the bed. The chair should be on the resident's stronger side. For example, if he or she had a stroke that affected the left side, put the chair on the right side. If he or she had a hip fracture on the right side, put the chair next to the left side.

▶ The walker or cane, if used, is next to or in front of the resident.

▶ Any brace or other special equipment is placed correctly on the resident.

▶ The bed height is at the lowest position in most cases, or raised as necessary for a tall resident.

▶ When transferring a resident out of bed, be sure to let him or her dangle his or her legs while sitting on the edge of the bed for a few minutes before standing. This minimizes any dizziness due to sudden postural change. If a resident complains of dizziness, help him or her to lie back down and call the charge nurse.

▶ Do not leave a resident unattended.

There are several types of transfers:

▶ Stand pivot transfer

▶ Assisted transfer with an assistive device

▶ Less commonly, sliding board and seated transfers

▶ Mechanical lift

▶ Dependent lift using two or more staff

The stand pivot transfer and assisted transfer with an assistive device are the most common methods and are described first.

Note: The same transfer is used for getting someone out of bed and into a chair or wheelchair or onto a bedside commode. A chair is used in the following descriptions.

The Stand Pivot Transfer

Remember:

▶ Resident preference
▶ Common preparation steps
▶ Equipment and supplies needed
▶ Environment preparation
▶ Resident preparation

Begin this transfer with the steps for moving a resident to a sitting position on the bed, described above.

1. Stand in front of the resident.
2. Place one of your legs between the resident's legs and the other outside close to the target you are moving toward. (This gives you better control over the speed and the direction of the movement.)
3. Hold onto the guard belt in the back slightly to either side. If you are not using a guard belt, put your arms around his or her waist (Fig. 13-24A).
4. Ask or assist the resident to push down on the bed with his or her hands, leaning the trunk forward and standing up (Fig. 13-24B). If he or she does not understand, you can have him or her hold around your waist during the transfer. Do not let him or her hold you around the neck, as this can cause injury.
5. Count to 3 and help the resident stand by leaning your body back and up and thereby bringing his or her trunk forward. Ask him or her to lean forward and stand up (Fig. 13-25).
6. Once the resident is standing, keep your back straight and body facing forward, and pivot (turn on your feet or take small steps) to turn him or her until his or her back is to the chair.
7. Ask the resident to reach back for the arm of the chair with one or both hands if possible (Fig. 13-26).
8. Help the resident to bend the knees and sit, as you assist (Fig. 13-27).
9. Once the resident is sitting, ask or help him or her to push back in the chair by pushing down with the feet on the floor and arms on the arm rests.

Remember:

▶ Meet resident needs
▶ Common completion steps
▶ Clean and put away equipment and supplies
▶ Environment completion (Is it safe? Is it clean?)

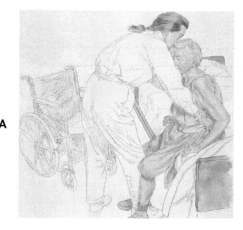

A

Fig. 13-24. **A,** Hold the guard belt.

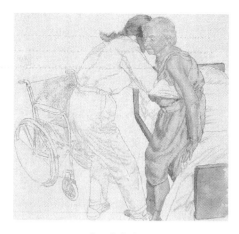

B

Fig. 13-24. **B,** While the resident pushes down on the bed to stand.

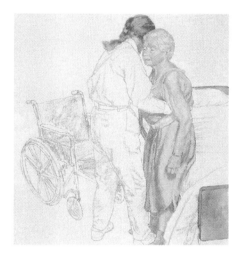

Fig. 13-25. Help the resident to stand.

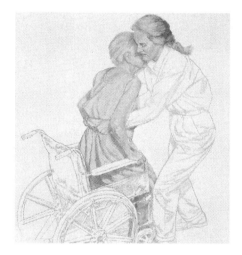

Fig. 13-26. Help the resident to pivot until his or her back is to the chair and ask the resident to reach back for the arm of the chair with one or both hands.

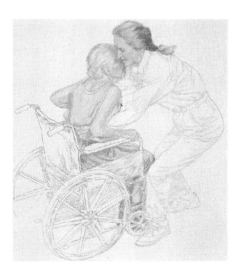

Fig. 13-27. Assist the resident to sit down.

Remember:

▶ Resident preference
▶ Common preparation steps
▶ Equipment and supplies
   needed
▶ Environment preparation
▶ Resident preparation

Remember:

▶ Meet resident needs
▶ Common completion steps
▶ Clean and put away
   equipment and supplies
▶ Environment completion
   (Is it safe? Is it clean?)

Assisted Transfer with an Assistive Device (One Person)

1. Once the resident is sitting on the side of the bed without difficulty, place the assistive device in his or her hand (with a cane) or in front of him or her (with a walker).
2. Stand to the side of the resident, usually on the side opposite to the chair (Fig. 13-28).
3. Ask and help the resident to push down on the bed with his or her hands and stand on the count of 3. You can help him or her by pulling up and forward on the back of the guard belt with one hand and stabilizing (pushing down on) the walker or cane with the other while he or she stands.
4. Help the resident put both hands on the walker, if used, and stand (Fig. 13-29A). *Note:* Have the resident stand for a few minutes before trying to move, especially if he or she is dizzy (Fig. 13-29B).
5. Assist the resident to move toward the chair. Guide him or her by saying, "Turn, turn, take a step toward me, now back up" (Fig. 13-30A).
6. Assist the resident to the chair by backing up to it (Fig. 13-30B). Ask the resident if he or she can feel the chair against the back of his or her legs. Explain that the resident cannot sit until he or she feels this.
7. Once the resident is in front of the chair, ask him or her to reach back and put one hand on the armrest.
8. Help the resident reach back with the other hand for the arm of the chair and slowly sit down (Fig. 13-31).

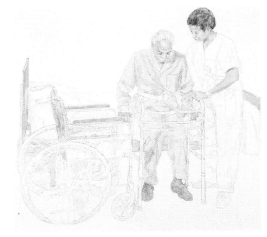

Fig. 13-28. Stand next to the resident and help him to stand using the guard belt.

Fig. 13-29. A, After the resident puts his or her hands on the walker, help him or her to stand. **B,** Allow the resident to stand for a few minutes before beginning to move.

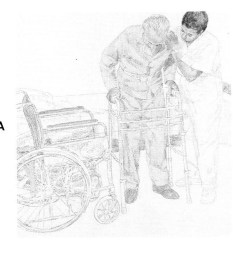

A

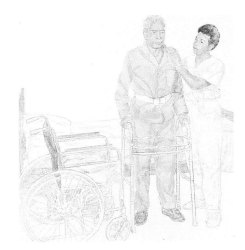

B

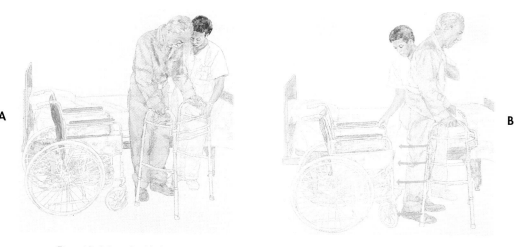

Fig. 13-30.   **A,** Help the resident to move toward the chair. **B,** Back up to the chair.

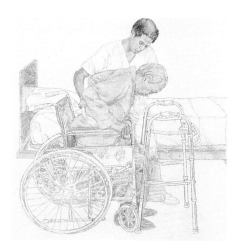

Fig. 13-31.   Once the resident is in the front of the chair, ask him to reach back and slowly sit down.

Transferring a Resident from a Chair to the Bed, Commode or the Toilet

Whether you are helping a resident to move from a chair back to bed or to the toilet or commode, you can use the stand pivot method or an assistive device transfer if he or she can help with the transfer. If a resident cannot help, use the mechanical lift or have a co-worker help with the transfer. Follow these steps:
1. Position the chair with the resident's stronger side closer to the bed.
2. If the resident is in a wheelchair, ask him or her to move his or her feet off the footrests. Raise up the foot pedals.
3. Ask the resident to slide forward to the edge of the chair. This is often difficult, and he or she may need help.
4. Use either the stand-and-pivot or assistive device transfer procedures in reverse to move a resident out of the chair and into bed.

Remember:
▷ Resident preference
▷ Common preparation steps
▷ Equipment and supplies needed
▷ Environment preparation
▷ Resident preparation

Remember:
▷ Meet resident needs
▷ Common completion steps
▷ Clean and put away equipment and supplies
▷ Environment completion (Is it safe? Is it clean?)

Two-Person Assistive Device Transfer

Decide first how the second person can best help you. You may want the second person on the other side of a resident holding onto the guard belt and walker. Or you may want the other just to hold the chair in place during the transfer and be there in case a resident gets dizzy or another problem occurs.

Mechanical Lift Transfer

If a resident cannot help with any of the transfers described above, he or she needs to be lifted from the bed to the chair and back. You can do this with two or more staff or a mechanical lift.

There are various types of mechanical lifts. Some require more work than others. Used properly, all lifts help keep residents safe during a transfer and decrease the stress on you when moving a dependent resident from one surface to another.

Most lifts consist of a base and frame on wheels that can be locked and unlocked, a sling in varying sizes that is placed under a resident, and four chains or straps on hooks that attach the sling to the lift. You control the lift with a crank, button, or lever pump control. At least two people are needed to transfer a resident with a mechanical lift. Follow these steps.

Moving a Resident with a Mechanical Lift

Remember:

▶ Resident preference
▶ Common preparation steps
▶ Equipment and supplies needed
▶ Environment preparation
▶ Resident preparation

1. Adjust the head of the bed as flat as possible if the resident can tolerate it. Place the sling under him or her by turning him or her toward you. Assist the resident to move toward you while the other staff member pushes the fanfolded sling under the resident as far as possible (Fig. 13-32). Then assist him or her back and toward the other side so that you can pull the sling under him or her.
2. The sling should be placed from under the resident's shoulders to the back of the knees, with an even amount of sling material on both sides.
3. Insert the metal bars into the sides of the sling evenly so that the holes in the bars are accessible. These bars provide a connection between the sling holding the resident and the chains of the lift.
4. Place the lift frame so that it faces the bed with its legs under the bed, and then lock the wheels on the base.
5. If necessary, elevate the head of the bed so the resident is partially sitting up.
6. Ask the resident to cross his or her arms over the chest before lifting him or her up in the lift. *Note:* If a resident cannot keep the hands in the lap or across the chest, try having him or her hold an object in the hands on the lap.
7. Attach the shorter chains to the top and the longer ones to the lower part of the sling. Attach the chains one by one from the frame to the sling holes, making sure that they are securely fastened (Fig. 13-33). Make sure that the metal hooks on the chains face away from the resident to prevent injury.
8. Follow the directions for the particular lift you are using to raise the resident up to a sitting position with the lift (Fig. 13-34). As you operate the lift, your helper should help you guide the resident.
    Note: Repeatedly ask if he or she is OK, and be sure to reassure the resident as this can be a frightening experience, especially the first time.
9. Once the resident is sitting, keep raising the lift until he or she is 6 to 12 inches over the bed and chair height.
10. Unlock the swivel, if the lift has one, or use the steering handle to move the resident directly over the chair. (You may need to guide his or her legs.) The base of the lift may widen to go around the chair on some models.
11. Tell the resident that you are now going to lower him or her slowly into the chair. Press the release button to slowly lower him or her down (Fig. 13-35).

12. Once the resident is securely in the chair, unhook the chains from the sling and remove the lift frame. Your helper will guide the resident into the chair by moving the sling.
13. Position the resident in the chair leaving the sling under him or her until it is time to return to bed. Be sure to pull the metal bars of the sling out so that he or she is not leaning against or sitting on these, because they could cause pressure sores on the skin.

Remember:
▸ Meet resident needs
▸ Common completion steps
▸ Clean and put away equipment and supplies
▸ Environment completion (Is it safe? Is it clean?)

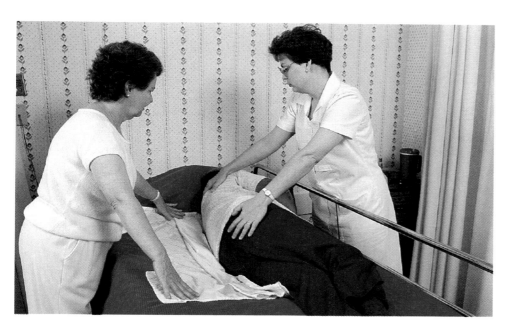

Fig. 13-32. The other staff member pushes the fanfolded sling under the resident while you steady the resident on his or her side.

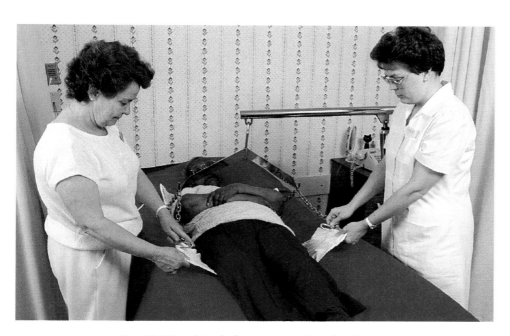

Fig. 13-33. Attach the straps to the sling holes.

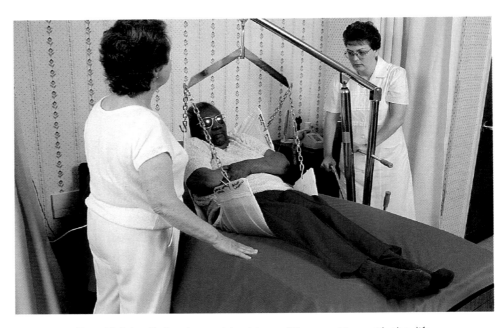

Fig. 13-34.   Raise the resident to a sitting position with the lift.

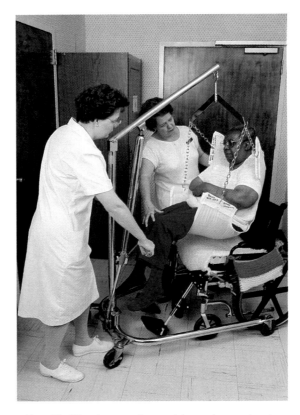

Fig. 13-35.   Lower the resident down slowly.

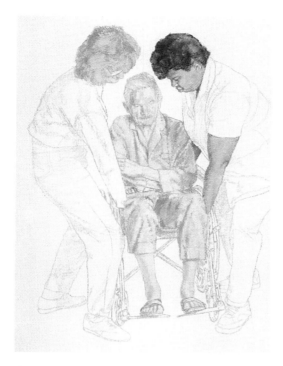

Fig. 13-36. Grasp the guard belt with one hand. Put your other hand under the resident's knees.

Moving a Resident Up in a Chair

Note: These steps are for moving a resident up in the chair following the transfer procedures to the chair. Two nurse assistants are needed for this procedure.

1. Place the guard belt on the resident.
2. Standing on both sides of the resident, each nurse assistant grasps the guard belt with one hand and under his or her knees with the other. Ask the resident to cross his or her arms in front of the chest (Fig. 13-36).
3. On the count of 3, breathe out and lift him or her back in the chair.

Remember:

▶ Resident preference
▶ Common preparation steps
▶ Equipment and supplies needed
▶ Environment preparation
▶ Resident preparation

Remember:

▶ Meet resident needs
▶ Common completion steps
▶ Clean and put away equipment and supplies
▶ Environment completion (Is it safe? Is it clean?)

Remember:

▶ Resident preference
▶ Common preparation steps
▶ Equipment and supplies
   needed
▶ Environment preparation
▶ Resident preparation

Remember:

▶ Meet resident needs
▶ Common completion steps
▶ Clean and put away
   equipment and supplies
▶ Environment completion
   (Is it safe? Is it clean?)

Returning a Resident to Bed Using a Mechanical Lift

The process for returning a resident to bed reverses the steps for transferring a resident from the bed:

1. Position the lift facing the chair.
2. Insert the metal bars into the sling sides.
3. Hook the chains into the sling holes as described earlier.
4. Crank (or raise) the resident up with the lift. Your helper will guide the resident by holding the sling.
5. Swing the frame of the lift over the bed and slowly lower the resident down onto the bed.
6. Unless the resident will spend only a short time in bed, roll him or her from side to side to remove the sling, because it could cause skin irritation if left under the resident.
7. Position the resident as preferred.

Positioning

When a resident cannot change positions, this becomes your responsibility. You must create a positioning schedule that assures proper blood flow to all body parts and comfort. This schedule is usually every 2 hours. Positions are described in the following sections. As you read these, think about a 24-hour period and how you would reposition a resident every 2 hours. You will find some positions are better for some residents, and some may even cause problems for a resident. For example, a resident who is short of breath may not tolerate being in a supine position (on back with head of the bed flat). Discuss all positions with the charge nurse to be sure they are allowed. As with any movements or positioning, consider body mechanics. Be sure also to remove any wrinkles from clothing before positioning a resident. Wrinkles can lead to pressure sores.

Positioning a Resident on His or Her Back

Items Needed
▶ Pillows
▶ Towel rolls

Lying on the back is the position often used for sleeping or resting in bed. Usually the arms and legs are out straight.

1. First move the trunk and lower body so that the resident's spine is straight (Fig. 13-37).
2. Begin to position the resident by working from the top of the body to the bottom.
3. Position the head and neck: Place a pillow under the resident's head and neck so the pillow extends to the top of the shoulders. Do not elevate the head too high. Keep it as close to even with the chest as possible or as is comfortable for him or her (Fig. 13-38).
4. Position his or her arms: The back of the shoulders and elbows are prone to pressure sores in residents who cannot change positions by themselves. Vary arm positions to prevent this. Keep the arms straight and resting on the mattress away from the resident's sides, or bend the arms slightly at the elbow and place a pillow between the inner part of the arm and the side so that the arm rests on the pillow on top of the abdomen. Always support the arms in two places when moving them, and move them gently (Fig. 13-39).
5. Position his or her legs: The sides of the hips, the buttocks, the sacrum and coccyx (tip of the spine at the buttocks, or "tailbone"), and the backs of the heels are all prone to pressure sores. Position his or her legs straight and slightly apart. Always support the legs in two places when moving them and move them gently (Fig. 13-40). You may wish to place a pillow between his or her legs for residents who tend to keep their legs tightly together or crossed.
   Note: If a resident has sores on the sides of the hips, place a towel roll along the hip between the hip and the mattress on the affected side. If a resident has redness or sores under the heels, support his or her legs with a pillow lengthwise to raise the heels off the bed or place a towel roll under his or her legs just above the heels (Fig. 13-41).
   Note: Support casts, splints, or swollen arms or legs by placing on a pillow lengthwise under the limb to support the hand or foot higher than the rest of his or her arm or leg.

Remember:
▶ Resident preference
▶ Common preparation steps
▶ Equipment and supplies needed
▶ Environment preparation
▶ Resident preparation

Remember:
▶ Meet resident needs
▶ Common completion steps
▶ Clean and put away equipment and supplies
▶ Environment completion (Is it safe? Is it clean?)

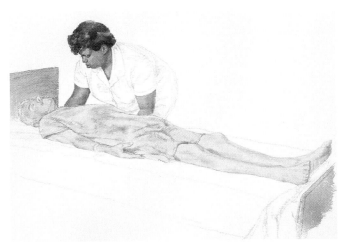

Fig. 13-37. Move the resident's trunk and lower body until the spine is straight.

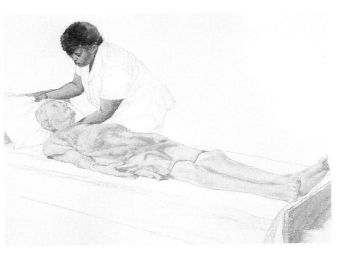

Fig. 13-38. Lift the resident's head and neck.

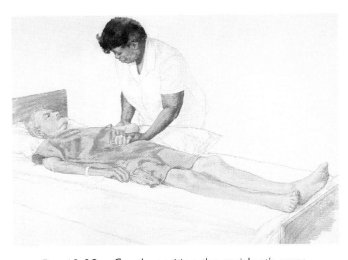

Fig. 13-39. Gently position the resident's arms.

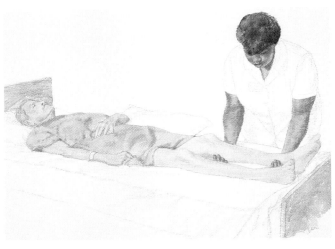

Fig. 13-40. When moving the resident, support the legs in two places.

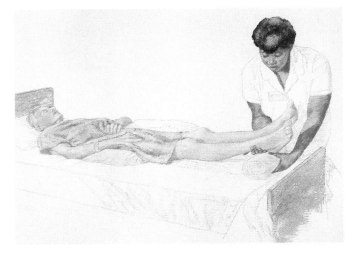

Fig. 13-41. Support the legs with a pillow or rolled towel to raise the heels.

Fowler's Position

Some residents have breathing problems caused by obesity, pulmonary disease, heart disease, or other causes. For these, the Fowler's position is often ordered by the physician or suggested by the charge nurse. The head, neck, and trunk are raised by elevating the head of the bed 45 degrees to the Fowler's position (Fig. 13-42) or up to 90 degrees (high Fowler's). When the resident is raised up only halfway (45 degrees), this is called the semi-Fowler position. This position is reached by elevating the head of the bed or placing pillows under the back, head, and neck. If possible, keep the head and neck only slightly higher than the resident's chest.

You can use this position also when you want to feed a resident or assist a resident with some personal care procedures.

Positioning a Resident on His or Her Side (Side-Lying Position)

1. Position yourself on the side on which the resident will be turning. Lower side rail (if used).
2. Help the resident to bend his or her knees up (Fig. 13-43).
3. Place one hand on the resident's shoulder furthest from you and the other hand on the hip furthest from you. On the count of 3, assist the resident to roll toward you, raise the side rail (if it is used), position him or her for comfort and proper body alignment (Fig. 13-44).
4. Position the head and neck: Place the pillow under the head so that the top ear is almost level with the top shoulder (Fig. 13-45).
5. Fold a pillow lengthwise and place it behind the resident's back, gently pushing the top edge of the pillow under his or her side and hip (Fig. 13-46).
6. Position his or her arms: Gently pull the bottom arm out from under the resident's body if it is not already in front of the body. Place a pillow diagonally under the top arm between the arm and the side. Bend the top arm at the elbow and shoulder to rest the arm on the pillow (Fig. 13-47).
7. Position his or her legs: Bend the top hip up and rotate it slightly forward. Place a pillow lengthwise between the resident's knees to separate his or her legs down to their ankles (Fig. 13-48).

Remember:

▷ Resident preference
▷ Common preparation steps
▷ Equipment and supplies needed
▷ Environment preparation
▷ Resident preparation

Remember:

▷ Meet resident needs
▷ Common completion steps
▷ Clean and put away equipment and supplies
▷ Environment completion (Is it safe? Is it clean?)

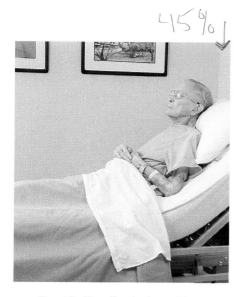

Fig. 13-42.   Fowler's position.

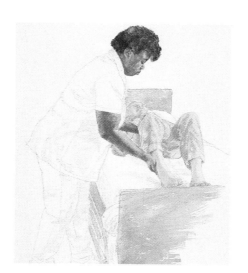

Fig. 13-43.   Assist the resident to bend his knees.

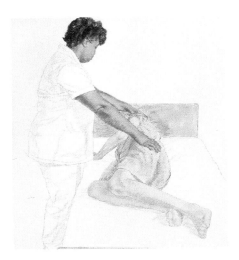

Fig. 13-44. Assist the resident to roll toward you.

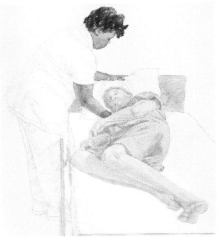

Fig. 13-45. Position the head and neck.

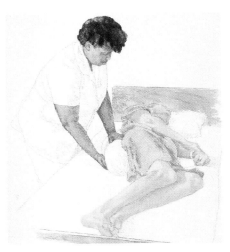

Fig. 13-46. Place a folded pillow behind the resident's back.

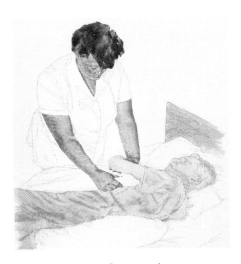

Fig. 13-47. Position the arms.

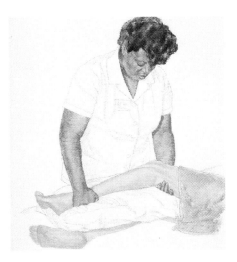

Fig. 13-48. Position the legs.

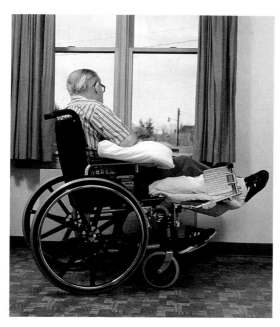

Fig. 13-49. In a wheelchair the leg rests should be positioned to the proper height as necessary.

Positioning a Resident in a Chair

Anytime you position a resident in a chair, follow these guidelines:

▶ Look at how a resident sits and then watch his or her sitting posture throughout the day. You can prevent skin problems and pressure sores by padding with sheets or pillows any areas a resident leans on, such as elbows, calf, heels, one side of body, back of thigh, or buttocks. If a resident in a wheelchair is prone to skin problems, such as with redness or pressure sores on the buttocks, ask the physical therapist to assess this resident for a wheelchair cushion if this is not already being used.

▶ A resident's legs and feet must always be supported. In a wheelchair, put the feet on the footrests and position the calf pads of the leg rests down behind the calves. The knees should be at the same height as the hips. Ask maintenance or the physical therapist to adjust the leg rests to the proper height if necessary (Fig. 13-49).

Note: If a resident is in a regular chair and his or her feet do not reach the floor, put a stool or pillow under the feet to support them, because dangling feet are uncomfortable and can cause swelling in his or her legs.

▶ Support the resident's arms and back with the chair's armrests and chair back.

▶ If a resident has a leg cast or a swollen leg, his or her leg needs to be elevated. To do this, elevate the leg rest of the wheelchair, recline the resident in a recliner chair, or prop his or her leg up on a stool or chair.

▶ If a resident has a swollen hand, place a pillow on the lap and armrest under the forearm and hand to support the hand higher than the elbow.

▶ If a resident has had a hip fracture and tends to bring the knees together or cross his or her legs, put one or two pillows between the knees. If this does not work, discuss the situation with the physical therapist, because this resident may need a special pillow to hold the knees apart.

▶ If a resident has a rounded back and is sitting in a recliner, support the head with pillows such that the ears are directly above the shoulders. Sitting with the head and neck extended is very uncomfortable and dangerous because the blood supply to a resident's brain can be obstructed.

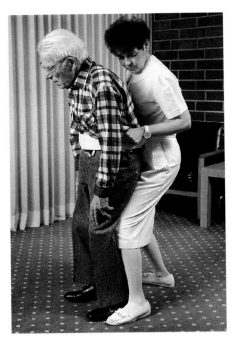

Fig. 13-50. To cushion a resident's fall, get behind the resident, hold onto the guard belt, and support the resident on your knee.

Stopping a Fall

If you are transferring or walking a resident and he or she starts to fall, what do you do? This can be a frightening experience for both of you. Be prepared for a possible fall, and use these steps to help a resident:

1. First try to pull up on the guard belt and ask the resident to try to stand back up.
2. If you cannot prevent a resident from continuing to fall, get behind him or her, hold onto the guard belt with both hands or gently hold him or her around the chest, and support him or her on your knee. Remember good body mechanics and call for help (Fig. 13-50).

If you cannot hold a resident up until help arrives and he or she is falling to the floor:

1. Gently lower the person to the floor as best you can and as slowly as possible to avoid injury to both of you.
2. Once the person is lowered to a safe stable position such as sitting or lying on the floor, call again for help. Do not leave a resident, because he or she is likely to be frightened and may feel helpless. Always ask if he or she is OK and reassure that help is on the way.
3. If you must leave a resident to get help, first ask if he or she is OK, and lie the resident down with his or her head supported. Explain you are going to get help and will be right back. Try to keep an eye on him or her as you seek help. In a busy area, be sure the person is not in anyone's path or ask someone else to get help so you can stay.

If a Resident Falls and Seems Injured

If a resident appears to be hurt or you are unsure if he or she is injured, DO NOT MOVE HIM OR HER. Leave him or her on the floor until a nurse or physician does an examination. Do not leave the person alone unless absolutely necessary, such as you feel he or she is in serious condition and no one is answering your call for help.

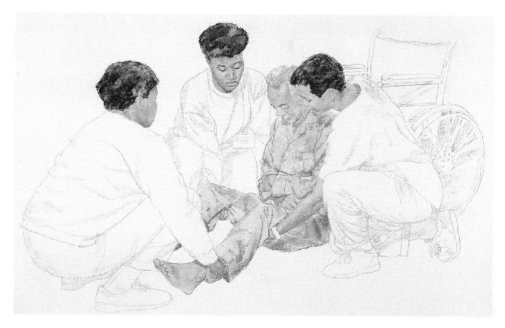

Fig. 13-51. Prepare for the lift.

Once help arrives and it is OK to move the resident, help him or her back to a sitting position on the floor. If the person can walk fairly well, help him or her stand with one staff member on each side, pulling up on both sides of the guard belt.

If a resident can be moved or you need to move him or her into a chair for further examination, you may need to lift him or her onto a stretcher or back into the chair. Follow these steps to lift a resident up from the floor:

1. Get at least two other staff to help.
2. If you do not feel that your back can take heavy lifting, get more staff or ask other staff to do the lift instead of you. (If so, you can still help by instructing them what to do if they have any questions, telling medical personnel about the circumstances of the fall, and holding the chair and comforting the resident.)
3. Prepare for the lift by first getting the resident to a sitting position on the floor with the knees bent up and feet flat on the floor. Ask him or her to fold his or her arms across the chest (Fig. 13-51).
4. When preparing to lift the resident, have each person kneel down by the resident's side and hold onto the guard belt with one hand and under his or her leg with the other hand. The third person holds under both of the legs while kneeling down in front of the resident facing him or her. You may need a fourth person to hold the chair or stretcher.
5. As team leader, you ask if everyone has a good grip and is ready. When everyone is ready, say "On the count of 3, lift. Ready? 1, 2, 3 and lift" (Fig. 13-52).
   Note: You may find that doing the lift in two steps may work well. For example: "1, 2, 3 and lift to stand," and then "1, 2, 3 and lift into the chair" or onto the stretcher (Fig. 13-53).
   Note: Anytime a resident falls, be sure to report the situation to the charge nurse.

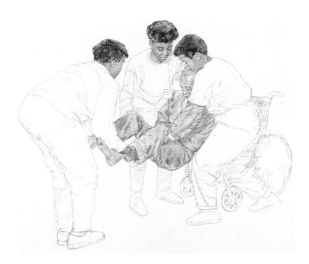

Fig. 13-52. Each person holds the guard belt with one hand and places the other under the resident's leg.

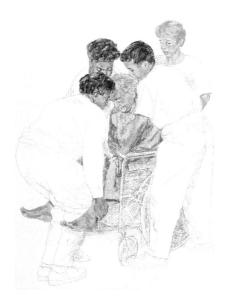

Fig. 13-53. A fourth person can assist by holding the wheelchair.

PERSONAL CARE

Think about the following statements:
▶ Most people care how they look.
▶ When you like the way you look outside, you feel good inside.
▶ Everyone has his or her own style and preferences.
▶ What you like may be very different from what others like.
▶ The way people style their hair is a very personal matter.
▶ Bathing daily is important to most people.
▶ Clean teeth and a nice smile are inviting to look at and they feel good.

Remember these ideas when you assist residents with personal care. This is care that involves cleanliness and appearance, including bathing, mouth care, and dressing. How much help you give a resident depends on his or her needs. You help residents create who they are on the outside, depending on how they view themselves on the inside.

In this chapter you will learn how the word "personal" relates to the care you give and how to make routine activities mindful. You will learn how to give personal care while respecting residents' autonomy and individuality.

WHAT IS PERSONAL CARE?

Think about the word "personal." What does personal mean to you? Some people think of "personal" as meaning private, something you do for yourself, something no one else sees or knows about, or something you wouldn't want anyone else to touch or invade. When you give personal care, keep in mind that residents think and feel as you do about personal things (Fig. 14-1). Remember that some residents have to let you help them with things they always did on their own, in private, with no help.

Every person has the right to be treated as an individual. If a resident wants to wear a red dress, help her put on that dress. If a resident wants to comb and style his or her hair a certain way, assist in doing so. Your responsibility is to provide individualized care to improve the quality of life for each resident you care for.

Making Routine Activities Mindful

Long term care facilities call daily care activities routine care. This means the care is given every day. Even so, the care you give should not become "routine" or unvarying. Instead, give routine care based on each resident's individual needs. Look back to the section on providing care in Chapter 4. As you read this chapter, think about mindfulness and discovering each resident's needs. Apply these principles in this chapter.

When you give care every day, think of what you can do for a resident to prevent it from seeming mundane or routine. For example, ask a resident what he or she would like to do first: "Would you like to read today for an hour before taking a shower?" or "Would you like to have a foot soak before or after physical therapy today?" Just by asking simple questions and encouraging residents to participate and make choices, you are more mindful in your everyday care. Plan your day according to each residents' preferences, not your own.

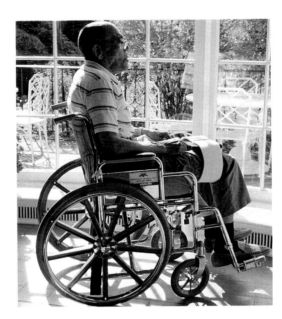

Fig. 14-1. Residents think and feel as you do about privacy and personal things.

Incorporating Personal Preferences into Daily Routines

Before you give personal care, you need to know each resident's likes and dislikes. Gather your information first to help meet each individual's needs. One resident may like to style her hair very differently from another. One resident may enjoy bright, dressy clothes while another may prefer casual clothes in pastels.

Think about how you yourself like to dress, bathe, brush your teeth, and style your hair. Now think about someone else—your best friend, your spouse, or a relative. Does this person do things exactly the same as you? The same hair style and the same clothing? Chances are the other person has different preferences, unique and individual. Residents too have different ideas about dressing, cleanliness, and grooming. Always incorporate a resident's personal preference into the personal care you give (Fig. 14-2).

Assessment and Observation while Providing Personal Care

As you learn to provide personal care, you are learning about oral hygiene, bathing, and grooming. However, your job involves much more than just this. You need to assess a resident's situation before each task and observe him or her while you're giving care. This means looking at the situation to see how best to do the task. For example, you need to know if a resident needs help with bathing or only needs you to help him or her out of the tub. If a resident does need help, you need to determine how much help and exactly what to do.

By doing an assessment you will be better prepared and organized. Residents too will find the experience more pleasant and will appreciate your attentiveness. Following are two other examples of assessment:

▶ You are assisting a resident with a tub bath, and he or she cannot stand without assistance. You assess this situation ahead of time and arrange for another nurse assistant to help you assist this resident into and out of the tub.

▶ You are giving a complete bed bath to a resident whose legs are paralyzed. You assess the situation and realize you need another nurse assistant to help you turn this resident for back care and perineal care.

Observation is the other major component of personal care. You observe residents' for physical and psychological changes during care. Think of your observa-

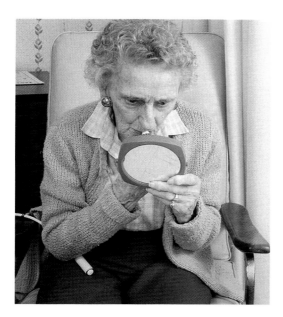

Fig. 14-2. Everyone has unique and individual preferences about how they want to look.

tion as a head to toe look at a resident, or you can do a quick check of each body system to see, hear, smell, or feel any changes (Fig. 14-3). You have the best opportunity to observe residents. Any changes you observe must be reported and recorded, such as these examples of changes:

▷ During a bed bath you notice a quarter-sized reddened area on a resident's left hip.
▷ You notice a resident is more quiet than usual.
▷ When helping a resident shave, you notice a rash on his neck.
▷ Shampooing a resident's hair, you see a dry flaky scalp.
▷ When assisting with brushing and flossing you notice a resident's gums are bleeding more than usual.

What you do with your observations is very important. Start by writing down your observations so you do not forget to report and record them. You must communicate any change in a resident to the charge nurse so correct treatment can be given. You must also report any resident complaints. Remember to be clear which information is subjective or objective. Never consider a change you observe as insignificant. All changes are important.

Assessments and observations are your responsibility when you give personal care. Residents depend on you to see changes so that they receive the best possible care.

BATHING

Bathing helps keep skin healthy and prevents skin problems. There are three main purposes of bathing:

▷ To remove dirt, perspiration, and microorganisms (germs, bacteria) that build-up on the surface of the skin
▷ To increase circulation to the skin
▷ To make the resident feel better and more comfortable

If a resident can leave the bed, use a bathtub or shower. Facilities have a schedule for residents needing assistance with bathing, based on residents' hygiene needs and comfort. Bathing too often may cause excessive skin dryness, which can cause skin breakdown. Give partial baths between complete baths as needed.

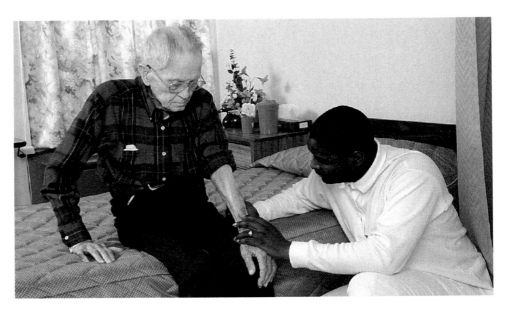

Fig. 14-3.   Observe residents for any changes during care.

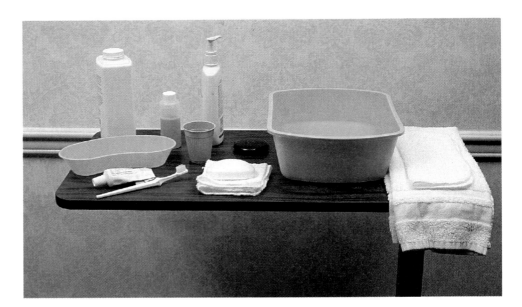

Fig. 14-4 .   Honor requests to use specific personal care products.

Remember, bathing is a very personal activity, and a resident may feel very uncomfortable being assisted. Help the person be more comfortable by providing privacy during bathing and encouraging him or her to make choices about how to bathe.

Using a Resident's Personal Products

A resident or family member may want to use certain bathing and personal hygiene products during personal care (Fig. 14-4). Honor their requests and become familiar with these products, such as bathing oils, special fragrance soaps, deodorants, powders, special lotions for dry skin, perfumes, and aftershave lotions. Most products come with directions for use. Check the directions and talk with the resident about how he or she likes to use them.

Personal Care Routines

The next sections describe many personal care skills. You will do these on some regular schedule that you and your residents determine. Some days you may do them all, and on other days only a few. These changes are based on residents' preferences and facility policies. You may also do some of the skills at different times of the day and in preparation for different activities. For example, some facility staff may call care provided to residents before breakfast "A.M. care." This may include assisting a resident with washing his or her face and hands, toileting, and oral hygiene. This care helps prepare for the day's activities. P.M. care helps prepare for bedtime. Assisting with washing a resident's face and hands, oral hygiene, back rubs, undressing, and toileting are common P.M. care skills. Keeping a resident's preferences in mind at all times will help you determine what skills to do, how to do them, and when.

Complete Bed Bath

Items Needed

- 2 Washcloths
- Towels
- Bedpan
- Basin half filled with water
- Soap
- Gloves

- Plastic trash bag
- Lotion
- Plastic covered pad or protective covering
- Bath blanket

Remember:
- Resident preference
- Common preparation steps
- Equipment and supplies needed
- Environment preparation
- Resident preparation

Some residents need bed baths because they cannot get in and out of bed. Below are the steps for a complete bed bath.

Note: Before beginning bath, remove the blanket and spread from the bed and place them on a clean surface. Place a bath blanket over the top sheet, then pull down the top sheet to the foot of the bed, leaving the bath blanket over the person. Expose only the part of the body you are cleansing. This gives the person privacy. Remove clothing the same way. The best position is flat in bed. Always wash, rinse, dry, and inspect each body part. Be sure to be gentle. Start by making a bath mitt.

Making a Bath Mitt

Make a bath mitt with the washcloth to cushion the washing. This provides a soft surface for the person's skin and is easier for you to work with than an unfolded washcloth.

1. After wringing out the wet washcloth, place your hand in the center of the washcloth.
2. Fold the side of the washcloth over from your little finger and secure the fold with your thumb (Fig. 14-5).
3. Fold the remaining cloth over and hold it firmly with the thumb (Fig. 14-6).
4. Fold the top edge of the cloth down and tuck it into your palm. Hold it with your thumb (Fig. 14-7).
5. The mitt is now ready to use. Rinse the cloth and refold the mitt as needed.

Giving a Complete Bed Bath

1. Begin with the eyes, using only water—no soap. With one corner of the washcloth, wash from the inner corner of the eye outward toward the ear. Start with the eye that is farthest from you. Use another corner of the washcloth to wash the near eye. Be sure to move the washcloth from the inner corner of the eye outward.
2. Wash the resident's face. Some residents prefer not to use soap on the face—if so, use water only. Rinse, dry, and inspect the area.

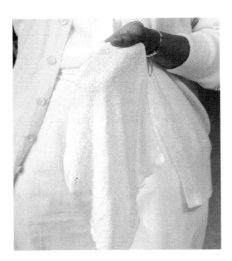

Fig. 14-5. Fold the side of the washcloth and secure with your thumb.

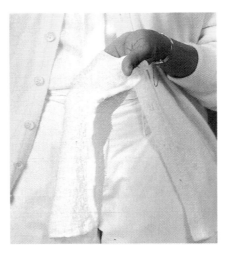

Fig. 14-6. Fold the remaining cloth over. Use your thumb to hold it in place.

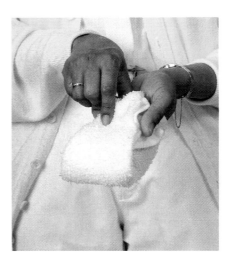

Fig. 14-7. Fold the top edge down. Tuck it into your palm and hold it with your thumb.

Note: To wash with soap, wet the face cloth and apply a small amount of soap to it.

3. Wash the resident's ears and neck. Rinse, dry, and inspect the area.

4. Wash the arms, underarm, and hands, and use soap sparingly. (Remember, soap is drying to the skin.) Wash the side away from you first, then the side near you, so that you are moving from a clean area to a dirty area, unless you feel you have to stretch too far and might injure yourself. Rinse, dry, and inspect the area. You may wash one side of the resident's body and then the other.

5. Wash the chest and abdomen. Rinse, dry, and inspect the area. Pay particular attention to the skin under the female residents' breasts, a common area for skin irritation and breakdowns. Note any redness, odor, or skin breakdown.

6. Wash the legs and feet. Don't forget between the toes. Rinse, dry, and inspect the area. Check between the toes for any redness, irritation, or cracking of the skin. Note any swelling of the feet and legs.
Note: Change the water at any time during the bath if the water gets too cold, soapy, or dirty. Be sure to pull side rails up (if used) before leaving the resident to change water, and lower them when you return.

7. Help the resident to turn to one side (see procedures for moving residents).

8. Wash the resident's back and buttocks. Rinse, dry, and inspect the area.

9. Give the resident a back rub. Rub a small amount of lotion into your palms. Starting at the resident's lower back, gently move your hands up toward the shoulders, then downward to the lower back and continue the back rub for at least 3 minutes (Fig. 14-8). Back rubs are comforting and relaxing and stimulate circulation, preventing skin breakdown.
Note: You may also give a back rub on request or as P.M. care.

10. Assist the resident to move back into the supine position.

11. Provide perineal care (wash the genital and anal area of the body), as described below.
Note: After the back rub and before perineal care, put a plastic-covered pad under the resident to absorb any extra water used to wash the perineal area, and

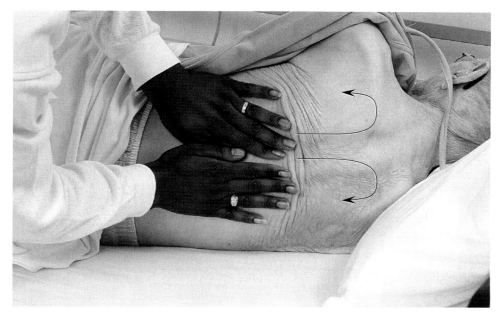

Fig. 14-8. During bathing, give the resident a back rub for at least 3 minutes.

put on gloves. You can also use a bedpan when providing perineal care. The bedpan allows a good view of the perineal area because it raises the pelvis and lets you use more water for washing and rinsing. Since this might be uncomfortable for a resident, ask first. Sometimes a fracture pan or a folded towel under the buttocks can also elevate the pelvis. Remember these guidelines:

▶ Always change the water before perineal care
▶ Always change the washcloth and towel
▶ Always wear gloves when giving perineal care

Note: Perineal care is part of giving a complete bed bath. If it is performed separately, you need to perform preparation and completion steps before and after the perineal care.

Perineal Care for Female Residents

1. Help the resident onto the bedpan or pad.
2. Put on gloves.
3. Drape the resident by folding back the bath blanket to expose only her legs and perineal area. Ask the resident to bend her knees.
4. Wash the pubic area first, moving from the pubic area to the anal area. Separate the labia and wash downward on each side of the labia using different corners of the washcloth. Wash downward in the middle over the urethra and vaginal openings. Always wash downward toward the anus to prevent infection (Fig. 14-9).
5. If you use a bedpan, help the resident off the bedpan onto her side. Wash the anal area, moving up toward the back.
6. Rinse, dry, and inspect the perineal area and then the anal area.

Perineal Care for Male Residents

1. Put on gloves.
2. Drape the resident to expose only his legs and perineal area, by folding back the bath blanket.
3. Wash the penis from the urethral opening at the tip of the penis down towards the bottom of the penis and then wash the scrotum. Take care to wash, rinse, and dry between any skin folds (Fig. 14-10). Pull back the foreskin on uncircumcised males and clean under it. Remember to return the foreskin.
4. Help the resident to turn onto his side. Wash, rinse, and dry the anal area well, moving upward toward the back.

Remember:

▶ Meet resident needs
▶ Common completion steps
▶ Clean and put away equipment and supplies
▶ Environment completion (Is it safe? Is it clean?)

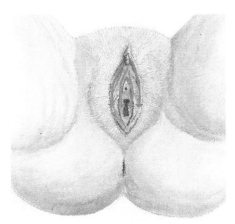

Fig. 14-9. Always wash downward.

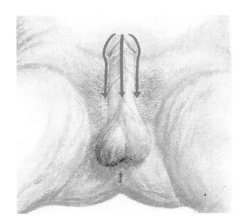

Fig. 14-10. Wash the penis from the urethral opening downward.

Tub Bath

Items Needed

- Gloves
- 2 Washcloths
- 3 Towels
- Clothes for resident to wear
- Soap, lotion, shampoo, etc.
- Bath mat

1. Assist the resident to the tub room with all supplies.
2. Help the resident sit on the chair. Fill the tub halfway with warm water (Fig. 14-11). Remember, always turn the hot water off first.
   Note: The tub water should be no more than 105° F. (40° C.). Use a thermometer if available, or test the water temperature with the inside of your wrist. The resident's doctor may order special medication to be added to the bath water, such as bran, oatmeal, starch, sodium bicarbonate, epsom salts, pine products, sulfa, potassium permanganate, or salt. Always check with the charge nurse about the proper use of any of these substances.
3. Help the resident to remove his or her clothing.
4. Check that the bath mat is in place. Help the resident into the tub.
5. Assist with bathing as needed. (Put gloves on if you will be assisting with perineal care.)
   Note: Never leave the resident alone while bathing in a tub. Always encourage residents to use safety rails.
6. Place a clean towel on the seat of the chair and a clean towel on the floor in front of the tub.
7. Help the resident out of the tub. Encourage him or her to use safety rails. Cover him or her with a bath blanket.
8. Assist the resident with drying, applying personal hygiene products, and dressing.
   Note: You may give him or her a back rub now if desired.
9. Help the resident back to his or her room. Bring any of his or her personal hygiene products.

Remember:
- Resident preference
- Common preparation steps
- Equipment and supplies needed
- Environment preparation
- Resident preparation

Remember:
- Meet resident needs
- Common completion steps
- Clean and put away equipment and supplies
- Environment completion (Is it safe? Is it clean?)

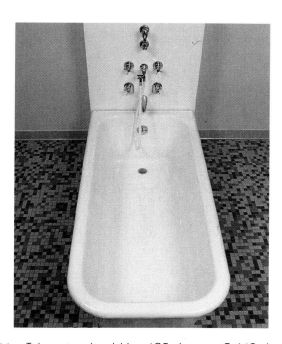

Fig. 14-11. Tub water should be 105 degrees F. (40 degrees C.)

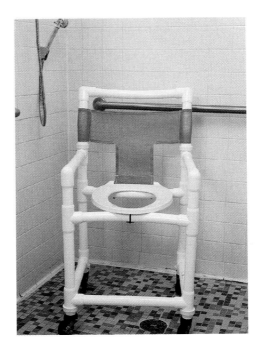

Fig. 14-12. Before use, check that the shower chair is locked in place.

Shower

Remember:

▶ Resident preference
▶ Common preparation steps
▶ Equipment and supplies
  needed
▶ Environment preparation
▶ Resident preparation

Items Needed

▶ Gloves
▶ 2 Washcloths
▶ 3 Towels (4 if shampooing)
▶ Clothes for resident to wear
▶ Soap, lotion, shampoo etc.

▶ Shower cap if needed
▶ Shower chair
▶ Shower mat
▶ Bath blanket

1. Help the resident to the shower room with all necessary supplies.
2. Help the resident sit on the chair.
3. Turn on the shower with warm water. Test the water on the inside of your wrist. Adjust the temperature as necessary.
4. Help the resident remove clothing.
5. Help the resident into the shower. Encourage him or her to use safety rails.
   Note: Most facilities have shower chairs that lock in place. If the resident needs to shower sitting down, be sure the shower chair is locked before he or she sits down (Fig. 14-12).
6. Help the resident with showering as necessary. (Remember to wear gloves if you will be assisting with perineal care.)
   Note: If resident is not shampooing, use a shower cap to prevent the hair from getting wet.
7. Place a dry towel on the chair.
8. Assist the resident out of the shower and onto the covered chair. Cover him or her with a bath blanket.
9. Turn off the shower. Turn the hot water off first, then the cold to prevent a burn.
10. Help the resident with drying, applying personal hygiene products, and dressing.
    Note: You may give a back rub at this point if desired.
11. Assist the resident back to the room. Bring his or her personal hygiene products.

dress ctin his or her room

Remember:

▶ Meet resident needs
▶ Common completion steps
▶ Clean and put away
  equipment and supplies
▶ Environment completion
  (Is it safe? Is it clean?)

A whirlpool bath is a special therapeutic bath a resident's doctor may order for a specific treatment. The person may have a wound that needs daily cleaning or poor circulation that needs stimulation. Whirlpool baths move the water to achieve these goals. Some whirlpools have a mechanical lift to move residents into the tub. Follow the facility's guidelines for using the whirlpool there, including cleaning guidelines and infection control measures before and after using the whirlpool (Fig. 14-13). You will learn these guidelines on the job.

Whirlpool Bath

Items Needed

▶ Gloves
▶ 3 Towels
▶ 2 Washcloths

▶ Personall hygiene products
▶ Clothes for resident to wear
▶ Bath blanket

1. Help the resident to the whirlpool room with all supplies.
2. Help the resident to sit on a chair.
3. Turn on the water in the whirlpool according to your facility's procedure. The water temperature should be 105° F. (40° C.). Test the water temperature on the inside of your wrist.
4. Help the resident remove clothing.

Remember:

▶ Resident preference
▶ Common preparation steps
▶ Equipment and supplies needed
▶ Environment preparation
▶ Resident preparation

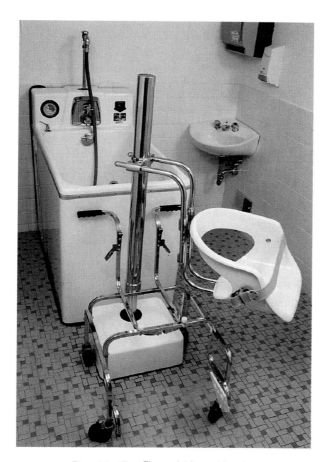

Fig. 14-13.   The whirlpool bath.

5. Help the resident into the whirlpool bath. Encourage use of safety rails.
   Note: Remember to follow the manufacturer's and facility's guidelines. If a mechanical lift is used, be sure you know how to use it properly.

6. Assist the resident with bathing. (Remember to wear gloves if you will be assisting with perineal care.)
   Note: If the resident has a dressing over a wound, ask the nurse to remove it before the bath and replace it with a clean one afterward. If the doctor has ordered an antiseptic solution in the whirlpool bath, the nurse will add the solution or give you specific instructions.

7. Place a dry towel on the chair.

8. Help the resident out of the whirlpool bath and onto the covered chair. Encourage use of safety rails. Cover him or her with a bath blanket.

9. Help the resident with drying, applying personal hygiene products and dressing.
   Note: You may give him or her a back rub at this point if desired.

10. Help the resident back to his or her room.

Remember:

▶ Meet resident needs
▶ Common completion steps
▶ Clean and put away equipment and supplies
▶ Environment completion (Is it safe? Is it clean?)

Partial Bath

A partial bath is used to cleanse certain body parts only. On days a resident is not having a complete bed bath, tub bath, shower, or whirlpool bath, you often provide a partial bath. When giving a partial bath, you help a resident wash his or her face, hands, and underarms, then provide perineal care.

Shampooing and Conditioning

Shampooing can be done in the shower, tub, or sink. Shampooing once a week is usually enough to keep a resident's hair and scalp clean, although some prefer to shampoo more often.

Many facilities have a beauty parlor and hairdresser who shampoos and styles hair. Some may also have a barber shop or bring in an outside barber to give haircuts to men. But often you are the one who shampoos a resident's hair, especially those who are unable to go to the beauty or barber shop.

Shampooing and Conditioning

Remember:

▶ Resident preference
▶ Common preparation steps
▶ Equipment and supplies needed
▶ Environment preparation
▶ Resident preparation

Items Needed

▶ Comb or brush
▶ 1 or 2 Towels
▶ Shampoo
▶ Conditioner (if used)
▶ Face cloth

1. Help the resident into a chair.
2. Comb or brush out any tangles before shampooing.
3. Turn on the water to a warm temperature: no more than 105° F. (40° C.). Test the water temperature on the inside of your wrist.
4. Help the resident remove clothes for showering or tub bathing. Wash the resident's hair as a resident prefers (some residents want it done first, and some last). If a resident is shampooing at the sink, put the back of the chair against

the front of the sink. Protect his or her clothes with a towel draped over the shoulders.

5. Wet the hair entirely. Put a face cloth over the eyes to prevent shampoo from getting into the resident's eyes.

6. Pour a small amount of shampoo in your palm and apply it to the resident's wet hair. Massage the shampoo gently throughout hair and scalp.

7. Rinse the hair well with warm water.

8. Apply conditioner, if used.

9. Rinse the hair well with warm water.

10. Help the resident out of the shower or tub into the chair. Cover him or her with a bath blanket. Wrap a towel around his or her hair. Dry the resident and assist with dressing.

11. Dry the hair thoroughly and quickly to prevent chilling. Use a hair dryer if available.

12. Style the resident's hair as he or she likes it. Look for any flaking, reddened areas, or other problems on the scalp.

   Note: Some residents may need to use special shampoos or conditioners, often with medicine ordered by the doctor for a specific condition. Ask the nurse for instructions and read the labels carefully before using them.

13. Help the resident back to his or her room.

Remember:
▶ Meet resident needs
▶ Common preparation steps
▶ Clean and put away equipment and supplies
▶ Environment completion (Is it safe? Is it clean?)

ORAL HYGIENE

Mouth care is important for preventing gum disease and tooth loss. Mouth care improves a resident's sense of well-being, appearance, appetite, and ability to chew food properly.

Brushing and Flossing

Help a resident brush at least twice a day and floss his or her teeth at least once a day. Always encourage a resident to do his or her own mouth care if possible. While brushing and flossing, inspect the gums for any paleness, discoloration, bleeding sores, or irritation. Inspect the teeth for decay or looseness. Flossing stimulates the gums and removes particles of food from between the teeth that brushing alone cannot remove.

Brushing and Flossing

Items Needed

▶ Towel
▶ Soft bristled toothbrush
▶ Toothpaste
▶ Paper cup half filled with cool water
▶ Mouthwash, if desired

▶ Dental floss
▶ Emesis basin
▶ Towel
▶ Gloves
▶ Plastic trash bags

Remember:
▶ Resident preference
▶ Common preparation steps
▶ Equipment and supplies needed
▶ Environment preparation
▶ Resident preparation

Note: You can assist with brushing and flossing at the bedside table or the resident's sink, as he or she prefers.

1. Apply a small amount of toothpaste to the wet toothbrush and set it aside. Mix water and mouthwash in a cup. (A solution of half water, half mouthwash is best. Set this aside. Mouthwash is strong and could be harmful to sensitive gums.)

2. Break off at least 18 inches of floss. Set this aside.
3. Put on gloves.
   Note: If it is known that the resident's gums bleed, discuss with the charge nurse other personal protective equipment that may be needed.
4. Put a towel over the resident's chest to protect clothing.
5. Give the resident a small amount of mouthwash solution to swish around in his or her mouth to rinse it. Place the emesis basin under the resident's chin so he or she can spit the solution out.
6. Brush the resident's upper teeth and gums first, moving the brush from the gums to the teeth downward, then the lower teeth and gums moving again from the gums to the teeth upward. Be sure to brush the back of the teeth. Inspect the teeth and gums while brushing.
7. Brush the tongue gently.
8. Rinse the resident's mouth with a little mouthwash solution.
9. Wrap the ends of the floss around your middle fingers on each hand to get a good grip. Gently insert the floss between each tooth and the next. Move the floss to the gum line and down. Advance the floss around your fingertips to a clean section as you move in between teeth (Fig. 14-14).
10. Have the resident rinse his or her mouth thoroughly.
11. Dry any solution around the resident's mouth or chin.

Remember:

▶ Meet resident needs
▶ Common completion steps
▶ Clean and put away equipment and supplies
▶ Environment completion (Is it safe? Is it clean?)

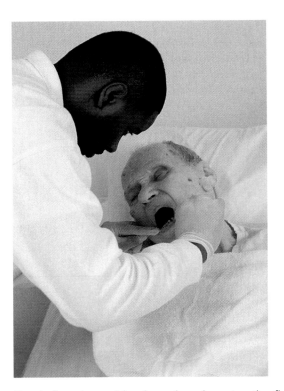

Fig. 14-14. Gently floss the resident's teeth, advancing the floss as necessary.

Dentures

Dentures (false teeth) are worn by people who have lost some or all of their natural teeth. A resident may have full dentures (both upper and lower replacements) or partial plates that replace some teeth. Partial plates are usually held in place by an attachment to remaining teeth. Dentures and plates are expensive and must be handled carefully to prevent breakage. Encourage residents to wear their dentures as often as possible to avoid gum shrinkage, to improve speech, to help chew food, and to improve their appearance. Dentures should be cleaned at least twice daily. When dentures are removed for a time, always store them in a denture cup in cool water or a commercial denture cleansing solution if a resident prefers.

Caring for Dentures

Items Needed

- Denture cup (paper cup half filled with cool water)
- Lemon glycerin swabs
- Plastic bag for disposable items
- 1 or 2 pairs of gloves
- Towel

- Denture adhesive (if used)
- Tissue or paper towel
- Toothbrush
- Toothpaste
- Emesis basin
- Mouthwash

Remember:

- Resident preference
- Common preparation steps
- Equipment and supplies needed
- Environment preparation
- Resident preparation

1. Put on gloves (optional).
2. Ask the resident to remove his or her dentures and place them in the denture cup. If the resident cannot remove his or her own dentures, follow these steps:
   a. Place a towel over the resident's chest.
   b. Rinse the resident's mouth with mouthwash solution to moisten it. Ask him or her to swish the solution around, and place the emesis basin under the chin so the resident can spit out the solution.
   c. Remove the upper denture using a tissue or paper towel for a better grip. Loosen the denture by gently rocking it back and forth. Put it in the denture cup.
   d. Remove lower denture using a tissue or paper towel for better grip. Loosen it by gently rocking it back and forth. Place it in the denture cup.
3. Rinse the resident's mouth with mouthwash solution.
4. If the resident cannot rinse, use a lemon glycerin swab to clean inside the whole mouth, including the tongue and gums.
5. Explain you will clean the dentures and then return them.
6. Take the denture cup with dentures, toothbrush, and toothpaste to the resident's bathroom.
7. Apply toothpaste to the toothbrush.
8. Turn on cool water (hot water can damage dentures), place a small towel or face cloth on the bottom of the sink, and fill the sink half way (to prevent dentures from breaking if they slip from your hands).
9. Clean the dentures by brushing all surfaces while holding dentures over the sink (Fig. 14-15).
10. Rinse the dentures with cool water.
11. Return the dentures to the denture cup.
12. If the resident uses denture adhesive, apply it to dentures before putting them back in his or her mouth. If the resident does not want the dentures put back at this time, store them safely. Place them in a denture cup labeled with the resident's name and half filled with cool water.

Remember:

- Meet resident needs
- Common completion steps
- Clean and put away equipment and supplies
- Environment completion (Is it safe? Is it clean?)

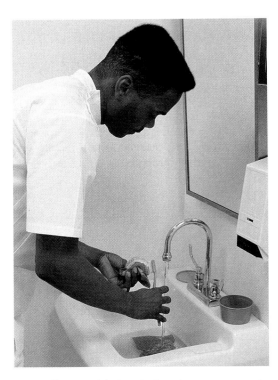

Fig. 14-15. Thoroughly brush the dentures over the sink.

Mouthcare for Comatose Residents

You may care for residents who are comatose. These residents are not aware of their surroundings and cannot respond. Comatose residents need mouth care every 2 hours, as they often breathe through the mouth, and the mouth and lips become dry.

Remember:

▶ Resident preference
▶ Common preparation steps
▶ Equipment and supplies needed
▶ Environment preparation
▶ Resident preparation

Mouth Care for Comatose Residents

Items Needed

▶ Towels
▶ Gloves
▶ 1 or 2 packages of lemon glycerin swabs
▶ Protective jelly or lip balm
▶ Plastic trash bag

1. Gently turn the resident's head toward you and elevate the head of the bed (if he or she can tolerate it) to prevent aspiration (inhaling fluid or food into the lungs).
2. Put a towel over the resident's chest to protect clothing.
3. Put on gloves.
4. Gently open the resident's mouth and, using a toothette dipped in mouthwash or a lemon glycerine swab, clean the inside of the mouth (gums, tongue, teeth, roof of the mouth, and insides of the cheeks) (Fig. 14-16).
   Note: Be sure to rid a toothette of excess mouthwash. Excess fluid can drip back and potentially cause aspiration.
5. Using a corner of the towel draped over the resident's chest, dry any solution from around the mouth and chin.
6. Dispose of swabs as you use them into the plastic trash bag.
7. Apply protective jelly to moisten the lips.

Remember:

▶ Meet resident needs
▶ Common completion steps
▶ Clean and put away equipment and supplies
▶ Environment completion (Is it safe? Is it clean?)

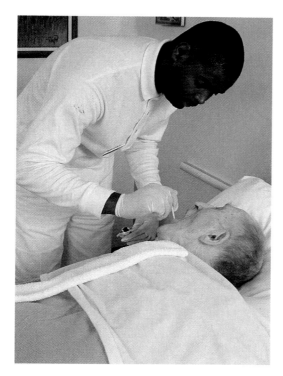

Fig. 14-16. Gently swab the inside of the resident's mouth clean.

GROOMING

Grooming care includes shaving, which may include face, legs, and underarms, trimming facial hair, hair care, and care of fingernails and toenails.

Shaving

Shaving is often a daily activity for male residents. Some female residents may want their legs and underarms shaved during a shower or bath. Male residents can use either an electric razor or a safety razor. Never share razors among different residents or recap disposable razors. Discard disposable razors in a sharp's container. Always check with the charge nurse before shaving a resident to learn of any special considerations for a resident. For example, some residents must use electric razors because their medication could cause excessive bleeding if they were accidently cut with a safety razor.

Shaving a Male Resident's Face

Items Needed

▶ Razor
▶ Shaving cream
▶ Aftershave (if used)
▶ Basin, half filled with warm water
▶ Towel

▶ Wash cloth
▶ Mirror
▶ Plastic bag
▶ Gloves

Remember:

▶ Resident preference
▶ Common preparation steps
▶ Equipment and supplies needed
▶ Environment preparation
▶ Resident preparation

1. Observe face for any moles, rashes, or cuts. Avoid shaving those areas or use extra care.
2. Place a towel over the resident's chest to protect clothing.
3. Put on gloves.
4. Using a face cloth, wet the entire beard with warm water and apply shaving cream with your hands.

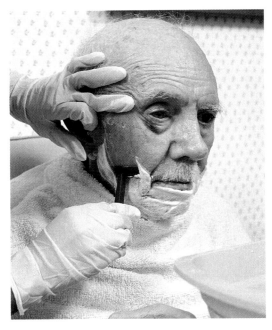

Fig. 14-17. Shave in the direction the beard grows.

5. When the beard is well lathered and softened, start shaving. Shave in the direction the beard grows. Hold the skin tight and smooth by pulling the skin upward with one hand and shaving with a downward stroke with your other hand. Use short, even strokes. Be particularly careful with the neck, chin, and upper lip area. Use upward strokes for the neck; downward and slightly diagonal strokes for the chin; and very short, downward strokes above the lip (Fig. 14-17).
6. Rinse the razor in warm water after each stroke.
7. Wash and rinse the resident's face with the washcloth, dry the face, and apply aftershave lotion if he prefers.
8. Supply a mirror for the resident to inspect his face.
9. Remove the towel from resident's chest.

Remember:
▶ Meet resident needs
▶ Common completion steps
▶ Clean and put away equipment and supplies
▶ Environment completion (Is it safe? Is it clean?)

Shaving the Resident's Underarms

Remember:
▶ Resident preference
▶ Common preparation steps
▶ Equipment and supplies needed
▶ Environment preparation
▶ Resident preparation

To shave a resident's underarm, follow these steps:
1. Raise her arm up along the ear to expose the underarm.
2. Wash the area with warm water.
3. Lather some soap and apply it over the area to be shaved.
4. Carefully shave the area, moving the razor downward from the arm toward the chest.
5. Be sure to rinse the soap thoroughly and pat the area dry.

Remember:
▶ Meet resident needs
▶ Common completion steps
▶ Clean and put away equipment and supplies
▶ Environment completion (Is it safe? Is it clean?)

Shaving the Resident's Legs

To shave a resident's legs, follow these steps:
1. Wash the part of the leg to be shaved with warm water.
2. Lather some soap or use shaving cream and spread it over the entire area to be shaved.
3. Carefully shave the area, moving the razor upward from the ankle to the knee. *Note:* Be sure to ask the resident if she wants the area above her knee shaved.
4. Be sure to rinse the soap thoroughly and pat the area dry.

Remember:
▶ Resident preference
▶ Common preparation steps
▶ Equipment and supplies needed
▶ Environment preparation
▶ Resident preparation

Remember:
▶ Meet resident needs
▶ Common completion steps
▶ Clean and put away equipment and supplies
▶ Environment completion (Is it safe? Is it clean?)

Trimming Facial Hair

Some female residents have facial hair. This is common on the chin, on the upper lip, and under the lower lip. Never shave this facial hair unless she requests it. Always check with the charge nurse before trimming facial hair.

Trimming Facial Hair

Items Needed
▶ Safety scissors
▶ Mirror

1. Using safety scissors, carefully trim the facial hair. Be careful not to trim too close to the skin (Fig. 14-18).
2. Supply a mirror for the resident's inspection.

Remember:
▶ Resident preference
▶ Common preparation steps
▶ Equipment and supplies needed
▶ Environment preparation
▶ Resident preparation

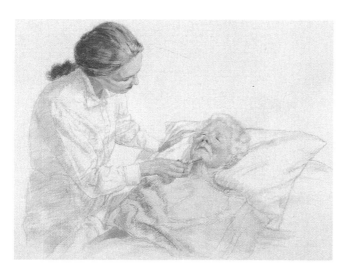

Fig. 14-18. Carefully trim the facial hair.

Remember:
▶ Meet resident needs
▶ Common completion steps
▶ Clean and put away equipment and supplies
▶ Environment completion (Is it safe? Is it clean?)

Hair Care

Hair care includes regular shampooing and daily brushing, combing, and styling. Daily brushing or combing along with good nutrition and adequate fluid intake promotes healthy hair and scalp. Hair style is a personal matter. Always ask a resident his or her preference for hair style. Encourage residents to brush and comb their own hair. If a resident cannot brush or comb his or her hair, follow this procedure.

Remember:

▶ Resident preference
▶ Common preparation steps
▶ Equipment and supplies needed
▶ Environment preparation
▶ Resident preparation

Remember:

▶ Meet resident needs
▶ Common completion steps
▶ Clean and put away equipment and supplies
▶ Environment completion (Is it safe? Is it clean?)

Hair Care

Items Needed

▶ Resident's own brush or comb
▶ Mirror
▶ Personal items for styling

1. Brush hair gently. If the resident's hair is long and has tangles, remove the tangles first with a comb, starting at the ends and working your way up to the scalp.
2. Gently brush and style the hair according to the resident's preference (Fig. 14-19). *Note:* Use any personal items that he or she may request, such as hair spray, clips, or gel.
3. Supply a mirror for the resident's inspection.

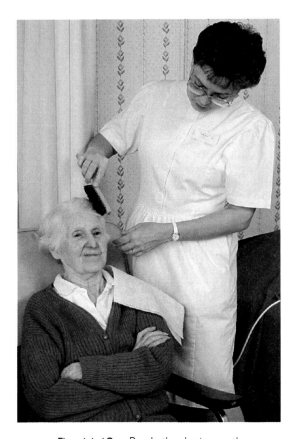

Fig. 14-19. Brush the hair gently.

Care of fingernails

Fingernail care includes daily cleaning and regularly trimming the nails. Although the visible part of the nail is not living tissue, the skin around and under it is, and this needs to be protected from injury and infection. Trimmed and smooth nails also prevent a resident from accidentally scratching and injuring other skin. If a resident cannot clean and trim his or her own fingernails, follow this procedure. You can do this as part of a resident's complete bed bath or tub bath.

Care of Fingernails

Items Needed

- Bath basin, half filled with warm water
- Towel
- Wash cloth
- Soap
- Lotion
- Orangewood stick
- Nail clippers
- Nail file (or emery board)

1. Place the basin with warm water on the overbed table.
2. Ask the resident to soak hands in basin 3-5 minutes.
3. Wash and rinse the resident's hands. Remove and dry the hands, and place them on a dry towel.
4. Clean under the nails with the orangewood stick (Fig. 14-20).
5. Inspect the hands.
6. Trim the fingernails using the nail clipper. Clip nails straight across. Shape and remove any rough edges using an emery board or nail file.
7. Apply lotion to the hands and gently massage the hands from fingertips toward the wrists to stimulate circulation.

Remember:

- Resident preference
- Common preparation steps
- Equipment and supplies needed
- Environment preparation
- Resident preparation

Remember:

- Meet resident needs
- Common completion steps
- Clean and put away equipment and supplies
- Environment completion (Is it safe? Is it clean?)

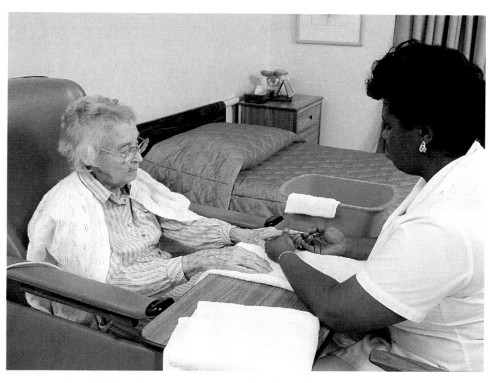

Fig. 14-20.   Use an orangewood stick to clean under the nails.

Care of Toenails

Toenails tend to be thicker than fingernails, particularly as one ages. Foot care is very important because older residents have a greater risk of infection if skin breakdown occurs, because circulation to the feet is often decreased. Skin care includes cleaning and trimming toenails. A podiatrist, nurse, or physician usually trims toenails. Follow your facility's policy. Inspect the feet and between the toes for the condition of the skin and the presence of any corns, callouses, or other problems. Report any signs of poor circulation, reddened areas, skin breakdown, or cracking of the skin between the toes.

Care of Toenails

Remember:

▶ Resident preference
▶ Common preparation steps
▶ Equipment and supplies needed
▶ Environment preparation
▶ Resident preparation

Remember:

▶ Meet resident needs
▶ Common completion steps
▶ Clean and put away equipment and supplies
▶ Environment completion (Is it safe? Is it clean?)

Items Needed

▶ Bath basin, half filled with warm water
▶ 2 towels
▶ Soap
▶ Wash cloth
▶ Orangewood stick
▶ Lotion
▶ Shoes and socks

1. Place a towel on the floor and the basin on the towel, for foot care for a resident sitting in a chair.
   Note: Foot care can be done while a resident is in bed or the bath, usually during a bed bath. Place a towel on the bed and the basin on the towel. Ask him or her to flex the leg and soak one foot at a time (Fig. 14-21).
2. Help the resident to remove socks and shoes.
3. Place the resident's feet in the basin of warm water.
4. Soak the feet for 3-5 minutes.
5. Wash, rinse, dry, and inspect the feet thoroughly.
6. Clean under the toenails with the orangewood stick to remove any dirt.
7. Help the resident put on clean stockings and shoes.
8. Report the need for toenail trimming to the charge nurse.

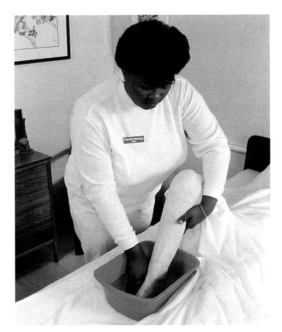

Fig. 14-21. Footcare can be performed when the resident is in bed.

ASSISTING THE RESIDENT WITH DRESSING AND UNDRESSING

Some residents can dress and undress independently, while others need assistance. This depends on the individual:

▶ A blind resident needs help choosing color-coordinated clothes and removing clothes from the closet.

▶ A resident with limited mobility of the shoulders needs help zipping up her dress.

▶ A resident who gets dizzy when bending over needs help putting on and taking off shoes and stockings.

▶ A confused resident may need help putting on clothes properly.

Always encourage a resident to choose the clothes he or she wants to wear.

Dressing a Dependent Resident

Items Needed

▶ Clothes, undergarments

▶ Plastic-covered pad (if resident is in bed)

▶ Stockings, socks, shoes

▶ Accessories resident wants to wear (belt, tie, jewelry)

Remember:

▶ Resident preference
▶ Common preparation steps
▶ Equipment and supplies needed
▶ Environment preparation
▶ Resident preparation

Note: If a resident has a weak or paralyzed arm, or has an IV in one arm, help him or her to put a shirt or dress on that arm first. With an IV you must place the solution through the sleeve first. Then hang the solution on the pole. Gently guide the arm through the sleeve, being careful not to dislodge the IV. Use the same method with a weak leg, dressing the weak side first.

1. Remove gown or pajamas.
   Note: For privacy and to prevent chill, remove the top portion of gown or pajamas first, dress the resident with clean clothes, and then move to bottoms.
2. Help the resident to put on a shirt, blouse, or dress.
3. Assist the resident with putting on underwear, stockings or socks, and pants or a skirt.
4. Always help the resident put on shoes before standing, to avoid slipping on the floor. Put a pad on the bed to protect bedding when you put shoes on in bed.
5. Help the resident stand so you can smooth out clothing and fasten and tuck clothing neatly.
6. Help him or her put on any accessories he or she wants to wear.
   Note: Residents are typically assisted out of bed after dressing for the day.

Remember:

▶ Meet resident needs
▶ Common completion steps
▶ Clean and put away equipment and supplies
▶ Environment completion (Is it safe? Is it clean?)

Undressing a Dependent Resident

Items Needed

▶ Clothes to be worn after undressing

Note: This procedure is easier if the resident is sitting at the side of the bed.

Note: If a resident has a weak or paralyzed arm or an IV, remove clothing from the other side first and then from the weak side. For residents with an IV in place, carefully guide the tubing and solution through the sleeve as the resident's arm is being moved.

1. Help the resident to remove upper garments (shirt, dress, blouse, then undergarments).
2. Help the resident put on top half of pajamas or nightgown.
3. Help resident remove shoes, stockings, pants, or skirt.
4. Help the resident put on lower night clothing if wearing pajamas.
5. Assist resident into bed.

Remember:

▶ Resident preference
▶ Common preparation steps
▶ Equipment and supplies needed
▶ Environment preparation
▶ Resident preparation

Remember:

▶ Meet resident needs
▶ Common completion steps
▶ Clean and put away equipment and supplies
▶ Environment completion (Is it safe? Is it clean?)

PREPARING FOR AN EVENT

Just as you like to look nice when receiving visitors or going out, residents too like to look good. You can help a resident feel good about a coming event by helping him or her get ready. If visitors are coming, help with grooming in advance. Remove any clutter and bring in extra chairs if needed.

If a resident is leaving the facility on an outing, communicate with the family in advance. A family member may want to help prepare a resident that day. If not, find out what time the resident needs to be ready. Find out what the outing is. Does he or she need to wear special clothes? With rainy or cold weather, be sure he or she has the right outer wear and accessories, hats, gloves, and boots, and so on (Fig. 14-22).

Preparing for a big event may be confusing for a resident. Remind him or her what is going to happen, especially those residents with memory loss. This prevents a resident from being surprised and gives something to look forward to. If a resident will be away overnight, prepare an overnight bag of essential items. Make a checklist to be sure you forget nothing.

The extra attention you spend with a resident preparing for a visit or an outing helps both the resident and family feel good. They will appreciate your effort.

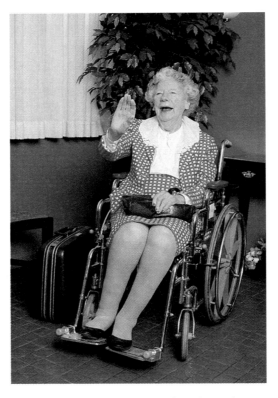

Fig. 14-22. Make sure that the resident has the right outer wear and accessories for the weather.

15

A RESIDENT'S ROOM

Have you ever moved from one house or apartment to another? What did you unpack first? How did you make your new space a home? How long did it take before you could call it home? At first you probably felt uncomfortable. You might have wondered, "Where will I put all my things? Will I make new friends? Will I ever become comfortable in this new place?" People have a great ability to adapt to change if they feel they have some control over their surroundings. If you can decide things about how you live and have familiar things around you, you feel more secure and in control and feel better about your life in general.

This chapter discusses how to help create a home for residents in a long term care facility. You will learn why it is important to respect residents' privacy. You will learn how to make a resident's bed and make his or her room more comfortable. The call systems used in residents' rooms are also described.

CREATING A HOME IN A LONG TERM CARE FACILITY

When an individual enters a long term care facility, he or she may feel many losses. Among these is the loss of home and many cherished belongings. Nurse assistants face the challenge of helping create and maintain a home for residents in the facility. To meet this challenge, you first learn how a resident wants the room arranged so that it feels like his or her own place. A resident may want pictures of grandchildren on the walls or a special spread on the bed. He or she may want personal things in a special place. Meeting a resident's wants is your number one priority. You must be sure each resident feels like the facility is his or her home.

You can promote a home-like feeling by encouraging residents and their families to bring in furniture (as space permits), wall hangings and decorative items, pictures and mementos of loved ones, plants, clothes, and personal grooming items. Familiar things help create a positive environment and the secure feeling of home. Follow these guidelines for residents' personal things:

▶ Treat a resident's belongings as if you are a visitor to the person's home.
▶ Comment positively on pictures and furniture.
▶ Encourage residents to use their own things.
▶ Help safeguard a resident's possessions.

Talk with every resident to see how he or she wants the room cared for, and together set a schedule that meets his or her needs as well as the facility's policy.

Residents may choose not to bring in personal items. If so, treat the furniture in the room as if it were resident's own, and encourage them to treat it like their own (Fig. 15-1).

RESPONSIBILITIES IN CARING FOR RESIDENT'S PERSONAL BELONGINGS

Although individual space is a concern in any long term care facility, residents have the right to bring with them and use personal items as space permits. Residents often bring things that are necessary (such as clothes, hearing aids, etc.) or of a special, sentimental nature.

If belongings are broken or otherwise damaged, misplaced, or stolen while in the facility, this can cause great distress for a resident and family, a feeling of greater loss, vulnerability, and lack of caring. Therefore, residents and family must be able

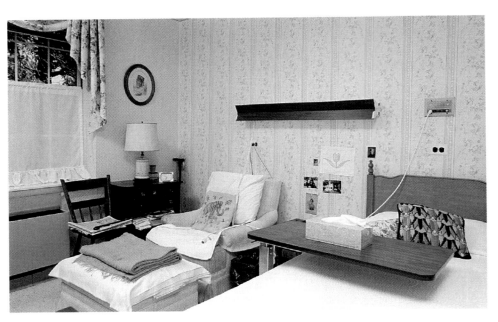

Fig. 15-1. Respect everything in the resident's rooms as if it were his or her own.

to count on staff to respect and protect special belongings to the very best of their ability. Always think this way: "How would I feel if that happened to me?"

A list or inventoried record of all resident's belongings becomes part of a resident's chart (Fig. 15-2). Additional items brought into a resident's room after admission must be recorded on the inventory list, and removed items noted on the record.

Keeping track of personal belongings is a responsibility for the whole team. For example, if a resident's eye glasses are missing, housekeeping, laundry, and dietary staff should all be informed. The glasses may have gone to the laundry in a shirt pocket, or were removed along with dirty dishes on a dining tray.

Care of a Resident's Clothes

A resident's clothing represents an important aspect of the person's self-esteem. Follow these guidelines:

▷ Ensure all clothing is labeled with a resident's name. The name should be where it can be easily seen but not on public display, such as on the inside on a tag (Fig. 15-3).

▷ Watch for new clothing family members and friends might bring to a resident, and make sure they are labeled. Be especially aware on special occasions, such as holidays or a resident's birthday. Imagine how a resident and family would feel if that beautiful gift blouse worn only once was sent to the laundry or misplaced and never seen again.

▷ All residents have the right to look good. As discussed in Chapter 14, encourage residents to choose their clothing.

▷ Try to keep residents' clothing from becoming very soiled and stained. If a resident tends to spill food, use a bib or large napkin to help avoid stains, at snacks as well as at meal time.

▷ If an item of clothing becomes very soiled, wash it in a sink as soon as possible to prevent staining. You may also contact the laundry department to treat the area, depending on facility protocol.

▷ Put laundry in the appropriate bag or container when soiled, following the protocol for the facility.

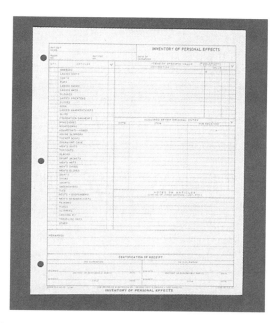

Fig. 15-2. Part of a resident's chart includes a complete list of the resident's belongings.

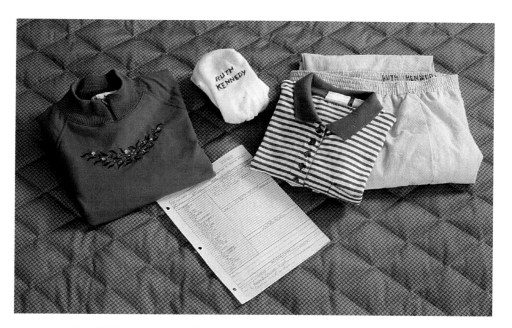

Fig. 15-3. Label all of a resident's clothing with his or her name.

Care of Other Resident Belongings

Belongings like hearing aids, eye glasses, and dentures are necessary for the well-being of residents. Follow these guidelines:

▶ These items should be labeled or marked with a resident's name. (There are kits available to mark dentures.)

▶ Keep these items in appropriate containers when not in use. Encourage residents to help with this.

▶ Record the serial number on hearing aids in a resident's record in case a problem develops.

▶ Routinely check pockets when bagging or collecting clothes or for the laundry. Try to prevent valuables such as a watch, hearing aid, and wallet from going through laundry machines.

▶ Keep an eye on bedding or food trays to make sure dentures, eye glasses, or hearing aids are not left on them.

Follow these guidelines for other personal belongings:

▶ Keep the attitude that a resident's things are important and valuable. Treat them like your own.

▶ Be careful when cleaning or tidying rooms not to break or damage special belongings. Open the closet and drawers only with the resident's permission.

▶ Whenever possible, valuable items such as cash, jewelry, heirlooms, etc. should not be kept in the facility. The family should take them home. However, if such items remain, check with the charge nurse and follow the protocol of the facility. These must be on the inventory list.

▶ If a belonging becomes lost or broken, report it to the charge nurse immediately.

It can be challenging to keep track of residents' personal belongings. Use your common sense and mindful care to limit the risk of loss or damage.

RESPECTING RESIDENTS' PRIVACY

Even though people frequently move in and out of residents' rooms, you and all staff must respect their privacy. Remember the facility is their home. You must remember that residents have private lives—they are not just part of your routine. As you become more familiar with residents, you must be careful not to let this familiarity become routine. You must always be mindful. Consider this example:

> You have been caring for Mrs. Jones for a month. You know her usual morning routine: she brushes her teeth, eats breakfast in her room, and then showers and dresses for the day. Once she is up and about, she likes her room straightened and her bed made before her daughter's daily visit. You have become familiar and comfortable knowing that everyday by 10 A.M., Mrs. Jones is out of her room.
>
> Today at 10:30 A.M., you walk into Mrs. Jones's room without knocking or speaking, pull the curtain open, and find Mrs. Jones having a very private conversation with a clergy member from her church. Everyone is embarrassed, and you have violated Mrs. Jones's right to privacy. In this situation, you did three things wrong:
> 1. Assuming Mrs. Jones's routine does not change
> 2. Not knocking on the door and not waiting for Mrs. Jones's permission to enter
> 3. Not announcing yourself

If you had not assumed that Mrs. Jones's routine never changed, you would have acted differently in this situation. You must remember that residents are people; never take their actions for granted. If you had knocked on Mrs. Jones's door, given your name, and said you were there to make the bed, Mrs. Jones would have had the opportunity to tell you that now is not a good time and ask you to return later. You would have respected Mrs. Jones's home and her right to have privacy.

To show respect for residents' privacy, always follow these principles:
1. Knock on the door (Fig. 15-4).
2. Ask permission to enter.
3. Ask how residents want their rooms.
4. Never move items without a resident's permission.
5. Encourage residents to help in their care and arrangement of their room (Fig. 15-5).

Maintain a resident's privacy with respect and clear communication in everything you do.

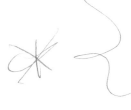

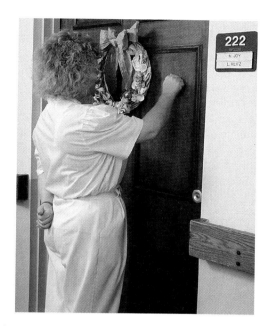

Fig. 15-4. Always knock on the resident's door before entering the resident's room.

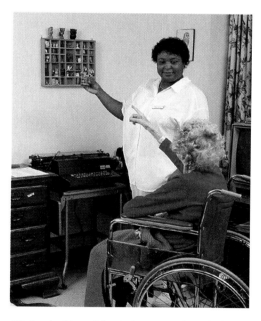

Fig. 15-5. Assist residents in arranging their rooms.

BED MAKING

As a nurse assistant you are responsible for all the items in a resident's room, especially the bed. Some facilities have hand-crank beds, and others electric ones. The difference is that crank beds need effort for raising and lowering the entire bed, or the head or foot. A resident is more likely to ask for your help with a crank bed. The cranks are at the bottom of the bed and are pulled in and out for use. Be careful to always return the crank after use, as you or a resident can bump into or trip over one. Electric beds have either foot pedals or controls on the side of the bed. The electric bed is easier for residents to use with simple instructions.

Making a neat, wrinkle-free bed for residents is important for comfort and dignity. It also helps prevent skin irritation and breakdown. Most residents can get out of bed while you make it. This is called making an unoccupied bed. Some residents cannot get out of bed, and you will need to make an occupied bed. Follow these guidelines when making a bed:

▶ Raise the height to prevent a back strain.
▶ Making one side of the bed at a time reduces the number of steps you have to take.
▶ Never put linens on the floor.
▶ Keep soiled linens away from your uniform.
▶ Always roll a resident toward you, and use the side rail to support him or her when making an occupied bed.

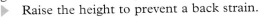

Making an Unoccupied Bed

Remember:

▶ Resident preference
▶ Common preparation steps
▶ Equipment and supplies needed
▶ Environment preparation
▶ Resident preparation

Items Needed

▶ 2 Flat sheets
▶ Draw sheet (if used)

▶ Blanket and spread, if needed
▶ Pillowcases

1. Look for any belongings. (Residents often fall asleep with personal belongings under their pillow or elsewhere in their beds.)
2. Flatten the bed and raise it to a comfortable position.
3. Remove soiled linen, including the pillowcase, loosen sheets from under the mattress, and then carefully roll them into a ball, keeping the soiled side inside the ball, and away from your body. (This keeps the cleaner side close to you. Rolling linens prevents the spread of organisms from dirty linens.) Put the sheets in the laundry bag.
4. Check the mattress for any soiling or wetness. (Wash and dry with a paper towel if necessary.) Change the mattress pad if it is soiled or scheduled for change.
5. Unfold the bottom sheet lengthwise down the bed's center. Do not shake the linen while unfolding. (Shaking the linen raises dust and organisms.) Put the hem seams toward the mattress. (This keeps rough edges from touching the person.)
6. Slide the sheet so that the hem is even with the foot of the mattress. Keep the fold in the exact center of the bed from head to foot. (You want the extra sheet at the top to tuck it under the mattress.) (Fig. 15-6).
7. Open the sheet from the fold so that the sheet covers the entire mattress and hangs evenly on both sides (Fig. 15-7).
8. Tuck the top hem in tightly under the mattress at the head of the bed. Carefully lift the head of the mattress and slide the sheet under the mattress. Make a square corner (also called a mitered or "hospital" corner):
   a. Face the side of the bed.
   b. With one hand, pick up the top of the sheet hanging down the side of the bed, and lay it on top of the bed (it looks like a triangle) (Fig. 15-8).
   c. Tuck the remaining sheet under the mattress (Fig. 15-9).
   d. Drop the section of sheet from on top of the bed over the side of the bed, and tuck it in (Fig. 15-10).
9. Tuck the remaining sheet under the mattress neatly, starting from the squared corner down to the foot of the mattress. If a draw sheet is used, place it in the center of the bed so it covers the middle part of the bed. Tuck in the draw sheet (Fig. 15-11). A draw sheet is often used for residents needing assistance with moving and positioning, or sometimes to keep bottom sheets clean and dry.
   Note: If you are using a fitted sheet (shaped to the mattress by elastic edging), use the following step instead of Steps 6-9:
      Starting at the top corner of the mattress, wrap the edge of the mattress with the corner of the sheet, then go to the bottom of bed on the same side and wrap

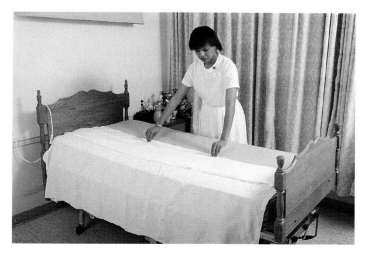

Fig. 15-6. Make sure bottom sheet is even with the foot of the mattress.

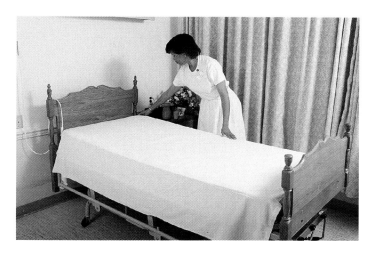

Fig. 15-7. Open the bottom sheet completely.

page 121
Shieli's

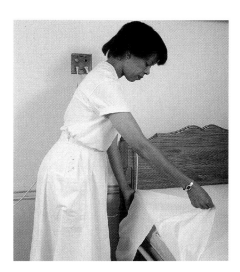

Fig. 15-8. Pick up the top of the sheet.

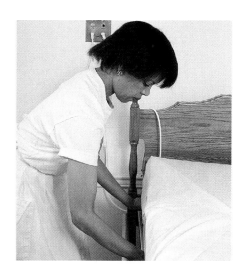

Fig. 15-9. The remaining sheet should be tucked under the mattress.

the edge. Go to the opposite corner, wrap that edge up to the top of the bed, and wrap the last edge over the last corner. The sheet should fit the mattress snugly.

10. Place the top sheet on the bed so that the fold is in the exact center. The wide hem should be even with the head of the mattress, with the seam on the outside. When you fold the hem over, the smooth side will be next to the resident's skin, preventing any rough edges from touching him or her (Fig. 15-12). The excess sheet will be over the foot of the bed.

11. Open the sheet from the fold so that the sheet covers the entire mattress and hangs evenly on both sides.

12. Place the spread on top of the sheet in the same manner. Make sure the sheet does not hang below the spread on the sides.

13. Tuck in the sheet and spread at the foot, and make a square corner at the bottom end, using the steps above (Fig. 15-13).

14. Smooth the sheet and spread from bottom to top of bed, and fold down the top hem of the sheet over the spread.

15. Move to the opposite side of the bed and finish in the same manner, starting with the bottom sheet and finishing with the top sheet and spread. Pull the bottom sheet tight before each tuck to remove wrinkles. (Tuck in the draw sheet tightly if used.)

16. Place a clean case on the pillow by grabbing the center of the closed end of the pillow case with your hand and turn it inside out over your hand (Fig. 15-14). Grab the pillow with the hand in the pillow case and slide the case over the pillow (Fig. 15-15). Make sure the corners of the pillow are fitted into the corners of the case. Place the pillow(s) at the head of the bed and fold the spread over the pillow(s) (Fig. 15-16).

17. Put the blanket at the foot of the bed or in the closet if a resident prefers.

18. Return bed to low position.

Remember:

▶ Meet resident needs
▶ Common completion steps
▶ Clean and put away equipment and supplies
▶ Environment completion (Is it safe? Is it clean?)

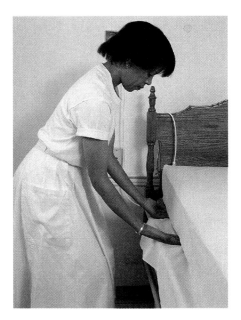

Fig. 15-10. Tuck the remaining section of the sheet under the mattress as well.

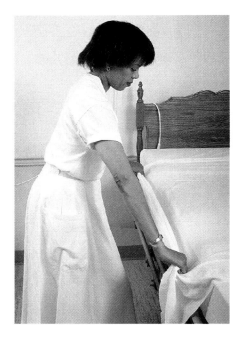

Fig. 15-11. If a draw sheet is used, tuck it under the mattress.

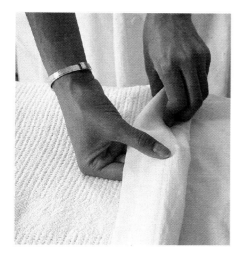

Fig. 15-12. When you fold the hem of the top sheet over, the smooth side should be next to the resident's skin.

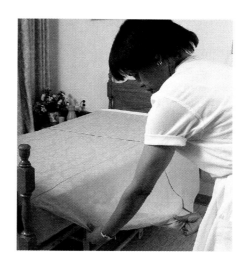

Fig. 15-13. When tucked in, the sheet and spread should form a square corner at the end.

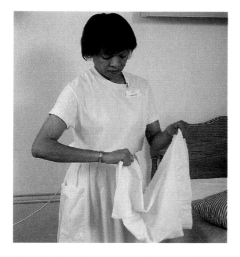

Fig. 15-14. Turn the pillowcase inside out over your hand.

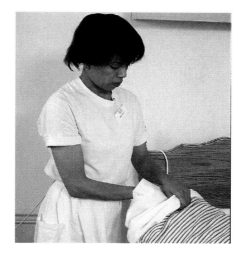

Fig. 15-15. Slide the pillowcase over the pillow.

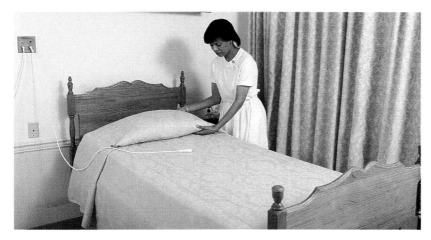

Fig. 15-16. At the head of the bed cover the pillow with the spread.

Remember:

▶ Resident preference
▶ Common preparation steps
▶ Equipment and supplies needed
▶ Environment preparation
▶ Resident preparation

Items Needed

▶ 2 Full sheets
▶ Draw sheet (if used)

▶ Blanket and spread, if needed
▶ Pillowcases

1. Put the bed in a flat position, and remove the pillow from under the resident's head. (Do this only if he or she is comfortable in a completely flat position.)
2. Remove the spread and any blankets, and fold them on the chair.
3. Loosen the top and bottom sheets from under the mattress.
4. Help the resident to roll over to one side and turn toward you. Raise the side rail and ask him or her to hold onto it for support. Go to the other side of the bed. *Note:* Be sure to get help in advance if you will need it.
5. Check for the resident's belongings in the bed.
6. Roll lengthwise (top to bottom) the bottom soiled sheet from the side of the mattress to the center of the bed. (If the linen is wet or soiled, place a barrier like a plastic-covered padding over the sheet.) Change the mattress pad if it is soiled or scheduled for changing.
7. Unfold the bottom sheet lengthwise, centered on the bed. Do not shake the linen while unfolding (shaking the linen raises dust and organisms). Be sure the hem seams face the mattress. (This prevents any rough edges from touching the resident.)
8. Slide the sheet so that the hem is even with the foot of the mattress. Be sure to keep the fold in the exact center of the bed from head to foot. (You want the extra sheet at the top so that you can tuck it under the mattress.)
9. Open the sheet and fan-fold it lengthwise so that one half of the sheet is next to the rolled dirty sheet (Fig. 15-17).
10. Tuck the top hem in tightly under the mattress at the head of the bed. Carefully lift the head of the mattress and slide the sheet under the mattress. Make a square corner:
    a. Face the side of the bed.
    b. With one hand, pick up the top of the sheet hanging down the side of the bed, and lay it on top of the bed (it looks like a triangle).
    c. Tuck the remaining sheet under the mattress.
    d. Drop the section of sheet that is lying on top of the bed over the side of the bed, and tuck it in.
11. Tuck the remaining sheet under the mattress neatly, starting with the squared corner down to the foot of the mattress. If a draw sheet is used, place it in the center of the bed so it covers the middle part of the bed. Fan-fold the excess and tuck it in with the sheet. Tuck in the draw sheet (Fig. 15-18).
12. Flatten the rolled or fan-folded sheets and help the resident roll over the linen toward you, using the procedure for turning him or her (see Chapter 13). Don't forget to tell the resident that the roll of linen is behind him or her.
13. Put up the side rail and ask the resident to hold onto it for support.
14. Go to the opposite side of the bed, lower the side rail, and remove the dirty bottom sheet (Fig. 15-19).
    Note: Never leave the resident unattended. Put the dirty sheet in the laundry bag (if it is in the room) or at the bottom of the bed between the mattress and footboard.
15. Pull the clean linen toward you until it is completely unfolded, and tuck the sheets in tightly in the same manner as you did on the opposite side (Fig. 15-20). (Tuck in the draw sheet if used.)
16. Help the resident roll back to the center of the bed.

17. Place the top sheet on the bed. Open the sheet from the fold so that the sheet hangs evenly on each side of the bed. The wide hem should be even with the head of the mattress, with the seam on the outside. When you fold the hem over, the smooth side will be next to the resident's skin, preventing any rough edges from touching him or her. The excess sheet is over the foot of the bed.

18. Ask the resident to hold onto the clean sheet, then carefully remove the dirty top sheet by placing your hand under the clean top sheet and rolling the dirty sheet down toward the foot of the bed. Remove it, and put it with the other dirty linen (Fig. 15-21).

19. Place the spread on top of the sheet in the same way you did the top sheet. Make sure the sheet does not hang below the spread on the sides.

20. Tuck in the sheet and spread at the foot of the bed, and make a square corner at the bottom ends:
    a. Face the side of the bed.
    b. With one hand, pick up the top sheet hanging down the side of the bed, and lay it on top of the bed (it looks like a triangle).
    c. Tuck the remaining sheet under the mattress.
    d. Drop the sheet lying on top of the bed over the side of the bed, and tuck it in.

21. Smooth the sheet and spread from the bottom to the top of the bed, and fold down the top hem of the sheet over the top of the spread. Be sure the top linens are not so tight that they would press downward on the resident's feet. To be sure, make a toe pleat. This is done by pulling the top linen up to form a pleat (Fig. 15-22).

22. Remove the dirty pillow case, and put a clean case on the pillow. Grab the center of the closed end of the pillow case with your hand, turn it inside out over your hand, and then grab the pillow with the hand in the pillow case and slide the case over the pillow. Make sure the corners of the pillow are fitted into the corners of the case. Put the pillow under the resident's head (Fig. 15-23).

Remember:

▷ Meet resident needs
▷ Common completion steps
▷ Clean and put away equipment and supplies
▷ Environment completion (Is it safe? Is it clean?)

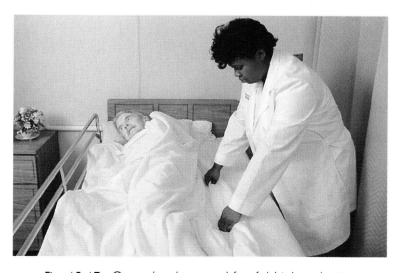

Fig. 15-17. Open the sheet and fan-fold it lengthwise.

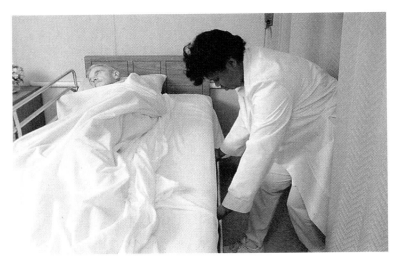

Fig 15-18. Tuck in the draw sheet.

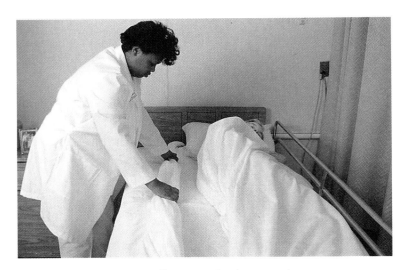

Fig. 15-19. Remove the bottom sheet.

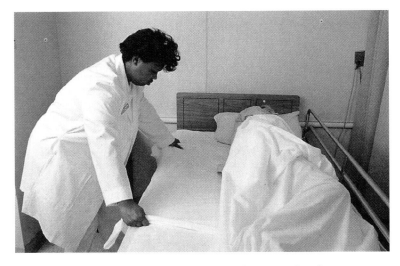

Fig. 15-20. Pull clean linen toward you and tuck it in.

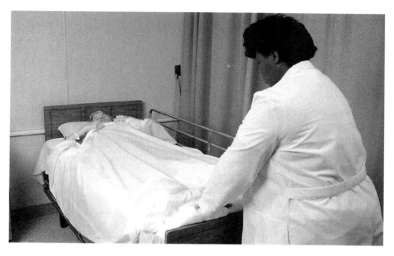

Fig. 15-21. Carefully remove the dirty top sheet.

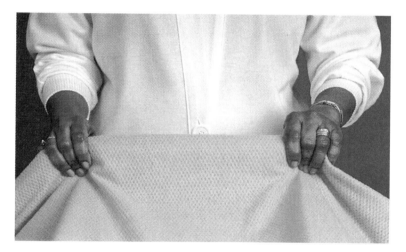

Fig. 15-22. Make a toe pleat, which allows ample room for the resident's feet.

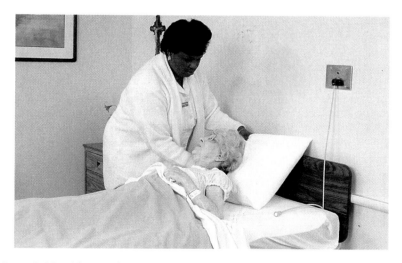

Fig. 15-23. After replacing the dirty pillowcase with a clean one, carefully place the pillow under the resident's head.

Finishing Touches

The bed is only one part of a resident's environment. You are also responsible for the bedside table, over-bed table, and any other furniture. Keep all a resident's belongings in mind when you consider the environment. Think also about finishing touches you can add to make a resident's room feel warm, friendly, and more comfortable, such as the following:

1. Eliminate clutter, like disposable cups, tissues, old newspapers, and magazines. Ask the resident before you throw anything away.
2. Adjust lighting as a resident prefers, such as drawing shades in the evening and raising them in the morning.
3. Consider the room temperature and ventilation.
4. Monitor noise levels.
5. Help care for residents' plants and flowers if needed.
6. Dust pictures and other mementos.
7. Hang up cards.

These simple things can really make a difference in the way residents feel about their home in the long term care facility.

CALL SYSTEM

You cannot be with every resident all the time. To make sure residents get help when they need it when you are not there, facilities have call systems for all residents.

The call system has these parts:

▹ An electrical call button on a cord plugs into an outlet over each resident's bed. A resident pushes the button when he or she needs help. The cord has a clip that can be attached to the pillow or sheet to keep the button from falling on the floor out of reach.

▹ A light outside each resident's door turns on when he or she pushes the call button (Fig. 15-24).

▹ A call board at the nurses' station has room numbers that light up (and may also buzz or ring) when a resident pushes the button. Some facilities may also have an intercom system from the station to residents' rooms (Fig. 15-25).

To help residents use the call system, you should:

▹ Explain the purpose of the call system (Fig. 15-26).

▹ Show how to use the call button. Then have a resident show that he or she can use the call button.

▹ Watch for call lights and answer quickly when you see one, even for residents you are not caring for that day. Turn off the light when you enter the room so that another nurse assistant does not also come.

▹ Make sure each resident's call light is always plugged in, working properly, and within reach when a resident is in bed or sitting near the bed.

▹ If a resident's call light is out of order, report it to the charge nurse immediately. A bell can be used until the light is repaired.

Note: Additional call buttons are often located in residents' bathrooms and shower areas. You should also instruct residents in how to use these safety systems.

If a resident does not understand the call system or cannot pull the cord or push the button, work with the charge nurse to find another means for residents to call for assistance.

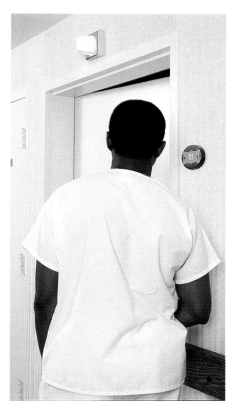

Fig. 15-24. When a resident pushes the call button, the light outside their door comes on.

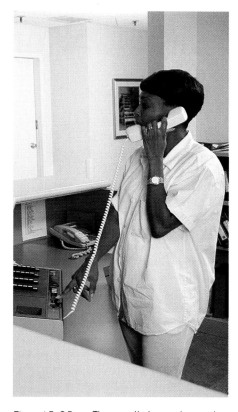

Fig. 15-25. The call board at the nurses' station will light up or ring when the resident pushes the call button

IN THIS CHAPTER YOU LEARNED TO:

▶ list three ways to make a resident's room home-like

▶ describe the nurse assistant's role in caring for a resident's belongings

▶ explain ways to ensure the resident's privacy

▶ demonstrate how to make an unoccupied and an occupied bed

▶ demonstrate the use of the call system

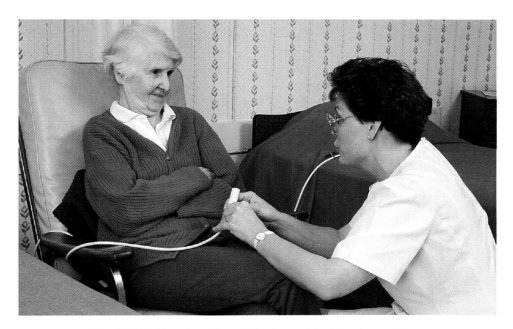

Fig. 15-26. You should explain the call bell to the resident.

16 *14 pages*

ASSISTING WITH NUTRITION

F ood and nutrition are an important part of life. Think about the emphasis on food on television and in magazines. Food gives pleasure and helps keep you healthy. Think about how you associate food with activities and how eating with others is a part of your social life. Food and nutrition are major factors in how most people stay healthy and happy. Each of us has different food preferences and customs. Why do we eat the way we do? People have different reasons. We eat partly because of:

▶ Taste: Your personal likes and dislikes for foods
▶ Cuture: The way you have been raised and your cultural practices
▶ Our state of health: We often eat less when feeling ill
▶ Our mental state: We often enjoy food more when happy and relaxed and less when sad or depressed
▶ Our ability to chew and swallow: One's appetite or ability to eat may change after dental work or with a sore throat
▶ Our social situation: Often people eat differently when alone than with friends and family

As you can see, our feelings about food and appetite for food are affected by many things. Each of us may be affected in different ways. This understanding can help you understand how residents' eating may be affected.

As a nurse assistant, you have a direct impact on the nutritional status of the residents you care for. This chapter discusses how you can help improve their nutritional health.

FUNCTIONS OF THE DIETARY DEPARTMENT

The dietary department of a long term care facility has many tasks. It provides food that is safe and appealing. It must also ensure that every resident receives the correct diet ordered by the physician in a form that meets the individual's needs. Most facilities use a cycle menu. Cycle menus vary in length, but are usually three to six weeks long. These menus are called cycle menus because the same meals are repeated, or cycled, over time (Fig. 16-1).

The dietary department also manages therapeutic and modified diets. For example, in a 100-bed nursing facility, the following diets may be ordered:

▶ Regular
▶ Diabetic, no concentrated sweets
▶ 1200-calorie diabetic
▶ 1500-calorie diabetic
▶ 1800-calorie diabetic
▶ Low-sodium
▶ 2-gm sodium
▶ Low-fat low-cholesterol
▶ Renal

These nine different diets must be prepared along with any special considerations for residents, such as food allergies and special preferences. The cook also grinds, chops, or purees some portions of each diet to meet individual consistency needs. As a nurse assistant, you will be working closely with the dietary department to meet the nutrition needs of each resident.

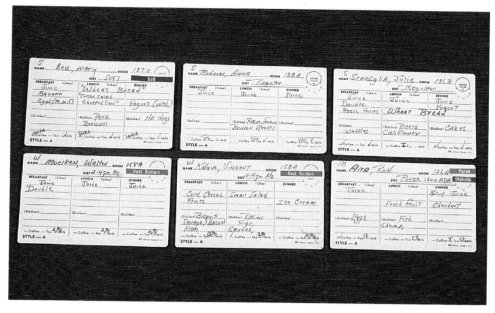

Fig. 16-1.   Examples of cycle menus.

WORKING TOGETHER TO PROVIDE THE BEST FOR THE RESIDENT

Like you, residents prefer familiar foods. Preferences may be personal, religious, regional, or ethnic. The best way to learn what a resident likes and dislikes is to ask. Ask questions that will provide you information about the following:

▷ A resident's personal preferences may be a simple like or dislike due to food appearance, familiarity, or taste. What foods do you like? Dislike?

▷ Religious preferences are guided by religious traditions. For example, some Catholics may still avoid eating meat on Fridays, and some Jews eat only kosher foods.

▷ Regional preferences are those characteristic to a certain area, such as grits in the south.

▷ A resident's ethnic preferences come from cultural heritage such as Latin American or Asian.

All these factors play a major role in how residents like their food prepared and when they like to eat (Fig. 16-2). You need to work with the resident, resident's family, and the dietary department to meet the resident's preferences.

Residents have a right to make choices and to express food preferences and dislikes. Responding to these needs requires a team approach between the dietary department and nursing. The dietary department asks about a resident's preferences soon after admission and arranges to substitute for foods he or she does not eat. If a resident refuses the food, you must offer to get him or her something else. This is especially important for a resident who is underweight or does not eat well.

Serving food at correct temperatures also involves a team approach. Food must be held at appropriate temperatures. Once it leaves the kitchen, you must serve it as quickly as possible while hot foods are still hot and cold foods cold.

HELPING RESIDENTS ACHIEVE HIGH NUTRITIONAL STATUS

Improving nutritional status can be accomplished by a combination of correct diet and proper assistance. While many residents receive a regular diet, some require special types of diets as part of therapy for a disease or a specific condition. These diets are called therapeutic diets.

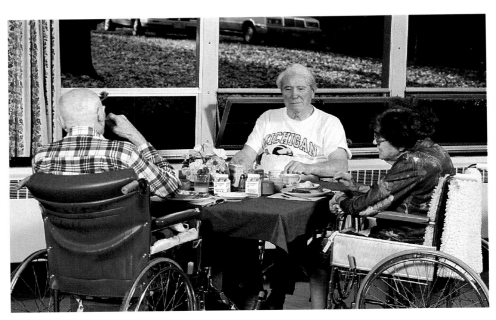

Fig. 16-2. The dietary department must be sure that the resident's food preferences are met.

A therapeutic diet is one that is ordered by the physician as a treatment for a disease or condition, such as a diabetic diet. A therapeutic diet can sometimes reduce or eliminate the need for medication. Any diet may be modified in consistency to meet individual needs. Food may be chopped, ground, or pureed for residents with problems chewing, such as those caused by a lack of or ill-fitting dentures or a poor condition of teeth or gums. Consistency alterations may be necessary due to difficulty swallowing caused by a stroke or other digestive difficulties (Fig. 16-3).

Because the facility is home and the diet may be long term, a resident's dietary needs should be met with as few restrictions as possible. Elderly residents often dislike restrictions if they can no longer have their favorite foods or seasonings. This may result in eating less. Balancing a therapeutic diet and its restrictions along with a resident's preference is a challenge. Discussions with residents can help in finding the balance.

Four commonly ordered diets are:

▷ *Calorie-restricted diets.* These usually range from 1000 to 2000 calories per day and are usually ordered for diabetics or for weight reduction. A liberal version of this diet is the "no concentrated sweets" diet (NCS), which only restricts foods high in simple sugars such as many desserts, foods prepared with sugar, and sugar packets.

▷ *Sodium-restricted diets.* This diet is usually ordered for residents with fluid retention or high blood pressure. Sodium is commonly restricted at different levels, such as the 2-gm sodium and the low-sodium (3-4 gms). The abbreviation for sodium is "NA," and you may see a diet written as "Low NA." These residents do not receive salt on their trays and do not receive foods with a lot of sodium such as canned soups, salted crackers, or corned beef.

▷ *Fat-restricted and/or cholesterol-restricted diets.* Fat-restricted diets may be ordered for residents with diseases of the liver, gallbladder, pancreas, cardiovascular system, or malabsorption syndromes (difficulty absorbing nutrients) where fat is not tolerated. Low-cholesterol diets are used to reduce blood fat levels. Foods high in fat such as bacon, sausage, cream, gravy, margarine, whole milk, and high-fat desserts are restricted.

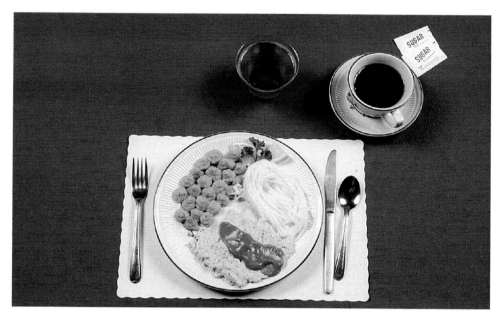

Fig. 16-3. Part of a resident's treatment may include a therapeutic diet.

▶ *Protein-restricted diets.* Protein restrictions are often necessary in treatment of renal or liver disease, sometimes along with other restrictions as well, such as sodium and potassium. These diets are often called renal diets and can be difficult for a resident to follow if the restriction is severe. But the renal diet may allow postponing dialysis or transplantation. Foods restricted include not only meat, eggs, and dairy products but breads and other foods that contain small amounts of protein. The renal diet is usually carefully calculated by the dietitian.

DIETARY SUPPLEMENTS

Many residents cannot eat enough food to furnish the calories and protein they need. This may be because of a physical change, like gastrointestinal problems or cancer treatments, or an emotional change such as depression. Supplements are often ordered. Supplements provide concentrated nutrition. Many kinds of supplements are available. Some provide calories and protein, and some are fortified with vitamins and minerals as well. Some facilities prepare their own. Some supplements come in forms such as shakes, puddings, and frozen bars or "pudding pops." They can also be in the form of supplemental feedings, such as a small sandwich between meals.

Examples of residents who benefit from supplements include:

▶ Residents who accept liquids better than food
▶ Residents who cannot consume large amounts of food
▶ Residents with an altered sense of taste and smell
▶ Residents who are very thin and malnourished

Although supplements can play an important role in maintaining the nutritional status of a resident, you should always think of the supplement as an addition to the meal. The meal is the first priority. Except in extreme cases, supplements do not replace the meal but are given in addition to it. Encourage residents to consume as much of the meal as possible before offering the supplement.

As with food and fluid intake, supplement intake is important. If a resident refuses a supplement consistently, report this to the nurse so that another supplement can be tried.

MAKING THE DINING EXPERIENCE PLEASANT

Mealtime is much more than eating. Mealtimes provide pleasure and enhance one's well-being. Think of what factors affect how you feel when you dine out. Attractive surroundings, pleasant company, and courteous service combine to increase your enjoyment. The dining experience in a nursing facility is similar. Many factors can influence a resident's feelings about the experience and affect his or her food intake. These factors can be grouped into three categories: environmental, service, and social.

Environmental Factors

These include the physical surroundings. Residents have a right to expect the dining room to be clean and uncluttered and free of unpleasant odors. Linens, if used, should be clean and pressed. Temperature should be comfortable. Lighting should be soft, not glaring, and the sun should not be shining in anyone's eyes.

Table height is also important to comfort. If a table is too high, residents must reach up. This can cause fatigue and decreased intake. Residents in wheelchairs should sit at tables high enough to allow wheelchairs under the table so that they are close to the table. Tables should be spaced so that residents can come and go freely, even with walkers or wheelchairs.

Soft music, flowers, and pretty dishes also add to the pleasure of dining. Distractions such as a loud TV or radio should be discouraged. Do not stack plate covers on the table or scrape dishes while residents are still eating.

These same factors hold true for residents eating in their room. Clean any clutter from the over-bed table, prevent any unpleasant odors, adjust the table height correctly, and remove food from the tray and position it properly on the plate.

Also avoid nursing measures such as taking vital signs during meals.

Service Factors

The second type of influence is service. Have you ever had a restaurant meal spoiled by a discourteous waiter? Your attitude toward residents similarly affects their response.

Speak to residents in a courteous, pleasant voice. A caring, patient attitude encourages enjoyment of the meal (Fig. 16-4). Encourage residents to take their time

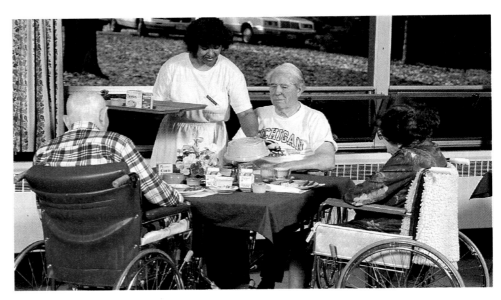

Fig. 16-4. Encourage enjoyment of the meal, by speaking in a courteous, caring, and pleasant voice and attitude.

to finish without hurrying or rushing. Some residents will stop eating if they think you are waiting for them to finish.

When serving the meal, report the menu in an enthusiastic manner. Your tone of voice and attitude can have a positive or negative influence on how residents view the meal.

Social Factors

Social factors also directly affect the dining experience. Encourage residents to sit with their own friends. If a resident has no friends, perhaps because he or she is new to the facility, always direct him or her to a table of residents of similar mental status. Avoid seating alert and oriented residents with confused, disruptive ones. Try to attain a pleasant, home-like atmosphere where residents will look forward to meals both for the food and for the enjoyment of the experience.

ASSISTING RESIDENTS WITH MEALS

One of your most important duties as a nurse assistant is to help residents with meals. Although you may at first think of this as a simple, common sense matter, it actually requires a lot of attention. Your ability to do it well directly impacts each resident's nutritional status.

Preparing Residents for Meals

Meals are enjoyed more fully when residents are properly prepared. Before the meal, comb a resident's hair as requested and assist female residents with makeup when desired. Do not forget to encourage use of dentures, glasses, and hearing aids. These devices increase residents' functional ability and help them be more independent. Also provide assistance as needed for hand washing and oral care. Good oral care before the meal may increase taste sensitivity to some food flavors. If a resident is to eat in bed, elevate the head of the bed to at least 30 degrees. Make each resident as comfortable as possible. Position bibs or napkins to protect clothing.

Tray Preparation

Before assisting with the meal, wash your hands thoroughly. This is an important part of infection control. Also try to pass trays as quickly as possible to preserve food temperature. You want to be sure cold foods are cold and hot foods are hot. Put yourself in the person's place. How would you feel if you were hungry and the trays were ready but no one came to serve them for 20 or 30 minutes?

When removing the tray from the cart, first check the diet card (Fig. 16-5). This tells you which tray goes to which resident. Do you have the right tray for the person you are serving? Does the diet appear correct? For example, there should not be a salt packet on a low-sodium diet.

Remove the food from the tray. Placing the plate directly on the table gives a more home-like appearance. Remove any covers and underliners from the plate unless the person is not ready to eat. Although it is preferable for residents to be ready for the meal before service, some residents may arrive late. Leave their plates covered to preserve food temperatures.

After removing plate covers and underliners, place them back on the tray and return them to the service cart or to another cart. Place the plate within easy reach. This is a good time to review the menu with a resident you are serving. Some residents have impaired vision and do not see well or may not be familiar with some items served. Remember to state the menu enthusiastically to increase anticipation. Think how you would feel if a restaurant waiter remarked "The chili looks terrible!" when serving you. Would you want to eat it?

Once the plate is within easy reach, remove any plastic wrap, lids, or foil. Open condiments and cartons. Ask residents if they want seasoning. Encourage residents to express their choices.

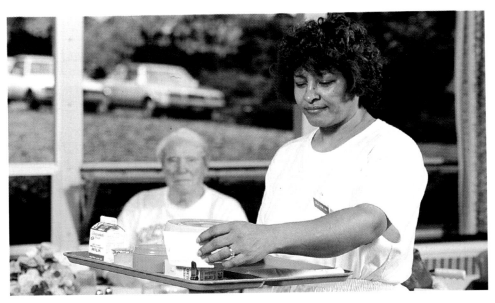

Fig. 16-5. Remember to check the diet card when removing the tray from the cart.

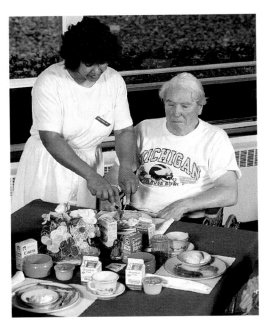

Fig. 16-6. You may have to assist a resident by cutting his or her food.

Serving Residents

Give any help needed, such as cutting meat or other food (Fig. 16-6). Always encourage residents to be as independent as possible, but be alert for residents who need help. If you do cut the meat, cut it in small pieces to prevent choking. When the first resident at the table is served, move on to other residents at the same table. Try to serve all residents at a table before moving on to the next. Again, think of yourself in a restaurant setting. Have you ever been the last at your table served? It is frustrating to watch others at the table eat and perhaps finish the meal while you continue to wait. This delay in service also detracts from the social pleasure of eating together.

Steps for Assisting Residents with Meals

1. Prepare residents before the meal by helping them with grooming, hand washing, and oral care.
2. Assist residents to the dining room or make them comfortable in their room.
3. Wash your hands.
4. Position napkins and bibs.
5. Pass trays quickly, making sure cold foods are cold and hot foods are hot.
6. Check tray cards: make sure the name matches the person and the diet appears correct and complete.
7. Place the plate on the table, open cartons, remove wrappings, cut meats, and season food if necessary.
8. While placing the plate, review the menu enthusiastically.
9. Make sure each resident is close enough to the table to reach food and utensils.
10. Encourage residents to feed themselves as much as possible.
11. Serve all residents at a table before moving to the next.
12. Check with residents frequently to offer assistance or substitutes for foods not eaten.
13. Be sure each resident has enough time to finish the meal.
14. Remove the tray and make sure each resident's hands and face are clean and that he or she is comfortable.

Once residents have been served, check with them frequently to offer further assistance or to encourage them to eat. Some residents respond to prompting. Always allow adequate time to finish the meal. Some residents eat much more slowly than others. If a resident does not eat well or rejects a particular food item, offer to get a substitute, especially for underweight or poorly nourished residents. A resident may have certain preferences and dislikes based on personal, religious, regional, or ethnic background, and each resident has the right to expect a substitute for an item he or she does not wish to eat. You must offer a substitute, and the dietary department must provide it. This policy is also a federal regulation. A resident should never leave the dining room hungry or receive food he or she cannot eat. Offering substitutes also conveys a caring attitude.

Feeding Residents

Some residents can eat independently or with minor help from the staff. Other residents, however, must be fed. These residents totally depend on the staff to meet their nutritional needs. Residents who are difficult to feed or who have special problems may be evaluated by a therapist, who can train the staff to use special feeding techniques to correct the problems.

Follow these general techniques for most residents who must be fed:

1. Prepare each resident for the meal. Provide oral care, wash hands, and make him or her comfortable. Check positioning. Elevate the head of the bed to at least 30-45 degrees. Cover him or her with a bib or a large napkin. Remember to preserve a resident's dignity at all times. Take food items off the tray and place them on the table (Fig. 16-7). Encourage residents to help in any way possible, such as by holding a cup. Report the menu and talk in a courteous conversational tone.
2. Choose a spoon with which a resident can easily remove the food. This is generally a teaspoon rather than a soup spoon. Avoid using a syringe unless instructed otherwise. Syringe feeding increases the risk of choking or aspiration. Feed residents in a manner as close to normal as possible to preserve their dignity (Fig. 16-8).

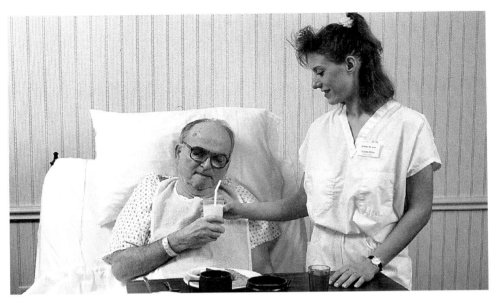

Fig. 16-7. Remove all food items from the tray, and place them on the table. Encourage autonomy.

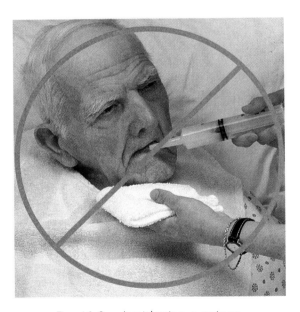

Fig. 16-8. Avoid using a syringe.

3. Be aware of food temperatures. If the food seems too hot, allow time for it to cool. Do not mix foods together unless a resident asks.

4. Encourage residents to eat more nutritious foods first. Save dessert until last if at all possible. Offer small bites, making sure each bite is swallowed before offering another. Do not rush. Offer liquids between bites to keep the mouth moist (Fig. 16-9).

5. Maintain a caring attitude.

6. Encourage residents to eat all of the meal. As with self-fed residents, offer to obtain a substitute if intake is poor or foods are refused.

7. When the resident is finished eating, remove food items and tray.

8. Provide oral care.

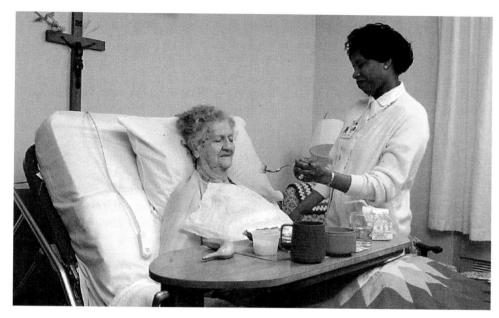

Fig. 16-9. Feed a resident nutritious foods first and do not rush the resident.

Remember this resident depends completely on you and others for his or her nutrition. Picture your own family member in this situation. Before leaving a resident, ask yourself:

▶ Have I done all I can to encourage this resident to eat?
▶ Have I provided the best nutrition possible?

Assisting Residents with Dysphagia

The term "dysphagia" refers to any problem chewing or swallowing food, beverages, or medications. It is not a disease but is rather a condition that affects swallowing. Dysphagia can be caused by stroke or head injury.

Residents with dysphagia may aspirate some of their food. This means that some of the food they eat falls into the lungs rather than through the esophagus into the stomach. Pneumonia or pulmonary infection may occur, which can be fatal. A resident may fear eating because of a fear of choking. As a result, inadequate intake and weight loss may occur.

Many problems caused by dysphagia can be corrected with proper diagnosis and treatment. The therapist may give you special instructions on feeding a resident to prevent problems. Positioning is very important. Follow instructions carefully to help the resident swallow without choking.

The therapist may also recommend a modified diet such as a pureed diet with thickened liquids to enhance swallowing ability. Some residents tolerate thick liquids better than thin. Products are available to thicken liquids, even water and coffee.

How do you recognize dysphagia? Observe residents for symptoms such as the following, and be sure to report any of these to the charge nurse:

▶ Coughing before, during, or after swallowing food, liquid, or medications
▶ Having to swallow 3 or 4 times after each bite
▶ Hoarse, breathy voice or gurgling breathing
▶ Drooling
▶ The feeling that something is caught in the throat
▶ Pocketing food in the side of the mouth
▶ A repetitive rocking motion of the tongue from front to back

A resident can be a "silent aspirator." This means that dysphagia may be present even without these symptoms. Indications of silent aspiration may include:

▶ Unexplained weight loss
▶ Decreased appetite
▶ A persistent low grade fever

If you have a resident with one or more of these symptoms, dysphagia could be a contributing factor. Discuss your observations with the charge nurse.

Important Observations while Eating

As you assist with meals, monitor residents' intake as part of good care. You may make observations that should be passed on to the nurse, such as:

▶ Avoidance of any major food groups, such as not eating meats or not drinking milk
▶ Consistently eating less than 75% (or 3/4) of meals, especially if a resident is underweight or losing weight
▶ Complaints of repeatedly receiving foods he or she does not like and will not eat
▶ A change in status such as needing more help with meals
▶ Changed behaviors such as playing with the food or taking food from other trays
▶ Choking easily
▶ Apparent difficulty chewing or swallowing
▶ Frequent complaints about the food or diet
▶ Trembling hands resulting in difficulty moving food or liquids to the mouth
▶ A changing attitude, becoming depressed or lethargic

Special Devices for Eating

Residents who have difficulty feeding themselves may benefit from special utensils, such as special spoons and forks, cups, and plates. Residents have to be taught to use these devices (Fig. 16-10). Usually the occupational therapist does this.

Residents with Feeding Tubes

Some residents cannot eat any food at all or enough food to keep them alive. Depending on the decision made by a resident or family member responsible, a

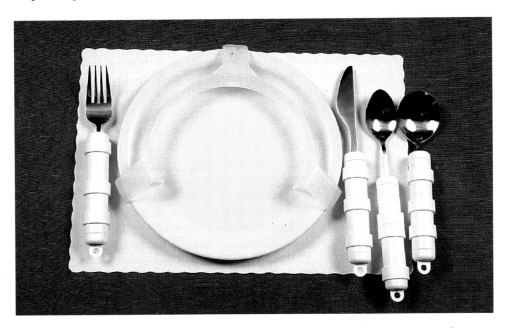

Fig. 16-10. Special eating utensils include spoons, forks, cups, and plates.

tube may be used to feed him or her. A special tube can be placed either directly into the stomach or into the stomach through the nose (Fig. 16-11).

The nurse feeds these residents, but you need to be sure that the resident is positioned with the head of the bed up at least 30 degrees, semi-Fowler's to Fowler's position, while the person is being fed and for about 1 hour afterward. This keeps the liquid from flowing back and causing him or her to choke and aspirate the fluid.

Assessing Good Nutrition

Nutrition and hydration affect residents' quality of life and quality of care in many ways. Nutrition and hydration:

▶ Maintain skin integrity, to prevent or heal pressure sores

▶ Help the body fight infections and disease

▶ Maintain overall strength, which is necessary to preserve functional abilities such as ambulation, independence in feeding, and ability to perform activities of daily living

▶ Maintain normal bowel and bladder functions

▶ Maintain normal weight and energy stores

Nutritional needs increase in conditions such as elevated temperature, recent fractures, surgery, and pressure sores. Fluid needs increase in cases of fever, urinary tract infections, and persistent vomiting and diarrhea. Hot weather increases fluid needs because of body fluid loss through perspiration.

Because adequate food and fluid intake are necessary for residents' health and well-being, intake measurements are important. These measurements help determine when and if to use nutritional intervention.

Evaluating Food Intake

Consider the following examples of two different residents:

▶ Resident #1 has lost 10 pounds in the past 2 months. He is eating 100% of his meals.

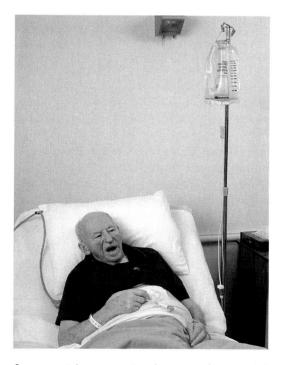

Fig. 16-11. Some residents require the use of a special eating tube because they are unable to eat food at all.

▶ Resident #2 has also lost 10 pounds in the past 2 months. He is eating less than 25% of his meals.

The food intake record tells us that these two residents may have totally different problems. Since Resident #1 is consuming all his meals, he may be losing weight due to a disease rather than insufficient calorie intake. Although additional calories will be added, further studies such as lab work may be necessary. Resident #2 does not appear to be getting sufficient calories. The focus will be on finding ways to increase his intake, such as supplements or tube feeding. Without accurate intake records, these residents could not be evaluated correctly.

Intake is usually expressed in percentage of food given: 100%, 75%, etc. This allows the dietitians to calculate the number of calories or amount of protein consumed. Many forms are available for recording dietary intake, depending on the facility. In general, evaluating intake is somewhat subjective because the nurse assistant observes the meal and judges the percentage eaten. Since it is impossible to actually measure the amount of food eaten, this method is often used. Take the time to evaluate the intake of each resident carefully and to record the percentage eaten immediately. It may help to use a pocket note pad and transfer the information to the flow sheet later.

Evaluating Fluid Intake

As with food, adequate fluid intake is vital. Fluid intake must be adequate to keep the body healthy. Diseases that cause mental or physical incapacity can reduce a resident's ability to recognize or express thirst. If a person does not drink enough, whether he is healthy or sick, a very serious condition can occur called dehydration. A person who is <u>dehydrated</u> may:

▶ Become suddenly confused
▶ Be more sleepy than usual
▶ Have skin that can be easily "tented," meaning you can pull up skin between your thumb and forefinger to form a "tent"
▶ Have dry eyes and dry mouth
▶ Be constipated

If you notice any of these things in a resident, <u>report it immediately</u>. This is an emergency that needs treatment.

The following examples help illustrate how quickly a person can become dehydrated:

▶ If a resident is thirsty yet shows few clinical signs of dehydration such as poor skin turgor, he or she may already need fluid replacement equal to 2% of body weight. A 70 kg (154 lbs.) man would need 1400 cc of fluid at this point.
▶ If this resident has consumed no water in 3-4 days, has a dry mouth, and little urine output, fluid replacement needed may be equal to 6% of body weight, or 4200 cc.

Although fluid requirements vary depending on a person's age, size, physical condition, and level of activity, most residents require 1500-2000 cc per day. Residents with diseases such as congestive heart failure (CHF) or renal disease may be restricted to a lower level. In these residents too much fluid can result in edema, causing too much fluid in places like their legs and ankles, which become swollen. The physician makes the decision and give instructions about how much fluid to allow.

Unless a resident is on a fluid restriction, fluids should be offered and encouraged frequently. To assist with adequate fluid intake, you should:

▶ Make sure every resident has a water pitcher. Place the pitcher within easy reach of a resident.
▶ Make sure the water is changed at least once each shift.
▶ Make sure there is a clean cup next to the water pitcher.

▶ Place a clean straw with a bendable neck next to the cup for those residents who may have difficulty drinking from a cup but have an easier time with a straw.

▶ Often remind everyone to have a drink, helping as needed (Fig. 16-12).

To record fluid intake, you need to know the capacity of common fluid containers. The guide in Table 16-1 may be helpful.

At times it is critical to monitor a resident's fluid intake and output (I & O). A person's output—amount of urine—depends on how much fluid has been taken in. The normal amount of urine put out is about 1500 cc per day. Recording on an I & O sheet is usually done after meals and immediately after serving fluids and assisting with toileting. A resident's I & O sheet is often kept in his or her room on the door or on the foot board. When recording intake and output, you should:

▶ Know how much fluid the commonly used glasses and cups in your facility hold.

▶ Accurately record all fluid intake in the appropriate space for your shift on the I & O sheet (Fig. 16-13). Remember to count any liquids given throughout the day.

Output may be difficult to measure. You should:

▶ Offer a bedpan or urinal.

▶ Pour the urine into a measuring cup and measure it. Record the output in the appropriate space for your shift on the I & O sheet.

If a person is incontinent, you will have to:

▶ Count the number of times he or she is incontinent and put an "X" on the output sheet for each incontinence. Describe volume: very small, moderate, or large.

▶ Check him or her frequently for wetness.

▶ Change him or her each time he is wet.

Note: If a resident is incontinent with diarrhea, it will be difficult to determine urine output. Discuss this situation with the charge nurse.

If a resident has an indwelling Foley catheter, the amount of urine is measured in the collecting bag at the end of each shift or when the bag is full.

Height and Weight

A resident's height is measured only on admission since this does not usually change. The weight is taken on admission and then at least once a month, or more

TABLE 16-1. Capacities of Common Containers

Container	cc
1 oz	**30 cc**
Water tumbler	240 cc
Iced tea glass	240 cc
Juice glass—4 fluid oz	120 cc
Coffee cup	180 cc
Individual coffee pot	240 cc
Individual pot of broth	240 cc
Ice cream—3 fluid oz	90 cc
Sherbet—4 fluid oz container	120 cc
Styrofoam cups—6 fluid oz, 3 1/4" tall	180 cc
4 oz juice cup	120 cc
6 oz can orange juice	180 cc
soup bowl—6 fluid oz	180 cc
cereal bowl—8 fluid oz	240 cc
carton of milk	240 cc
Jell-O—1/2 cup	120 cc

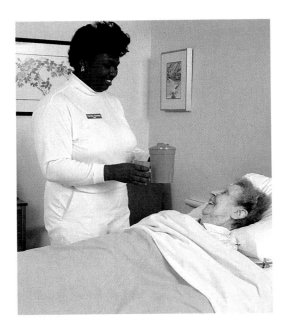

Fig. 16-12. Encourage residents to drink.

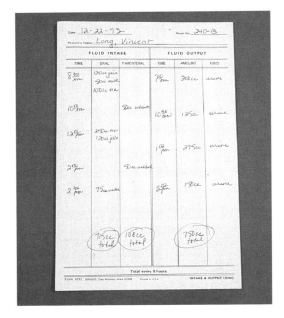

Fig. 16-13. Example of an input and output sheet.

often if ordered by the doctor. These measures help the nursing staff, dietitian, and doctor know if a resident's weight is normal for his or her height, sex, and age. The weight is taken regularly to see if the person is gaining or losing weight. Weight measurement is sometimes also used to calculate drug dosages and monitor diet and drug therapy success.

Weight is one of the most important indicators of nutritional status. One's weight status depends on one's height as well. Height is the most commonly used measurement for determining ideal body weight. For example, if a female resident is 5′5″ tall and weighs 130 pounds, this resident is considered neither obese nor underweight. But a resident who is 4′10″ and weighs 130 pounds is overweight.

Weight

Weight is interpreted in several ways. Weight is often calculated as either percentage of ideal weight or percentage of usual weight. Both of these are important. Percentage of ideal gives us a benchmark comparison for evaluating a resident's weight. For example, if a man is 30% above his ideal range, he is considered obese. We could not label him obese without first establishing a normal, or ideal, weight range. The dietitian or dietary manager calculates ideal weight.

Percentage of usual weight is also very important. If a female resident's normal weight is 120 pounds but she weighs 100 pounds when she is admitted to the facility, we see that she has lost 17% of her usual weight and so can be considered at risk for poor nutritional status. If, however, she has not weighed over 100 pounds for the last 10 years, we may accept this weight as normal for her and just monitor her weight closely.

Weight is usually measured each month, or more often if a resident has lost weight, is not eating, or is needed for other reasons like monitoring drug success. Accuracy is important because weight is an indication of a resident's health (Fig. 16-14). Underweight patients are less resistant to infection, have increased sensitivity to cold, and may have overall weakness. Weight loss should be called to the nurse's attention at once. A weight change is considered severe in these conditions:

▶ Loss of 5 pounds in 1 month
▶ Loss of 7.5% of body weight or greater in 3 months (for a 120 lb person, this would be a 9 lb loss)
▶ Loss of 10% of body weight or greater in 6 months (for a 120 lb person, this would be a 12 lb loss)

Because accuracy is so important, weight fluctuations of 5 pounds or more should be rechecked and confirmed before they are recorded and reported.

Weight can be measured in several ways, depending on a resident's status. If the person can stand, a scale is usually used. Scales for wheelchairs are also available. For residents confined to bed, lift scales are used. You will learn to use the type of scales used in your facility. Follow these guidelines:

▶ The scale should be checked periodically for accuracy.
▶ Always weigh a resident on the same scale. There may be slight differences between scales.

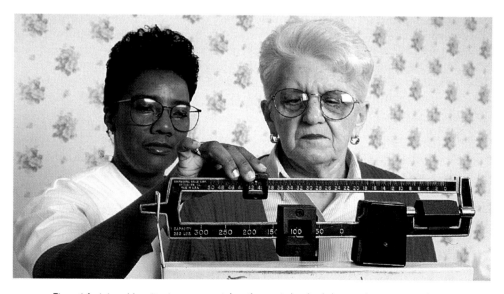

Fig. 16-14. Monitoring a resident's weight helps to determine how healthy a resident is.

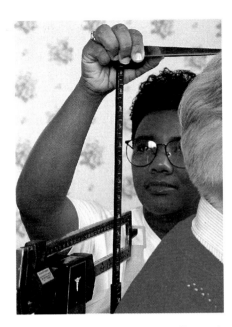

Fig. 16-15. Measuring a resident's height allows the staff to better evaluate a resident's weight.

▶ Try to weigh a resident at the same time of day and with the same amount of clothing.

▶ If a resident's weight has fluctuated more than 5 pounds over the previous month, reweigh him or her and report the weight change to the nurse.

Height

Weight cannot be properly evaluated without height. Height is difficult to measure for residents who cannot stand erect or with diseases such as arthritis or osteoporosis.

Asking alert and oriented residents to report their height provides a good guide for determining about what their height measurement should be. Height must still be measured, because it does progressively decrease with age. Knowing a resident's previous height will give you an idea whether your measurement is accurate. If, for example, Mr. Smith states his height as 5′8″ and your measurement is 5′7″, your measurement is probably correct. If, however, your measurement shows him to be 5′11″, you should measure again.

Height, like weight, is measured according to the person's status. Ambulatory residents should be measured standing, preferably without shoes. The measurement can be taken with a resident standing against the wall or standing on an ambulatory scale with a vertical measuring device (Fig. 16-15). If a resident is confined to bed, measure height with him or her lying flat on the mattress, face toward the ceiling. Using a tape measure, measure from the crown of the head to the bottom of the heel. Then calculate the height in feet and inches.

Residents with contractures may need to be measured by special means such as a knee-height caliper. This is usually done by the dietician. Discuss these residents with the nurse.

Height and weight measurements made at the time of admission are used as baseline data for the stay of a resident in the facility. If these baseline data are wrong, this can affect the person's assessment and plan of care for months or years.

Measuring Height and Weight Using an Upright Scale

Items Needed
▶ Scale with a height measure
▶ Paper towel

1. Determine if the resident can walk to the scale or whether you need to bring the portable scale into his or her room.
2. Before he or she steps on the scale, adjust the height measure higher than the resident's height.
3. Ask the resident his or her height as a check for accuracy.
4. Clear the scale and make sure it is balanced by monitoring the weight all the way over to the left.
5. Place a paper towel on the scale platform and help the resident stand on the scale. Make sure he or she is not holding anything.
6. Have the resident stand up straight, with the arms by his or her side and the eyes looking forward. Slowly lower the height measure to the top of his or her head. Record the height in inches.
7. Proceed to measure the resident's weight by moving the weights to the right until the balance is centered. *Note:* If there is a fluctuation of 5 pounds or more, reweigh the resident before reporting it to the nurse.
8. Assist the resident off the scale.
9. Record the height and weight on your worksheet and report findings to the nurse. Example of charting: Ht. 5'6", Wt. 135 lbs *Note:* Your facility may have special scales that weigh residents while they are in a wheelchair or if they are confined to bed. Follow your facility's policy for these.

Remember:
▶ Resident preference
▶ Common preparation steps
▶ Equipment and supplies needed
▶ Environment preparation
▶ Resident preparation

Remember:
▶ Meet resident needs
▶ Common completion steps
▶ Clean and put away equipment and supplies
▶ Environment completion (Is it safe? Is it clean?)

IN THIS CHAPTER YOU LEARNED TO:
▶ explain the role of the dietary department and how the nurse assistant works with that department
▶ list ways to provide and encourage good nutrition
▶ give examples of ways to make dining a pleasant experience
▶ demonstrate the proper recording procedure for intake and output
▶ demonstrate the skills for measuring height and weight

[Handwritten notes:]

Theig - Dr order —

↑ protein for bed sores.

CIB?

CHF maybe on restrictution (liq)

90 dregess ↑ while eating

17

5 pages long

ASSISTING WITH ELIMINATION

Elimination is the term for ridding the body of urine and stool. We all do it, but usually we don't think about it much. When you feel the urge to go to the bathroom, you probably just meet this need by going to the bathroom. But have you ever been in the situation where you really had to go but couldn't find a bathroom? Being unable to go probably kept you from thinking about anything else until you took care of this very basic need.

Think about how you might feel if you could not get to the bathroom easily. How would you feel having to depend on someone else to help with something so private? Think about how residents you care for feel about this too. As we age, food passes through the digestive tract more slowly and digestion slows, resulting in slowed bowel pattern and decreased absorption of nutrients. These normal aging changes may result in a concern about constipation or appetite. Helping with elimination and talking about it with residents may not be one of your favorite tasks as a nurse assistant, but you need to keep in mind residents' feelings and make the situation as private, dignified, and comfortable as possible.

EQUIPMENT FOR ELIMINATION

Some residents need assistance with elimination. They may need to use special equipment. A toilet, bedpan, urinal, or bedside commode can be used. Using a bathroom toilet to urinate or have a bowel movement is the easiest and most familiar method of elimination. A resident who cannot get to the bathroom may use a bedpan, urinal, or bedside commode. When a resident uses any method other than the toilet, try to create an environment that feels as private and normal as going to the bathroom.

Bedpans are used by both male and female residents for elimination. The two types are the large regular bedpan and the small fracture pan used for residents with hip problems (Fig. 17-1). Urinals are used by male residents for urinating when in bed.

A bedside commode is a portable toilet. A resident needs only to move out of the bed to the commode positioned nearby. Most models are simply a chair with a seat cover and a container under the seat that catches the urine and stool (Fig. 17-2).

DETERMINING ELIMINATION PATTERNS

Every resident has his or her own pattern of elimination, involving the frequency of elimination and the usual amount of urine and stool. Some residents urinate more often than others. Some residents normally move their bowels daily, and others every other or every third day. You learn a resident's normal pattern so that you know when a problem or illness changes it. A change in elimination can result from a simple change in food or fluid amounts or a serious condition like cancer. Determine how and when a resident eliminates in the following three ways:

1. Talk to a resident about his or her usual pattern.

   ▸ Get to know each resident.

   ▸ Develop a trusting relationship. Elimination is a private act, but a resident who trusts you feels more at ease answering your questions (Fig. 17-3).

   ▸ Ask the following questions privately: How often do you have a bowel movement? What time of day do you normally have a bowel movement? Is

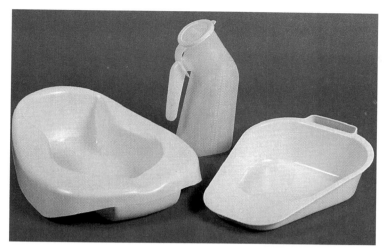

Fig. 17-1. The regular bedpan, fracture bedpan and urinal.

[handwritten notes:]
I) Constipation
A) ↑ Liq intake
↑ fiber
↑ exercise
↑ fresh veg.

routine bowel Reation
RBR~

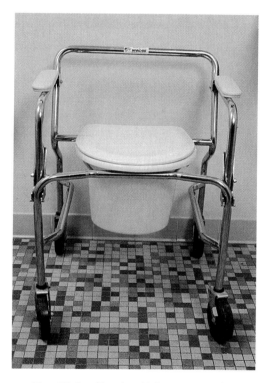

Fig. 17-2. The bedside commode.

there anything I should know that will help maintain your normal schedule? How often do you urinate? Do you urinate in large or small amounts? Do you have a pattern such as before breakfast, after lunch, before dinner and bedtime? Do you wake up at night?

2. Ask family members, if a resident can't tell you about how he or she eliminates.

3. Review a resident's chart to establish the patterns. The chart usually contains the following information:
   ▶ How often does the person have a bowel movement?
   ▶ What is the urine pattern and amount?
   ▶ On what shift does a resident usually have a bowel movement?

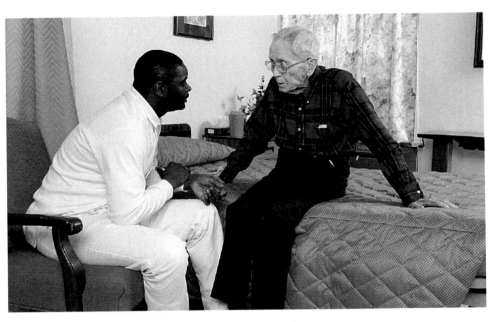

Fig. 17-3.   Get to know the resident in your care.

▶ What is the amount, color, and consistency of a resident's bowel movement?
▶ Is the resident incontinent? (When a resident is incontinent it means for some reason he or she is unable to control the flow of urine and or stool.)

Once you know a resident's normal bowel and urination patterns, do all you can to help these patterns stay normal. Changes in patterns can lead to problems, especially with the bowel, like constipation.

Tips for Promoting Regular Elimination Patterns

Promptly help residents to the bathroom when you are asked. If a resident cannot ask, help him or her to the bathroom upon awakening, before and after meals, at bedtime, when he or she wakes at night, and any time you think he or she may have to go, based on information you have.

Respond to call signals promptly.

Make sure residents eat a well-balanced diet and drink plenty of fluids, especially water.

Make sure you wash your hands before and after helping each resident so that you do not pass germs from one resident to another. Wear gloves when you assist with perineal care or emptying a bedpan, urinal, or bedside commode.

Make sure residents get adequate rest and exercise.

MAINTAINING RESIDENTS' DIGNITY WHEN ASSISTING WITH ELIMINATION

Elimination is a very private act. Consider that a resident's elimination, like bathing or grooming, is something he or she had always done alone and in private. Residents who now need your help still have the right to dignity, respect, and privacy. You can do several things to help maintain a resident's dignity when assisting with elimination:

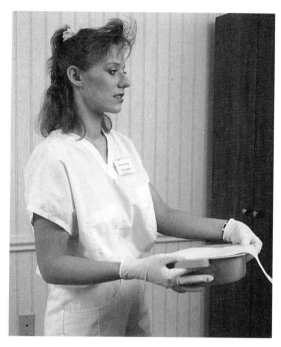

Fig. 17-4. Using gloves while assisting with elimination is for infection control.

1 ▶ Ask questions about elimination only in private.
2 ▶ Always maintain a professional attitude. Never use nicknames, slang words, or unprofessional gestures.
3 ▶ Help residents in a private setting. Close the door, pull the bedside curtains around the bed, and cover the person. Ask others to leave the room if possible.
4 ▶ Explain why you wear gloves during the procedure. Let residents know this is infection control that is used with all residents and that it protects them as well as you (Fig. 17-4).

ASSISTING WITH ELIMINATION

Assist a resident with elimination by helping with a bedpan, urinal, and portable commode. The item you use depends on the person's needs. For example, a male resident who is continent but does not want to walk to the bathroom at night may choose to use a urinal. Offering a male resident who cannot communicate his needs the use of a commode may be helpful. Do the best you can to determine a resident's need. Offer female residents use of a bedpan or commode. Offer male residents use of a urinal for urinating only and a bedpan or commode for both.

Using a Bedpan

Items Needed

▶ Bedpan and bedpan cover
▶ Wash basin
▶ 2 Towels
▶ Soap
▶ Toilet paper
▶ 2 Pairs gloves
▶ 2 Plastic-covered pads or protective covers

1. Put a pad or cover on the surface where you will put the bedpan after use.
2. Fold the spread and blanket down to the bottom of the bed, leaving the top sheet to cover the lower legs. Help the resident to lift nightgown or remove pajama bottoms and underpants.

Remember:
▶ Resident preference
▶ Common preparation steps
▶ Equipment and supplies needed
▶ Environment preparation
▶ Resident preparation

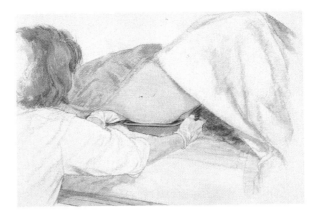

Fig. 17-5. Proper placement of bedpan under buttocks.

3. Place protective covering under the buttocks to protect the bed linen.
4. Ask the resident to bend both knees and lift buttocks up while you slide the bedpan underneath him or her. Adjust it for the person's comfort.
   Note: If the resident does not have the strength to lift his or her buttocks, ask or help him or her turn onto one side (as described in Chapter 13). Place the bedpan flush against the resident's buttocks. Then have him or her turn back over onto the bedpan (Fig. 17-5). (You may need help from another nurse assistant for this.)
5. Cover the resident with the top sheet for privacy.
6. Pull the side rail up, if used.
7. Elevate the head of the bed slowly until the resident is in a sitting position. (Remember, you are trying to create a normal setting.) Ask the resident if he or she is comfortable. Readjust the position of the bedpan until he or she is comfortable.
8. Provide toilet paper and position the call light for the resident. Tell him or her to call you when finished. *Note:* If a resident cannot tell you he or she is finished, check on him or her every 5 minutes. Because bedpans put pressure on the skin, do not leave a resident on a bedpan longer than necessary.

To remove a resident from the bedpan:
9. Put on gloves.
10. Lower the head of the bed. Ask the resident to raise his or her buttocks upward while you slide the bedpan out, or help him or her roll onto one side while holding the bedpan to prevent a spill. Move the bedpan to the covered surface.
11. If needed, assist in wiping the perineal area. *Note:* If you help with wiping, dispose of the toilet tissue into the used bedpan unless a specimen is needed. If a specimen is needed, dispose of the used toilet tissue into a plastic trash bag. You may need to wash the perineal area (remember to wash, rinse, and dry thoroughly). Remember to wash or wipe from front to back. Remove and dispose of the protective pad over the bed linen.
12. Help the resident to wash his or her hands.
    Note: If perineal washing was necessary, change the water and use a fresh washcloth and towel for hand washing.
13. Put the bedpan cover over the bedpan and dispose of the contents in the resident's toilet. Remove and dispose of the protective pad on which you put the bedpan.
14. Remove and dispose of your gloves in the disposable trash bag, throw trash bag away, and wash your hands.

Remember:

▶ Meet resident needs
▶ Common completion steps
▶ Clean and put away equipment and supplies
▶ Environment completion (Is it safe? Is it clean?)

Using a Urinal

1. Put a pad or cover on the surface where you will put the urinal after use.
2. If the resident can stand beside the bed to use the urinal, help him to stand and provide privacy and then continue with Steps 7-13 following.

If a resident uses the urinal while in bed, follow these steps:
3. Remove the top linens and assist with lowering bottom clothing.
4. Put on gloves.
5. Place the urinal between the resident's legs at an angle to avoid urine spillage. Gently place the penis into the urinal (Fig. 17-6).
6. Cover the resident with the top sheet and give him the call light. Tell him to call you when he is done. Check in a few minutes if he does not call you.
7. When the resident is finished, remove the urinal and place it on the covered surface.
8. Assist the resident in wiping off excess urine with toilet tissue. Dispose of tissue in the plastic trash bag.
9. Assist the resident with washing, rinsing, and drying hands.
10. Take off gloves and put them in disposable trash bag.
11. Put new gloves on.
12. Empty the urinal, clean it, and replace it at bedside table.
13. Remove and dispose of gloves in the disposable trash bag, and wash your hands.

Remember:
▶ Resident preference
▶ Common preparation steps
▶ Equipment and supplies needed
▶ Environment preparation
▶ Resident preparation

Remember:
▶ Meet resident needs
▶ Common completion steps
▶ Clean and put away equipment and supplies
▶ Environment completion (Is it safe? Is it clean?)

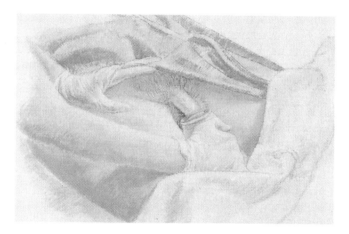

Fig. 17-6. Proper placement of urinal.

Using a Portable Commode

1. Help the resident out of bed to a standing position (as described in Chapter 13). Help pull down the resident's lower clothing and help him or her sit on the commode positioned by the bed.
2. Provide toilet paper and put the call light within reach.
3. When the resident is finished and is unable to wipe:
   a. Put on gloves.
   b. Assist with wiping and throw the tissue into the commode or the plastic trash bag.
   c. Take off gloves and put them in the plastic trash bag.
4. Help the resident pull up clothing and get back into bed or chair.
5. Help the resident wash, rinse, and dry his or her hands.
6. Put on new gloves.

Remember:
▶ Resident preference
▶ Common preparation steps
▶ Equipment and supplies needed
▶ Environment preparation
▶ Resident preference

7. Remove the container and empty its contents.
8. Clean, dry, and replace the container.
9. Remove and dispose of the gloves in the plastic bag.

**IN THIS CHAPTER YOU
LEARNED TO:**

▶ identify equip-
   ment used for
   elimination

▶ determine resi-
   dents' elimination
   patterns

▶ list ways to main-
   tain a resident's
   dignity when as-
   sisting with elimi-
   nation

▶ demonstrate the
   correct way to as-
   sist a resident in
   using the bedpan,
   urinal, and
   portable com-
   mode

▶ identify changes in
   residents' elimina-
   tion patterns

PROBLEMS WITH ELIMINATION

When you are helping a resident with elimination, watch for anything unusual or any problems a resident reports. Be especially watchful for the signs and symptoms of a urinary tract infection. If you observe any of the following, report them immediately to the charge nurse:

▶ Pain or burning sensation when urinating
▶ Foul-smelling urine
▶ Blood in the urine
▶ A resident often uses the bathroom, bedpan, urinal, or commode, but produces only a small amount of urine
▶ Lower abdominal discomfort

In addition, you may note and must report any other unusual observations. Report any of the following to the charge nurse:

▶ A resident has not urinated during your shift.
▶ A resident is incontinent.
▶ A resident who has never been incontinent suddenly has an accident.
▶ A resident has difficulty moving his or her bowels.
▶ A resident strains more while having a bowel movement.
▶ There is blood in a resident's stool. This can be bright red blood or black.
▶ A resident has frequent, watery stools.
▶ A resident's stool smells foul.
▶ The urine is not a light amber color but dark and concentrated.
▶ Stool is not brown and soft but greenish, black, hard, or watery.
▶ A resident's abdomen is bloated or swollen and he or she has not had a bowel movement recently.
▶ A resident has swollen, bleeding tissue around the anus.
▶ A resident has more difficulty getting to the bathroom.

Some of these situations may have a simple solution, but others require immediate medical attention. For example, a change in color of a resident's stool from brown to black can be a sign of gastrointestinal bleeding, a serious problem that must be reported immediately. You must know what is normal for residents you care for so that you will notice and report situations when things are not normal.

Common chronic illnesses and problems of the urinary and gastrointestinal system are described in detail in Chapter 24.

18

ADDITIONAL RESPONSIBILITIES

Gaining knowledge and responsibility is an important growing experience. As you become more comfortable in your job, your capabilities and responsibilities will grow. You will be asked to perform new tasks to meet the needs of individual residents. Some of these skills you will likely use every day, and some you will not use very often. The needs of residents in your facility determine what skills you will need. This chapter is a reference guide for additional responsibilities that you may take on in your career as a nurse assistant. The information here is organized in three general parts:

1. General information on how to admit, discharge, and transfer a resident
2. Special skills such as taking vital signs, specimen collection, use of nonsterile bandages and dressings, use of support hose and elastic stockings, application of topical preparations, hot and cold applications, and ostomy care
3. Emergency procedures such as what to do in the event of a cardiac arrest or seizure, as well as finding a wandering resident, helping a choking resident, and other emergencies

While you are learning this knowledge and these skills, you will see how versatile your career really is. Use every opportunity you have to learn more about meeting the needs of your residents. The skill information in this chapter applies to meeting the needs of residents with the common chronic illnesses, diseases, and problems covered in Chapter 24.

ADMISSION OF RESIDENTS

As you learned early in this text, residents are admitted to a long term care facility when their physical or mental abilities make it too difficult to remain at home. At that point a determination is made that 24-hour nursing care is required. Needless to say, this often becomes a very stressful situation for both a resident and the family (Fig. 18-1).

Sometimes a resident is admitted from his or her own home or a family member's. Sometimes a resident comes from the hospital or another facility. Each resident who is admitted has individual needs and concerns. From the minute a person begins the process of admission, use the six total quality management (TQM) skills you learned in Chapter 1 for the individual resident who is your customer. Remember how you want to be treated when you are a customer and treat each resident with the same respect.

Being admitted to a long term care facility is a very emotional and anxiety producing experience. You can make this experience much less difficult and trying. Remember the following when a resident is being admitted:

▶ A resident often is upset about being admitted. A friendly, home-like, caring, and welcoming atmosphere may help to make him or her feel more comfortable.

▶ A resident may feel fearful about the unknown and have many questions like, "Will staff know who I am and what I need?"

▶ How will I know what I can do in this place?

▶ Will my family and friends visit me here?

▶ Can I keep doing the things I have enjoyed doing?

▶ Can I get up in the morning and go to bed when I want? Can I bathe when I wish? Can I eat what I like and when I like?

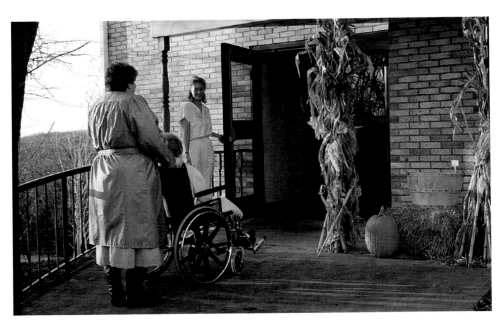

Fig. 18-1. When it is determined that 24-hour care is required for a person, it may cause stress to the resident and the family.

The Interdisciplinary Approach for Admission

The admission of a resident is a complex effort. Examples of how the departments might become involved include:

▶ *Social worker.* This individual may work as an admissions coordinator with a resident, the family, perhaps the social worker in another facility, and the staff in your facility. The social worker also helps complete admission paperwork and do a social history. The social worker is the front line person initially.

▶ *Housekeeping.* They help clean and set up the new room. They might also assist in helping residents move in.

▶ *Dietary.* They interview residents or family to find out what food preferences they have.

▶ *Maintenance.* They may assist moving residents into the facility and putting in a phone for residents who want one.

▶ *Front Office.* They assist with financial concerns and payment schedules. They might also give appropriate information on how to apply for Medicaid.

▶ *Nursing.* The charge nurse makes sure all equipment and medication needs are ready and available for a resident on admission. She or he must assess each resident carefully and document all findings. The charge nurse initiates the Resident Assessment Instrument (RAI) (Chapter 12). The charge nurse answers questions a resident and family might have and helps make them feel as comfortable as possible. The nurse also obtains or confirms orders with the physician. All team members work closely together to make the admission a successful experience for your new customer.

What Can You Do to Prepare for the New Resident?

▶ Check that the bed is made, a pillow is on the bed (with the opening on the pillow case away from the door), and a blanket is available in the room or in the unit's linen closet (Fig. 18-2).

▶ Check that a chair and reading light are in place and that the light is working.

▶ Check that the call light is in place and working properly.

▶ Check that the bed's electric or manual cranks are working.

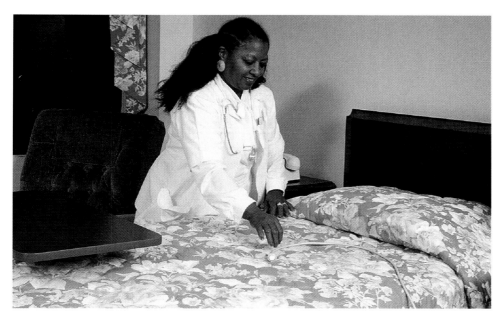

Fig. 18-2. Make sure that the room is ready for the new resident.

▷ Check that bed siderails are working properly.
▷ Check that personal care supplies such as washcloth, towel, soap, and soap dish, are in place (if you already know the person cannot get to the bathroom, have a clean bed pan, and a urinal for a male resident, in the bedside table.)
▷ Check that a water glass and water pitcher are ready to fill after a resident has been admitted.
▷ Be sure the resident's name is on the door.

A room that is properly prepared gives a sense of welcome to each resident and family. It shows that you are ready, organized, and capable of giving good care.

Greeting Residents

Greeting a resident warmly when he or she first comes to the facility can help make the admission more pleasant. Introduce yourself in a way that inspires confidence in the family and resident and a sense of well-being. Remember how you like to be treated when you are the customer.

To help a resident feel comfortable, you should:

▷ Greet him or her by name, e.g., Miss or Mrs. Smith. Some residents may prefer to be called by their first name. Ask what name they wish you to use, to let the person know you care about who he or she is as an individual (Fig. 18-3).
▷ Appear poised and assured, but warm. Remember, you are one of the first impressions of your facility for residents and their family.
▷ Introduce yourself by name, and let the person know you are a nurse assistant and will be helping him or her get settled. Assure the person someone is there to help if questions come up.
▷ Introduce the new resident to the roommate if the room is shared. This helps both residents feel more comfortable.
▷ Greet any family or friends with the person. This is a good time to begin to know them. Remember, this is most likely a very difficult time for this resident and the family. This process, although routine to you, is not routine to them. Mention to them that the charge nurse on duty can also answer their questions related to care.

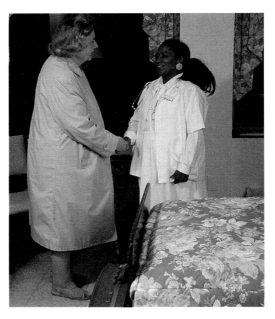

Fig. 18-3. Greet the resident by his or her preferred name or title.

After a resident has unpacked and you have finished filling out forms, such as a personal item inventory list and the basic assessment of the person, start orienting him or her to specific areas and equipment in the facility. This should include:

- Bathroom facilities
- Nurse's call light
- Television and/or radio equipment
- Dining area and mealtime
- Visitors' and/or residents' lounge
- Location of the nurse's station
- Location of the telephone

If a resident cannot leave the room or bed, orient him or her to everything in the room and describe other areas in the facility that he or she can visit at another time (Fig. 18-4).

It may take a while, sometimes as long as six months, for a resident to feel comfortable in his or her new home. It can be very frightening to come from a familiar home to a new environment with many strangers. Plan to spend extra time with and pay special attention to a resident during this time.

DISCHARGE OF A RESIDENT

Discharge is the process that occurs when a resident is leaving the facility. Many emotions come into play. Often the discharge is a very joyful occasion, such as when a resident has improved enough to go home or to a less restrictive facility. Sometimes, however, discharge may not be a happy occasion. We must do our best to help residents and family feel good about the decision made by the things we say and the way we respond to them. The most likely reasons that a resident is discharged are:

- A resident's condition has changed and a different setting is required.
- A resident has improved enough that he or she can go to a less restrictive setting.
- A resident or family dislikes or has a problem with the facility and desires a move.
- The facility a resident is moving to is closer to family and would be more convenient for them to visit.

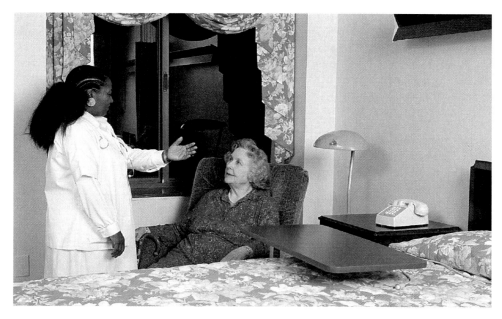

Fig. 18-4. Orient the resident to the room.

Many team members are involved in the discharge planning. For some residents, discharge planning begins the day a resident is admitted to the facility. This is most common for those residents admitted for rehabilitation and subacute care.

Interdisciplinary Approach for Discharging a Resident

The discharge of a resident from a long term care facility impacts other disciplines besides nursing. Examples of how other disciplines become involved might include:

▷ *Social services.* The social worker arranges a discharge planning meeting to help decide what is in a resident's best interest. If a resident goes home, the social worker helps set up community services to meet the person's needs. If a resident is moving to another facility, the social worker networks with it so that the discharge is handled smoothly. The social worker also needs to communicate to the rest of the facility when the discharge will take place.

▷ *Housekeeping.* Housekeeping may be involved in packing up residents' belongings. They help clean and prepare the room after the discharge has taken place.

▷ *Nursing.* The nurse works closely with the physician, resident, family, and social worker to determine the appropriateness for discharge. The nurse obtains the necessary discharge order from the physician. She or he must communicate carefully with this resident and family regarding care instructions. If a resident is going to another facility, the nurse must work closely with the nursing staff in that facility to ensure continuity of care. She or he must write a discharge note, coordinate the discharge plan of care, and send appropriate medications and records.

Helping Residents Adjust

If a resident is going home to a less restrictive setting, be encouraging and let him or her know you are happy with this. If for some reason you feel negatively about the discharge, don't let your feelings impact your attitude or how you carry out this procedure. Remain professional and warm. You may be the last impression a resident and family have of the facility.

Going to a different place will be a change for a resident, even when it's a positive move, and change can be frightening. A resident may be anxious and more demanding of your attention before the change happens. He or she may also feel sad because of leaving other residents and staff, or may feel angry if the change is not to his or her liking. To help a resident with feelings about change, you can:

▶ Accept that a resident may have feelings such as sadness, anger, or fear. Don't try to convince him or her that these feelings are not OK or will go away.

▶ Keep a positive attitude. Even if a resident is leaving because of not liking the facility, you can say, "Another facility may be better able to meet your needs."

▶ Encourage the person to say goodbye to residents and staff.

Ask the social worker to tell the person about the place where he or she is going, if it is unfamiliar. Include:

▶ The name of the place

▶ How big it is

▶ Where it is

▶ Services available

▶ What it looks like

Day of Discharge

When it is the day for a resident to leave, you should:

▶ Have a wheelchair or cart available if needed.

▶ Have personal belongings packed and ready. (Ask the person for permission first.) He or she may wish to do it himself. Have a cart ready to transport belongings (Fig. 18-5).

▶ Be sure you have checked the personal items inventory list, and that each item is accounted for.

▶ The person should be appropriately dressed and groomed.

▶ Go with the person to the exit of the facility.

▶ Do not forget to say goodbye and wish him or her well.

After a resident has left, the room needs to be prepared for the next resident. Usually housekeeping cleans and disinfects the room, but you assist in the preparation of the room for another resident (Fig. 18-6). You should:

▶ Take all the bedding off the bed and place the soiled linen in the laundry bag.

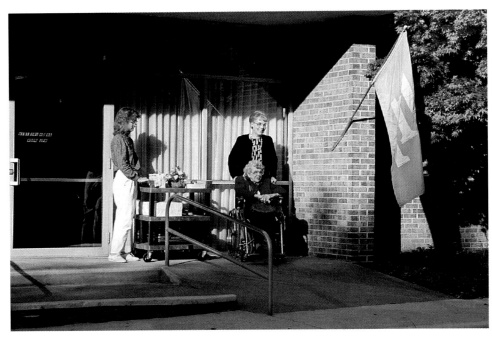

Fig. 18-5. Assist the resident to prepare for discharge from the facility.

▶ Take away all unnecessary articles, including disposable personal care items. Throw any trash away. Take any utensils kept at the bedside table, such as the wash basin and bedpan, to the service room.

Housekeeping will:

▶ Remove the mattress

▶ Clean the bed springs

▶ Wash the frame of the bed and all furniture

▶ Replace the mattress

After the room has been cleaned, you should:

▶ Make the bed with clean linen.

▶ Arrange the bedside table. Put everything in it that should be there for the next resident.

You are now ready for the next resident to be admitted. Note that this same cleaning is done regularly while a resident is in the facility. The charge nurse will show you how to move the resident out of the unit so that it can be cleaned. As always, be careful to see that a resident's belongings are not lost or broken. Treat them as if they were yours. Never throw away anything belonging to a resident without asking first.

TRANSFERRING RESIDENTS

Residents are often transferred to a different unit or wing in a facility for a variety of reasons. A resident, family, and doctor decide this in consultation from the other team members. A common reason is a change in a resident's level of needs or care. For example, a resident is admitted for rehabilitation after having had a stroke. Initially this resident is admitted to a more skilled area in the facility where licensed professionals such as physical therapists, speech therapists, and occupational therapists work closely with residents along with nursing staff to help the person regain as many personal needs skills as possible. After he or she regains lost skills or levels out in abilities, there is less need for such intense work. At that point, another wing or unit might meet a resident's needs just as well, and a transfer would be initiated.

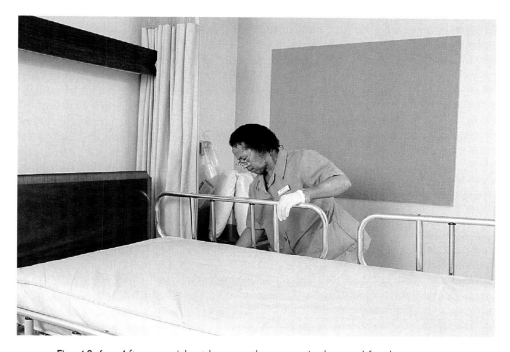

Fig. 18-6. After a resident leaves, the room is cleaned for the next resident.

Even though a person who is being transferred is already a resident in a facility, it can still be a difficult transition with anxiety, concerns, and questions. You can help minimize the trauma through proper communication and a caring attitude.

Interdisciplinary Approach for Transferring a Resident

It can be an involved procedure to transfer a resident within a facility. Nursing has a role, but so do many other departments in the nursing facility. The following are examples of how the departments work with each other.

▶ *Social worker.* The social worker must get permission from a resident and family before a transfer or a room move can take place. The social worker also communicates with other departments and staff involved, such as dietary, front office, medical records, etc.

▶ *Housekeeping.* Housekeeping cleans the new room to prepare it for the new resident. Housekeeping, at times along with the nursing staff, helps pack the new resident's belongings and actually moves them to the new room.

▶ *Nursing.* The charge nurse helps the new unit or wing become knowledgeable about the new resident. The nurse writes a note in the nursing record about his or her mental and physical condition on transfer. The nurse assists in transferring him or her and taking all treatments and medications to the new wing or unit.

Keep the following things in mind when you are transferring a resident to another unit, wing or room. As with a discharge, a resident may have feelings of loss.

▶ A resident may be upset and concerned about the move. He or she often has gotten used to and attached to the staff, other residents, and even the environment. A resident may not want to leave his or her roommate.

▶ A resident may be concerned that the new unit or wing may not be as accommodating as the former one.

▶ It can be very confusing to switch environments.

▶ This type of procedure is usually very routine to staff, but we must remember it is very stressful to residents.

How You Can Prepare for the Transfer of a Resident

Just as the nurses on the two different wings will communicate about the involved resident, the nurse assistants must do so also (Fig. 18-7). Share information about a resident's likes and dislikes and those ideas and techniques that have proven helpful in caring for him or her. Try to think of any information that would make the transition from one wing to another easier. Be sure before the transfer is actually underway that the right person in your facility has the resident's and family's permission. Be sure that the new room is ready just as for a new admission. Do all this before a resident is transferred. It often is helpful, if a resident is moving off the unit or wing, to call ahead and have representatives from the new staff come over to meet this resident before the transfer.

Transferring Residents

This should be handled professionally and warmly. If you are the nurse assistant conducting the transfer, reassure this resident and alleviate any fears or concerns. If you are the nurse assistant receiving the new resident, greet him or her warmly and genuinely. Use the name he or she is most comfortable using and introduce yourself. Introduce him or her to the new roommate. This helps both residents feel more comfortable. Treat this resident as if he or she were a new admission to the floor or unit. Help unpack and orient him or her to the new room:

▶ Bathroom facilities
▶ Nurse's call light
▶ Television and/or radio
▶ Dining areas and mealtimes

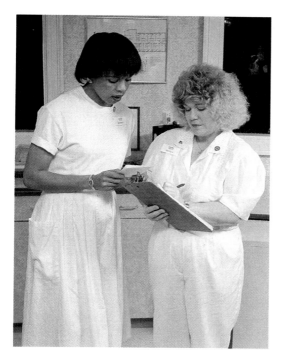

Fig. 18-7. Nurse assistants should communicate about a resident who is transferred.

▶ Visitors' and/or residents' lounge
▶ Location of the nurse's station
▶ Location of the telephone

Orient a resident to these areas even if he or she cannot leave the room or bed, because he or she may be able to in the future. Also make sure that all personal belongings and medical records are transferred.

SPECIAL SKILLS

The following sections describe various skills you may perform on a daily basis. Become familiar with these because they are an important aspect of your role as a nurse assistant. You should always ask for help or get a second opinion if you ever find you're unsure about any of these skills.

VITAL SIGNS

"Vital signs" is a term used for the following:
▶ Temperature
▶ Pulse rate
▶ Respiratory rate
▶ Blood pressure

You must take vital signs carefully and record them accurately. Even the term "vital signs" shows their vital importance. Nurses and physicians rely heavily on accurate records to decide how best to treat a resident's condition. Medications are often ordered based on vital signs records. If a resident's vital signs change or seem abnormal to you, report this immediately to the charge nurse. Vital signs provide objective information about the health of residents.

If ever you are unsure about taking vital signs, get help from your supervisor.

Vital signs are always taken on admission, and at least monthly or as ordered by the doctor. Vital signs are always taken if there is any change in a resident that might indicate illness. Facilities often have a protocol to follow on how often vital signs are taken. Vital signs are recorded in a resident's chart on a special form each time they are taken so that the nurse and doctor can evaluate any changes or abnormalities.

Temperature

Temperature is a measurement of body heat. It can vary slightly sometimes and still be considered normal. Temperature changes during the day, from the lowest in the morning before a person awakens to the highest in the late afternoon and evening.

A higher than normal temperature indicates a fever and possibly an infection. Often, an older person's temperature does not change as much as a younger person's, even with an infection. When a fever occurs there can be other noticeable signs and symptoms. Chapter 23 discusses fever in detail.

There are three ways to measure body temperature with a thermometer:
- Oral (temperature taken in the mouth)
- Rectal (temperature is taken in the rectum)
- Axillary (temperature is taken under the armpit)

The normal range for an oral temperature in an adult is 97.6° F. to 99.6° F. (the F means Fahrenheit scale). The average is 98.6° F. This temperature, using a glass thermometer, is taken for 5 minutes. The normal range for an axillary temperature in an adult is 96.6° to 98.6° F. The average is 97.6° F. This temperature measurement, using a glass thermometer, is taken for 10 minutes. The normal range for a rectal temperature is 98.6° to 100.6° F. The average is 99.6° F. This measurement, using a glass thermometer, is taken for 3 minutes.

There are different types of thermometers commonly used:
- *Oral glass.* This is a glass thermometer with a blue top and long narrow or small rounded tip.
- *Rectal glass.* This is a glass thermometer with a red top and a more rounded tip to prevent injury to rectal tissue.
- *Electronic thermometers.* These may be used in long term care facilities to take oral, rectal, and axillary temperatures. These thermometers are battery charged instruments with removable probes. If an oral or axillary temperature is to be taken, the probe has a blue tip. If a rectal temperature is taken, it has a red tip.
- *Ear Probe:* This thermometer measures the body temperature with a probe in the ear. The body temperature is measured by the heat from blood vessels in the eardrum.

The method you use determines which probe to use and what type of cover to use to protect the probe (Fig. 18-8). You use a lubricated cover for a rectal temperature to avoid discomfort and possible injury to the rectal tissue. Use a nonlubricated cover for an axillary or oral temperature.

Electronic thermometers are quick and easy to use. After the thermometer is inserted, you wait for a beep that indicates the thermometer is ready, and a digital display of the temperature appears on the top. These thermometers need to be recharged to work, so remember to return them for recharging.

Before you can take a resident's temperature, you must understand three skills: how to clean a thermometer, how to shake it down, and how to read it. These three skills are part of the skill of taking a temperature.

How to Clean a Glass Thermometer

To clean a glass thermometer before using it, you should:
1. Hold the stem end under cold running water to rinse off the disinfectant. Use cold water instead of hot water because hot water can break the thermometer. *Note:* This procedure is used if the thermomter is stored in a disinfectant.
2. Wipe the water off the thermometer with a tissue. Wipe from the stem toward the bulb end.

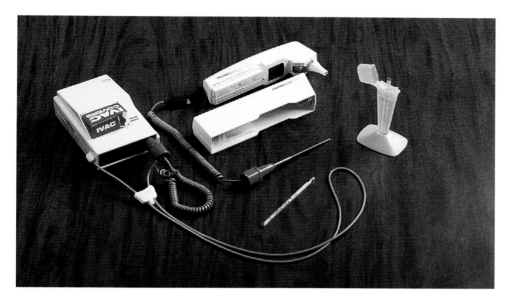

Fig. 18-8.   A resident's temperatures can be measured using one of several types of thermometers.

To clean a glass thermometer after use, you should:
1. Wipe the thermometer with a gauze that has been soaked in a cleansing or disinfectant solution.
2. Wipe the thermometer from the stem end to the bulb end. The bulb end is considered dirty, the part that goes into the mouth; and the stem end is considered cleaner. Twist the thermometer as you wipe it off to ensure full cleaning. Be sure to rinse thoroughly.
3. Replace the thermometer in the dirty/used container in the utility room or follow your facility protocol.

How to Shake Down a Glass Thermometer

You must shake down the mercury in the thermometer to be accurate. Hold the thermometer by the stem. With a quick wrist motion shake the thermometer as if shaking something off the bulb or metal end. Take care to avoid hitting the thermometer on anything. Shake the thermometer down to 95 degrees or lower.

How to Read a Thermometer

The glass thermometer is marked with lines that indicate degrees. Between large lines showing single degrees are five small lines, indicating 0.2. To read the thermometer, follow these steps:
1. Hold the thermometer at eye level to clearly see the lines.
2. Slowly rotate the thermometer until you can see the place when the mercury (silver or red) has stopped.
3. Read the temperature and write it down (Fig. 18-9).

Oral Temperature *5 min*

An oral temperature is the most common and least invasive method used. An oral temperature should *not* be used when:
▶ A resident is on continuous oxygen with a mask or has trouble breathing
▶ A resident is confused or combative
▶ A resident has a mouth disorder or gum disease or has had recent mouth surgery

Handwritten margin notes:
Waite 10 min After eat / Drinking r Smocking

C - Dif taken in the ear.

No g-tube

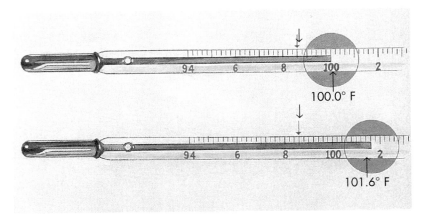

Fig. 18-9. Slowly rotate the thermometer until you can see where the mercury has stopped. Read the temperature and write it down.

> A resident has had a stroke with paralysis on one side of the mouth and cannot hold the thermometer in place

Ask the nurse if you have any questions. Follow this procedure:

Taking an Oral Temperature

Remember:
- Resident preference
- Common preparation steps
- Equipment and supplies needed
- Environment preparation
- Resident preparation

Items Needed
> Glass thermometer and cover
> Watch
> Paper and pencil

Note: Check with the person to make sure he or she has not just eaten something hot or cold or smoked a cigarette. Such activities alter mouth temperature and can give you a false reading. If so, wait 5-10 minutes before proceeding.

1. Shake the thermometer down to 95° F or lower and apply the plastic cover.
2. Insert the bulb end of the thermometer under the resident's tongue, and ask him or her to close the lips around the thermometer (Fig. 18-10). A resident may want to keep the thermometer in place by holding onto the end. A resident should not walk with the thermometer in his or her mouth.
3. Wait 5 minutes and remove the thermometer. As you wait, you can take the pulse and respiratory rates. Wipe off any mucus or remove the plastic cover and read the temperature.
4. If using an electronic thermometer, wait until it beeps.

Remember:
- Meet resident needs
- Common completion steps
- Clean and put away equipment and supplies
- Environment completion (Is it safe? Is it clean?)

Rectal Temperature

The rectal method is used when:
> A resident is confused or very restless and may bite the thermometer if placed in the mouth
> A resident can only breathe through the mouth
> The doctor orders a rectal temperature

A rectal temperature should *not* be used when:
> A resident has diarrhea
> A resident has had recent rectal surgery
> A resident has hemorrhoids

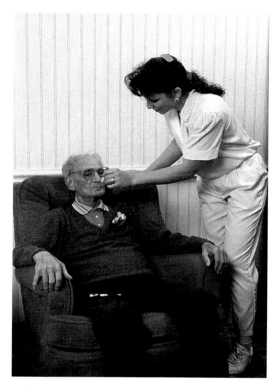

Fig. 18-10.   Insert the thermometer under the resident's tongue.

Check with the nurse to make sure the temperature should be taken rectally. Be sure to use a rectal thermometer (usually with a red stem and short, and rounded bulb). Some facilities use disposable thermometer covers.

Taking a Rectal Temperature

Remember:

1. Be sure to wear gloves for this procedure.
2. Position the resident on either side. Raise the side rail on the side he or she is facing so he or she can hold on to it. Have the resident bend up the upper leg as far as possible.
3. Put a plastic cover (if used) over the thermometer and lubricate it. Insert the bulb or metal tip 1 inch into the rectum while you separate the buttocks with your other hand.
4. Hold the thermometer in place 3-5 minutes, remove it, wipe it off, remove the cover, and read the thermometer. *Note:* Always cover a resident and never leave him or her while taking a rectal temperature because he or she may roll back from the side lying position and be injured with the thermometer. Talk with the person while waiting for the temperature reading to take his or her mind off the procedure.
5. Wipe any excess lubricant from a resident's rectum with a piece of tissue paper.

- Resident preference
- Common preparation steps
- Equipment and supplies needed
- Environment preparation
- Resident preparation

Remember:

- Meet resident needs
- Common completion steps
- Clean and put away equipment and supplies
- Environment completion (Is it safe? Is it clean?)

Axillary Temperature

An axillary temperature is the least reliable method. Use it only when the other two methods are not feasible (such as a confused resident with a new colostomy). To take an axillary temperature, use an oral thermometer in the armpit.

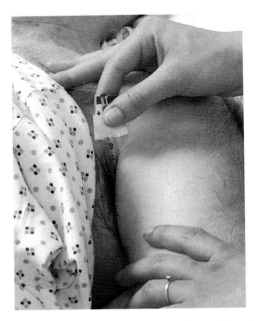

Fig. 18-11. Place the thermometer in the resident's armpit.

Taking an Axillary Temperature

1. Shake down the thermometer to 95° F or lower.
2. Dry the resident's armpit. Loosen clothing to allow access.
3. Place the thermometer in the resident's armpit. Have him or her place the arm down along his or her side (Fig. 18-11).
4. Wait 10 minutes and remove the thermometer; read the temperature.

Pulse Rate

You also take the other vital signs: pulse, respirations, and blood pressure. A pulse rate is the number of times the heart beats in a minute. The pulse can be felt in various body areas.

Usually you take a radial pulse. It is quick and easy to take and in most situations gives an accurate reading. You may be asked to take an apical pulse, however, if the physician or the nurse feels that exact accuracy of the pulse reading is critical for the resident's care. Often, irregular heart beats can only be measured by taking an apical pulse. This may be done to determine whether a heart medication should be given.

A pulse is felt as a throbbing sensation in a superficial artery located over a bony prominence each time the heart pumps blood through the body (Fig. 18-12). The normal rate in an adult at rest is 60-90 beats per minute. A normal rhythm is regular, with the pulse beating at regular intervals with pauses between.

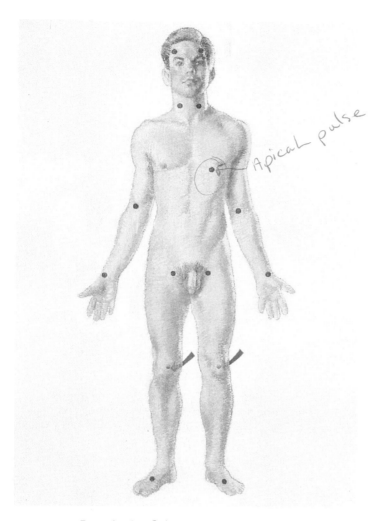

Apical pulse

Fig. 18-12. Pulse points in the body.

A pulse might be increased by such things as:
▶ Exercise
▶ Anxiety or anger
▶ Condition of the heart
▶ Some medications

A pulse rate can be decreased by such things as:
▶ Condition of the heart
▶ Some medications
▶ A pacemaker
▶ A calm resting state

Things to note when taking a pulse:
▶ The person needs to be calm and resting.
▶ Note any irregularities in the rhythm or pattern of beats of the pulse.
▶ Note how strong the pulse is. If the pulse feels like it is pounding under your fingers, you would say it is strong. If the pulse feels very faint under your fingers, you would say it is weak. The best way to identify the strength of a pulse is to practice on many people.
▶ Note the rate or how many beats per minute the pulse has.
▶ Do not use your thumb for taking a pulse because your own pulsations could be confused with a resident's pulse.

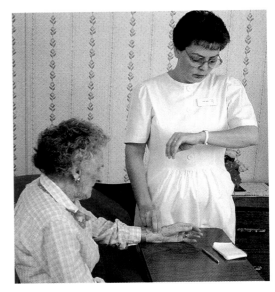

Fig. 18-13. Take a radial pulse by placing your second and third fingers over the resident's radial artery.

Taking a Radial Pulse

Remember:

▶ Resident preference
▶ Common preparation steps
▶ Equipment and supplies needed
▶ Environment preparation
▶ Resident preparation

Items Needed

▶ Watch with second hand
▶ Paper and pencil

1. Place your second and third fingers gently over the radial artery and note the rhythm of the pulse (Fig. 18-13).
2. Look at your watch, and when the second hand is on the 12, start counting the pulse for 1 minute. Count each beat you feel. You can count for 30 seconds and then multiply it by 2, if you prefer. Check for abnormalities in the rhythm.

Remember:

▶ Meet resident needs
▶ Common completion steps
▶ Clean and put away equipment and supplies
▶ Environment completion (Is it safe? Is it clean?)

Taking an Apical Pulse

Remember:

▶ Resident preference
▶ Common preparation steps
▶ Equipment and supplies needed
▶ Environment preparation
▶ Resident preparation

Items Needed

▶ Stethoscope
▶ Paper and pencil

To take an apical pulse, you will need a stethoscope. A stethoscope is a medical instrument with which you to listen to a resident's heart, lungs, and bowel sounds. The stethoscope is a tube with ear pieces on one end and a diaphragm on the other. Some may have both a diaphragm and a bell on the other end.

1. Place the stethoscope earpieces in your ears.
2. Place the diaphragm of the stethoscope just below and to the inside of the left nipple.
3. Look at your watch, and when the second hand is on 12, start counting the pulse for 1 minute. Listen for any abnormal rhythm (Fig. 18-14).

Remember:

▶ Meet resident needs
▶ Common completion steps
▶ Clean and put away equipment and supplies
▶ Environment completion (Is it safe? Is it clean?)

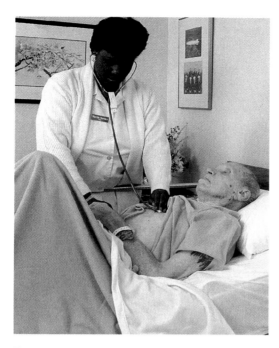

Fig. 18-14. Take an apical pulse by placing the stethescope below and to the inside of the left nipple; count the pulse for 1 minute.

Respiratory Rate

Counting respirations is part of taking a resident's vital signs. Respirations are the act of breathing air into the lungs (inhalation) and breathing air out of the lungs (exhalation).

The respiratory rate is counted by watching a resident breathe in and out. One respiration is equal to one inspiration (breathing in) and one expiration (breathing out). The respiratory rate changes with physical and emotional activity and with sleep but does not usually change with normal aging. The normal respiratory rate for an adult at rest is 12-20 breaths per minute. When counting a resident's respiratory rate, also observe depth and regularity. Is the resident taking in deep slow breaths or shallow rapid breaths? Are the breaths in a regular pattern or are some deep and slow and some shallow and rapid?

Taking a Respiratory Rate

Items Needed

▶ Paper and pencil

1. Count the respiratory rate immediately after counting the pulse rate.
2. Keep your fingers on the resident's radial pulse, but watch the chest go up (inspiration) and go down (expiration). Keep your fingers on the wrist because most people become self-conscious if they know you are counting their breathing and may try to control their breathing rate (Fig. 18-15).
3. Count the respiratory rate for 1 minute.

Remember:

▷ Resident preference
▷ Common preparation steps
▷ Equipment and supplies needed
▷ Environment preparation
▷ Resident preparation

Remember:

▷ Meet resident needs
▷ Common completion steps
▷ Clean and put away equipment and supplies
▷ Environment completion (Is it safe? Is it clean?)

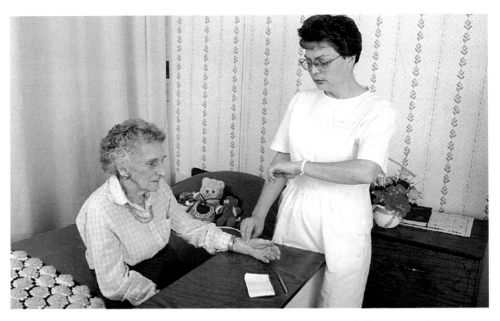

Fig. 18-15. To count a resident's respiratory rate, watch his or her chest move up and down while your fingers remain on the resident's radial artery.

Blood Pressure

Blood pressure, abbreviated BP, is the last of the vital signs. It is a challenging skill to learn, and accuracy is important. Blood pressure is an important indicator of some diseases. Too high a blood pressure can lead to such problems as strokes or heart attacks. If the blood pressure is too low, it can lead to such conditions as fainting, fatigue, or weakness.

Blood pressure is the pressure of blood in the arteries. Two numbers are recorded for a blood pressure, such as 170/80. The top number (systolic pressure) is the pressure in the artery when the heart is pumping. The bottom number (diastolic pressure) is the pressure when the heart is at rest.

The normal range for blood pressure in an adult is:

Systolic: 90-140
Diastolic: 60-90

Blood pressure differs from person to person and time to time. Various factors affect a person's blood pressure, such as:

▶ Stress
▶ Medications
▶ Weight and diet
▶ Family history
▶ Exercise

Obviously, some of these factors can be controlled and some cannot. For example, a resident's BP might be higher on admission because of the anxiety at that time. A resident's BP and other vital signs are often taken more often during the first week to determine what is normal for this person.

The systolic BP in older adults tends to be higher than in younger individuals because the arteries become narrower and more rigid with age. An older adult may have a high acceptable BP range of:

Systolic: 140-160
Diastolic: 90

Another term for high blood pressure is hypertension. Low blood pressure is called hypotension. Blood pressure is best measured when a resident is sitting or ly-

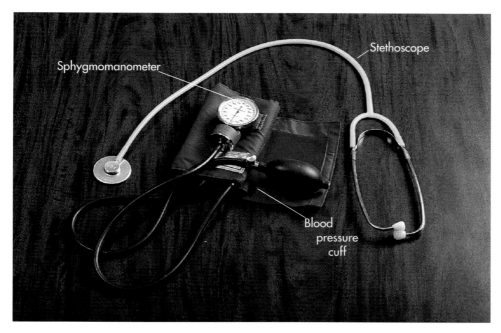

Fig. 18-16. The blood pressure cuff, sphygmomanometer, and stethescope are used to measure an individual's blood pressure.

ing down. You can take the blood pressure in either arm. Blood pressure should not be measured in an arm with intravenous fluid infusion or an injury. You use a stethoscope, a blood pressure cuff, and a sphygmomanometer (Fig. 18-16). You will learn the equipment used in your facility.

Taking a Blood Pressure

Items Needed
▶ BP Cuff
▶ Sphygmomanometer
▶ Paper and pencil

1. Have the resident place his or her arm on the bed, bedside table, or arm of the chair with the palm of the hand up and the elbow at the same level as the heart. If the arm is higher than the heart, the blood pressure could register too high. If the arm is lower than the heart, the blood pressure could register too low.
2. Expose the resident's arm by rolling the sleeve up to the shoulder, taking care that the sleeve does not become too tight on the arm and increase the blood pressure. Wrap the blood pressure cuff evenly around the upper arm 1 inch above the elbow. Make sure the arm is not lying on the tubing and the tubing is not kinked. (The tube that is attached to the bulb should be on the side closest to the resident's body. The tube to the sphygmomanometer gauge should be on the other side of the arm, away from the body.)
3. Close the valve in the air pump by turning it clockwise. (This is the little metal knob on the bulb.)
4. Place the stethoscope earpieces in your ears.
5. Locate the pulsation in the brachial artery by placing your second and third fingers over the area. When you find the pulse, place the diaphragm of the stethoscope firmly over the area and hold it in place with your left hand. (Use the right hand if you are left handed.)

Remember:
▷ Resident preference
▷ Common preparation steps
▷ Equipment and supplies needed
▷ Environment preparation
▷ Resident preparation

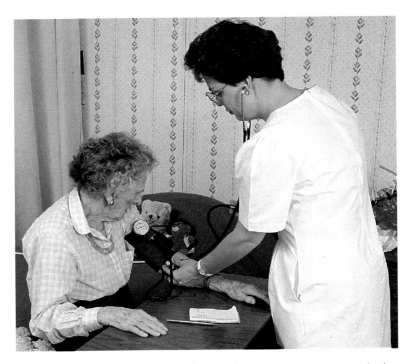

Fig. 18-17. Pump the bulb of the sphygmomanometer with the right hand.

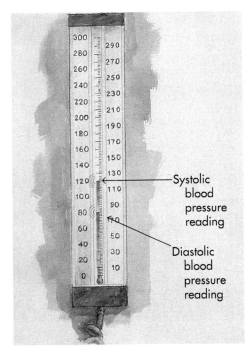

Fig. 18-18. The first sound is the systolic pressure. The last sound is the diastolic pressure.

6. With the right hand, pump air into the cuff by squeezing the bulb until the gauge measures 180-200 (Fig. 18-17).
   Note: If you hear the pulse immediately, you have to begin again and pump the cuff so the gauge reads higher than 200 mm Hg.
7. Slowly open the valve on the bulb and watch the cuff pressure decrease on the gauge.
8. Listen for the first sound and note the pressure reading and remember the number. This is the systolic pressure.
9. Continue to listen for a distinct change in sound (muffled sounding) or the last sound and note the pressure reading. This is the diastolic pressure (Fig. 18-18).

Remember:

▶ Meet resident needs
▶ Common completion steps
▶ Clean and put away equipment and supplies
▶ Environment completion (Is it safe? Is it clean?)

COLLECTING SPECIMENS

All people have bodily fluids and excretions. Excretions are wastes from the body, such as sputum, urine, and feces.

Sometimes these substances are analyzed in the lab or at the bedside to identify problems a person might be having. When used for this purpose, they are considered specimens. A specific physician's order is needed for each specimen collected.

Nurse assistants often collect and sometimes analyze certain specimens. For the specimen to be valid, correct collection and analyzing procedures must be followed. Learn about these procedures and ask your charge nurse if you have any questions.

Remember these key points:

▷ Always explain the procedure to a resident before collecting the sample.
▷ Specimens are considered "dirty" and should not be collected or stored in "clean" areas such as nurses' stations.
▷ Always wear gloves and wash your hands before and after obtaining a specimen.
▷ Never touch the inside of a specimen container.
▷ Many specimens need to be as fresh as possible, and some may need to be refrigerated if there will be any delay in getting them to the lab.
▷ Specimens need to be labeled correctly and promptly. Always put this resident's name, room number, and the date and time the specimen was collected. This is done to prevent any confusion regarding whom the specimen belongs to. Each facility has its own protocol for labeling.
▷ Lids on specimen containers must be put on securely to help avoid leakage.
▷ After obtaining and labeling a specimen, follow your facility's protocol if it needs to be transported to the lab. Place the specimen into a plastic bag as an additional barrier to prevent possible contamination that would occur if the specimen cup or container leaked.

URINE SPECIMENS
Urinalysis
60 cc

A urinalysis is often called a UA. You may periodically collect urine specimens for a urinalysis for some residents. A urinalysis is used to diagnose problems in the urinary system as well as other bodily problems. Usually the specimen should be as fresh as possible when analyzed.

Note: When collecting a UA, check with the charge nurse to find out what container and method to use. Ask to be shown the procedure if you are unsure. Follow infection control policies according to facility protocol. Sometimes urine is collected from a bedpan, urinal, or special device called a "hat" for toilet use. It must be as free of contamination as possible.

Collecting a Urinalysis Specimen

Items Needed

▷ Proper collection container
▷ Cleaning solution if needed
▷ Gloves
▷ Labels
▷ Disposable trash bag
▷ Testing equipment

1. Have the resident void or urinate into a bedpan, urinal (if male), or hat on the toilet.
2. Put on gloves.
3. Pour approximately 60 cc urine in the specimen container. Discard remainder.
4. Write the resident's name, room number, and date and time the specimen was collected on the label of the container.
5. Place the specimen container in a plastic bag and fasten it closed for infection control.

Remember:
▷ Resident preference
▷ Common preparation steps
▷ Equipment and supplies needed
▷ Environment preparation
▷ Resident preparation

Remember:
▷ Meet resident needs
▷ Common completion steps
▷ Clean and put away equipment and supplies
▷ Environment completion (Is it safe? Is it clean?)

Clean Catch Urinalysis

A clean catch urinalysis is often used to diagnose an infection in the urinary system. It is called a clean catch because the specimen must be collected after the urethral opening is cleansed. The cleansing will prevent contamination of the urine from organisms living around the urethral opening.

Collecting Clean Catch Urinalysis Specimen

1. For the female resident, use one wipe to cleanse one side of the labia, a second wipe to cleanse the other side of the labia, and a third wipe to cleanse down the middle. *Note:* Always clean in single strokes from front to back. Each wipe should be used only one time and then disposed of.
2. For an uncircumcised male resident, pull back the foreskin of the penis. Cleanse the penis following the same procedures used for perineal care.
3. Have the resident begin to urinate and then stop. Do not collect the first portion of the voiding.
4. Place the specimen container under the urethra, ask the resident to begin voiding again, and collect the remainder of the specimen.
5. Write the resident's name, room number, and the date and time specimen was collected on the specimen container.
6. Place the specimen container in a plastic bag and close it.

Collecting a 24-Hour Urine Specimen

A 24-hour urine specimen may be ordered by the physician to help diagnose various problems such as diseases of the urinary system. Check with the charge nurse for specific instructions as to how to best maintain the specimen. It may require a preservative to be in the bottle, or perhaps the bottle needs to be kept cool in a refrigerator.

A 24-hour urine specimen is a collection of all urine voided in a 24-hour period. Follow these principles:

▶ Place a sign in the bathroom to alert other staff or family and to remind a resident not to throw out any urine (Fig. 18-19). *Note:* Everyone involved needs to understand that if any urine is lost, the test may need to be restarted.
▶ All urine must be collected in the same container.
▶ The first voided sample of the day is discarded.
▶ Right after discarding the first specimen, the collection time for the 24 hours should begin.

Note: The test would be inaccurate if the first voided urine was not discarded because it contains urine that had collected in the bladder before the starting period.

Glucose and Ketone Testing

Checking urine for sugar/glucose and ketones or acetone is common for residents who are diabetic. Urine can easily be checked for extra glucose in the body. Fat burning also causes ketones or acetone in the urine. You may be asked to check the urine for glucose and ketones, often called an "S & A" (sugar and acetone). This test is done early in the morning before eating. The test uses specially designed strips to check for glucose and ketones. The strips bottle has a color chart to check the strip against. Sometimes a strip using + and 2 symbols is used to determine the presence or absence of glucose and ketones.

Testing Urine for Glucose and Ketones, or Sugar and Acetone

1. Have the resident void in the bedpan, hat on a toilet, or urinal.
2. Either dip the end of the strip in the fresh urine or pass it though the stream.
3. When removing the strip, pull its edge over the rim of the container you are collecting the urine in. This gets rid of excess urine.

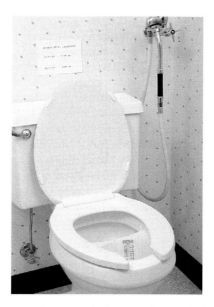

Fig. 18-19. A sign will remind the resident of the 24-hour urine specimen collection.

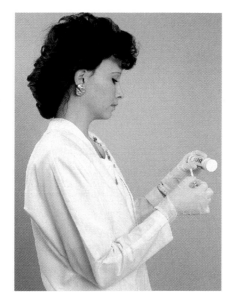

Fig. 18-20. Compare the glucose reading on the test strip to the chart on the test strip bottle.

4. Wait 15 seconds and compare the ketone portion of the test strip with the ketone color chart on the test strip bottle. This may also show up as a + or − symbol, depending on the type of test strip used.
5. Wait an additional 15 seconds and compare the glucose portion of the test strip with the glucose color chart on the side of the test strip bottle (Fig. 18-20). This may show up as a + or −, depending on the type of test strip used. (The total time for testing for glucose and ketones should not exceed 30 seconds. Ignore any color after this.)

Remember:

▶ Meet resident needs
▶ Common completion steps
▶ Clean and put away equipment and supplies
▶ Environment completion (Is it safe? Is it clean?)

Stool Specimens

Stool specimens are a valuable way for the physician to diagnose various gastrointestinal problems. Stool is also sometimes collected to check for parasites that could be causing a resident to be sick. The specimen is analyzed by a lab.

Bleeding in the gastrointestinal tract can be visible to the human eye. Occult blood is blood that is not visible to the human eye. Blood that is visible to the eye may be bright red, or the stool may appear black and sticky (called tarry stool), depending on where the bleeding is in the gastrointestinal tract.

Stool specimens are collected to check for occult blood. You may be asked to perform this procedure. This may be referred to as guaiacing the stool, or checking a guaiac on the stool (Fig. 18-21). Check with the charge nurse if you have any questions.

Remember:

▶ Resident preference
▶ Common preparation steps
▶ Equipment and supplies needed
▶ Environment preparation
▶ Resident preparation

Remember:

▶ Meet resident needs
▶ Common completion steps
▶ Clean and put away equipment and supplies
▶ Environment completion (Is it safe? Is it clean?)

Collecting Stool Specimen

Items Needed

▶ Bedpan
▶ Toilet paper
▶ Specimen collection application
▶ Gloves
▶ Container for specimen
▶ Testing materials

1. After the resident has defecated, obtain a small sample of the fecal material, using an applicator.
2. Apply a thin smear of the fecal material on the test slide for the kit in the designated area. *Note:* Sometimes there are two sections to place fecal material on the test slide so that you can obtain a thin smear from different areas of the stool.
3. After applying the smear to the slide, wait 3-5 minutes. This allows the slide to better absorb the fecal matter.
4. Apply two drops of the developer solution to the back of the slide directly behind the stool sample.
5. Read the results within 60 seconds of developing the sample. If any blue or blue-green color appears on or around the edge of the sample, it is positive for occult bleeding. *Note:* Often testing is done with three consecutive stools because bleeding may occur periodically rather than continuously and checking three stools at different times can better identify whether there is occult bleeding.

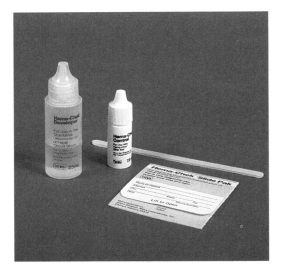

Fig. 18-21. The hemocult slide, developer, and wooden stick are used to check for occult blood in the stool.

Sputum Specimens

Sputum is a substance collected from a person's mouth. It contains saliva, mucus, and at times purulent secretions or infected drainage. Most often it is thicker than plain saliva. Sputum comes from further down in the lungs or bronchial tubes and is helpful in diagnosing diseases or conditions that affect the respiratory system.

✓ Collecting Sputum Specimen

Items Needed

▶ Specimen container and label   *easly in AM*

Note: Make sure a resident who chews tobacco has not done so before collection of a sputum specimen. If a resident has just eaten, ask him or her to rinse out the mouth. Try to collect the specimen in the A.M. Often large amounts of sputum are coughed up first thing in the morning.

1. Give the resident the sputum collection container or hold it yourself. Take care not to touch it inside.
2. Ask the resident to cough deeply from the chest. He or she may need to cough several times to get enough sputum for the sample. Tell him or her to try to avoid spitting saliva into the container.
3. Place the lid securely on the specimen bottle and label it with the resident's name, room number, and the date and time the specimen was collected.
4. Report to the charge nurse the color, amount, and consistency of the specimen.

Remember:

▶ Resident preference
▶ Common preparation steps
▶ Equipment and supplies needed
▶ Environment preparation
▶ Resident preparation

Remember:

▶ Meet resident needs
▶ Common completion steps
▶ Clean and put away equipment and supplies
▶ Environment completion (Is it safe? Is it clean?)

USE OF NONSTERILE BANDAGES AND DRESSINGS

Dressings are used for many reasons:
▶ Wound protection
▶ Protection of skin
▶ Keeping a medication or moisture in place
▶ Keeping an area clean
▶ Keeping a resident from picking at an area that could become an open sore

Dressings must be applied properly so that they do not irritate or hurt the skin by slipping or causing friction. Usually you place a sterile gauze over the affected area and carefully tape it in place (Fig. 18-22). If a resident's skin cannot tolerate tape, an elastic (Ace) bandage may be used. Elastic bandages can help hold dressings in place and support an injured limb. When applying an elastic bandage, begin above the dressing and carefully cover the area around with the elastic bandage, continuing over and slightly below the site. Elastic bandages can also help assist with circulation.

Elastic bandages should be put on securely enough to stay in place, but not so tight to impair circulation (Fig. 18-23). Make sure the person has feeling in the extremity below the bandage and the area is warm and "pink" after applying an elastic wrap. Check dry wraps every day to inspect progress of the affected area. If an area with a lesion is draining, the dressing should be changed often to prevent bacterial growth.

APPLICATION OF SUPPORT HOSE AND ELASTIC STOCKINGS

Residents often need support hose and elastic stockings. You may need to put them on the residents. Elastic stockings increase circulation in the legs and are beneficial in situations such as:
▶ To help prevent blood clots from forming in the legs
▶ To help prevent or decrease edema (fluid build-up) in the legs

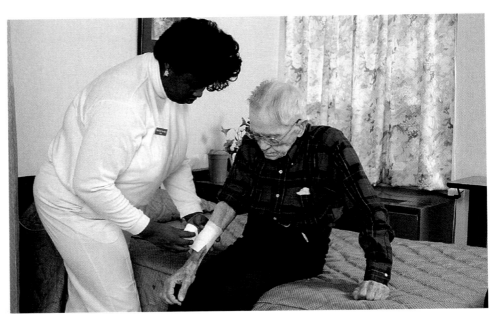

Fig. 18-22. Proper application of dressings helps prevent irritation of the skin.

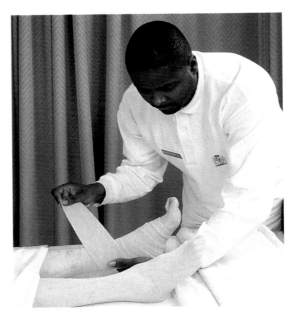

Fig. 18-23. Apply elastic bandages securely.

When applying elastic stockings, follow these guidelines:
- Be sure you have the correct size. The stocking should be snug enough to give support, but not really tight or really loose. If a person has gained or lost much weight, check for correct stocking size. Check with the nurse if unsure.
- Be sure that both the stockings and the resident's legs and feet are clean and dry.
- Explain to a resident what you are doing and see if he or she can assist.
- Put the stockings on before a resident moves the legs off the bed into a dependent position. Otherwise fluid may pool in the feet and be trapped there by the elastic stockings.

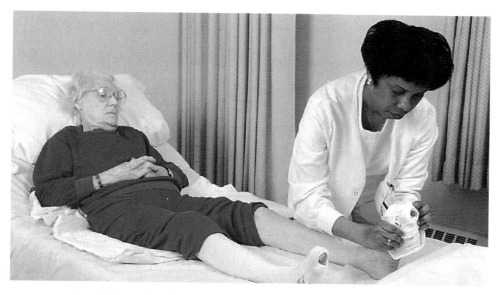

Fig. 18-24. Carefully put the support stocking on the resident.

▷ A small amount of talcum powder applied to the leg can minimize friction and help the stocking go on more easily.

▷ For proper placement, turn the stocking inside out except for the toe, securely put the toe in place, and slide the stocking up over the heel (Fig. 18-24). Be sure the heel is positioned properly in the stocking, and then carefully pull the stocking up and over the calf. Remember residents' skin may be thin and fragile and can tear easily.

▷ Make sure there are no wrinkles in the stockings. Wrinkles or twists can cause pressure and decrease circulation.

▷ Make sure residents know not to roll the stockings down. This could greatly reduce the circulation in the legs.

▷ Tell the resident to call you if he or she becomes uncomfortable. Check the toes every hour to ensure they are warm and a normal color. Also, check the stockings to make sure they stay wrinkle free.

▷ Remove elastic stockings at least twice a day. Check with the charge nurse on how long the elastic stocking should be off. This lets you observe the skin and lets the legs rest. Check with the nurse about any skin treatments required.

APPLICATION OF NONPRESCRIPTION TOPICAL PREPARATIONS

Applying topical (skin) preparations may be considered a treatment and thus must be done under the nurse's direction. Topical preparations include ointments, gels, creams, lotions, and pastes. Follow these guidelines and be aware of your facility's policies when applying a topical preparation:

▷ Always check the area where the preparation is to be used. If a rash, what does it look like? How large an area does it cover? Is there redness? Is there any discharge?

▷ Always wear gloves when applying topical preparations. Remember to change gloves between different procedures even with the same resident. For instance, if a resident has an area on the hip that needs a topical preparation and another on the face, use a clean set of gloves for each area. Always wash your hands between sets of gloves.

▷ Topical preparations often should be used somewhat sparingly and applied in

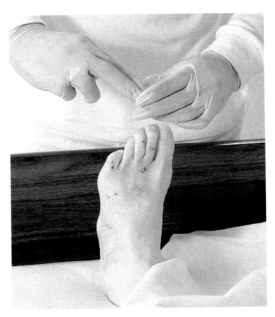

Fig. 18-25. When using a topical cream, apply it in thin, even layers to clean, dry skin.

thin, even layers on the affected area. Make sure the area is clean and dry before applying (Fig. 18-25).

▶ If the preparation comes out of a jar, use a tongue depressor to remove the needed amount and put it in a medication cup. When using a tube, squirt out what you need in a medication cup and take it to the person's room. Be careful not to contaminate the ointment in its container. Never put your fingers on the end of the tube.

▶ Each resident should have an individual tube or bottle of topical ointments, etc. to prevent cross contamination.

▶ Remember that privacy is very important when applying these preparations. Do it in the person's room.

▶ Never massage the calf of the leg with or without a topical preparation. Clots sometimes form there, and massaging could break them loose. Once loose, a clot could travel to the lungs, heart, or brain and block blood flow to the areas, causing a life-threatening situation.

HOT AND COLD APPLICATIONS

Hot or cold applications are used for treating specific diseases or conditions, as ordered by a resident's physician. Use these applications only on the nurse's direction.

Heat or cold may be applied to the entire body for a generalized effect. Usually, however, they are ordered for a specific or localized body area. Heat and cold may be applied dry or moist, depending on the situation and doctor's orders.

Hot Applications

Hot applications may be used for reasons such as:

▶ Heat helps speed up the healing process. Heat causes the blood vessels to dilate (get larger), increasing blood flow to the targeted area for healing.

▶ Heat eases pain for some individuals who may have inflammation or pain in an area. When the blood vessels become dilated, the increased blood flow often absorbs and carries away fluids. This is why warm water exercises can be so beneficial to some residents with arthritis.

▶ Heat can bring a boil or abscess to a "head." The doctor can then drain the area and reduce the person's discomfort.

▶ Heat helps reduce painful muscle spasms because it helps muscles relax.

▶ Some examples of heat applications include:

   ▶ Moist heat:

      ▶ Sitz bath—provides moist heat to the genitals or anal area

      ▶ Tub baths—provide moist heat to the whole body

      ▶ Hot moist compress—provides moist heat to a localized area using a cloth

      ▶ Soaks—provide moist heat to a localized area

   ▶ Dry heat:

      ▶ Rubber hot water bottle—provides dry heat to a localized area

      ▶ Electric pad—provides heat to a localized area (Fig. 18-26)

      ▶ Heat lamp—provides heat to a localized area using a light

      ▶ Consider these questions before applying heat:

▶ What method is to be used and what equipment do you need before starting?

▶ Where is the location? Is it localized or generalized?

▶ How long should the heat be applied?

▶ What safety rules should be followed for the hot application?

Safety Guidelines for Hot Applications

▶ If using a soak, be sure the person is in a position to prevent spilling the solution.

▶ Always double check the temperature of the heating device, to make sure it is not too hot. Check with the charge nurse if you are unsure. Ask the person if it feels too hot, then go back and check with him or her every 5-10 minutes. Note any area that seems red or discolored, which could indicate that a resident is being burned. If so, stop the treatment immediately and check with the charge nurse. It is especially critical to carefully evaluate residents with paralysis or a lack of or limited feeling in the area. These residents cannot feel if the heat becomes too hot and are therefore at a higher risk for burns. Also, residents who cannot express themselves should be checked closely.

▶ Never place an electric heating device over a wet dressing or compress. This could cause a burn as the moist heat may become too hot and intense. Moisture and electricity together also increase the risk of electrocution.

▶ The application should remain at the correct temperature. If it becomes too cool, it is not doing what it is supposed to do. After applying a hot compress, cover it with plastic to help prevent a loss of heat. A towel or other dry material should cover the plastic. You may use a hot water bottle along with the compress, but check with the charge nurse first and be sure that it is not too hot.

Cold Applications

As with hot applications, cold applications can be localized or generalized. Cold applications are used for a variety of reasons, such as the following:

▶ To reduce painful swelling in an area. Cold causes the blood vessels to constrict (become smaller), which decreases the blood flow to an area. This is helpful in the beginning stages of a bruise or sprained ankle.

▶ To help control bleeding. Again this is because the cold constricts the blood vessels. Cold applications are used immediately after some surgeries.

▶ To lessen pain sensitivity. Cold can act as an local anesthetic in certain situations.

▶ To help reduce a high temperature.

▶ Some examples of cold applications include:

   ▶ Moist cold:

      ▶ Cold compresses

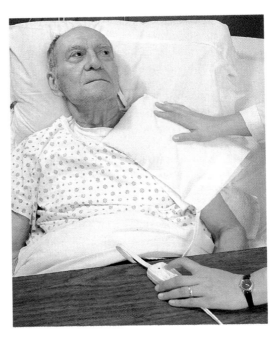

Fig. 18-26. An electric pad provides dry heat.

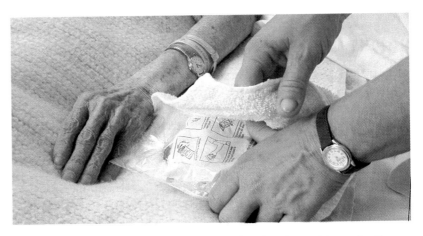

Fig. 18-27. An ice pack is an example of a dry, cold application.

- Cooling solutions
- Alcohol sponge baths
- Dry cold:
  - Ice cubes or collars
  - Ice packs (Fig. 18-27)
  - Consider these questions before applying cold:
- What method should be used and what equipment is needed?
- Where is the location? Generalized or localized?
- How long should the cold application be used?
- What safety rules should be followed?

Safety Guidelines for Cold Applications

- Use cubed ice rather than crushed in a cooling solution. Crushed ice melts too quickly and alters the temperature of the solution. Crushed ice, also, may stick to cloth and may be too cold for a resident.

▶ Take the person's temperature before and after the application. Report it to the charge nurse. If the application is for a fever, the body may not have cooled down enough and the treatment may need to be repeated.

▶ If a resident begins to shiver during the procedure, remove the cold pack and notify the charge nurse immediately. The nurse will give further instructions.

▶ Especially in the use of a generalized cold application there can be a danger of shock developing. Shock is caused by a significant decrease in the circulation of blood in the body. One sign of shock is a change in a resident's vital signs. Before using a cold application, take a resident's vital signs to make comparisons later. Observe the person frequently for:

   ▶ Gasping or labored breathing, often at a faster rate
   ▶ Faster and possibly irregular pulse rate
   ▶ Bluish or darker color (cyanosis) in such areas as the lips, fingernails, and even eyelids

If any of these occur, stop the cold application treatment immediately and inform the charge nurse. Shock is a life-threatening condition needing immediate treatment.

ASSISTING A RESIDENT WITH AN OSTOMY

Because you may care for a resident who has an ostomy, you need a working knowledge of what to expect and what your role may be.

Your attitude toward a resident with an ostomy is important. Treat this resident with respect and dignity. Be careful to avoid any facial expressions or untoward comments that could be considered offensive. These residents may be very sensitive about their ostomy and concerned about how others perceive them. They are often afraid of being avoided or treated differently.

Types of Ostomies

A *colostomy* is an opening of the colon or bowel on the surface of the abdomen. This surgical procedure is done for numerous reasons, such as cancer of the colon and diseases that involve inflammation of the colon. The bowel discharges its contents through this opening into an ostomy bag. The opening itself is called a stoma.

A colostomy can have one or two stomas, depending on the circumstances and future medical plans. Some colostomies are permanent, while others are reversible. The fecal contents from a colostomy may be semi-liquid or fairly well formed, depending on where in the intestine the colostomy is made (Fig. 18-28).

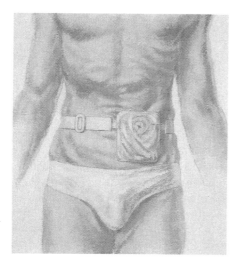

Fig. 18-28.   A colostomy and appliance.

An *ileostomy* is an opening of the ileum (a part of the small bowel) through the abdomen. The ileum is a part of the small intestine. The main difference between the care of a colostomy and that of an ileostomy involves the consistency of the stool. Ileostomy contents generally are much more liquid than a colostomy. More digestive juices are involved, and these can irritate the skin. An ileostomy is often permanent.

An *ileal conduit* procedure routes the urine into a section of the ileum and then through an opening or stoma on the abdomen. This procedure might be needed because of such illnesses as bladder cancer or congenital problems.

Your Functions in Working with Ostomies

Each facility has its own policies and procedures for working with ostomies. Your specific role is under the direction of the charge nurse.

Most residents with an ostomy use a bag apparatus, often called an appliance. Your observations of this are very important. When helping a resident with dressing, undressing, or bathing, take time to observe the appliance and area surrounding it. Report any of the following to the charge nurse:

- Is the appliance free of leaks?
- Is the seal around the stoma secure?
- Does the ostomy seem to be draining well?
- What is the consistency and color of the stool or urine?
- Do the stoma and surrounding skin appear intact, or is there redness, bleeding, or other skin breakdown?

Emptying an Ostomy Bag

You may be asked to empty and measure the contents from an ostomy bag. Follow the protocol in your facility. When emptying a ostomy bag, follow these guidelines:

1. Always wear gloves.
2. Measure the contents of the bag at least once a shift. To empty the bag, undo the clip on the bottom of the bag and empty the contents into a bedpan.
3. Rinse out the bag each time it is emptied. This may be done with a large irrigation syringe. Add deodorizers as needed.
4. Be sure to wipe off the end of the bag.
5. Reseal the bag with the clip.

YOUR RESPONSIBILITIES IN EMERGENCY SITUATIONS

Always be prepared for any situation that may occur. Don't let day-to-day activities become too routine, or you might not be ready to respond quickly enough if a crisis or emergency arises.

Emergency situations can happen anytime. You must know how to respond and be prepared for numerous emergency situations. Knowing how to respond prevents chaos and casualties. Keeping a cool head and having clear knowledge in these situations is crucial. Follow these general principles:

- Always know where the emergency equipment is located.
- When drills or mock emergencies are held, always treat the situation as you would a real emergency. If you understand what to do in an emergency, the appropriate steps will be second nature to you during a real crisis.

▶ Know the various "codes" that your facility uses to identify emergencies. When a code is called, all staff must know what is happening so that priceless time is not lost.

▶ Always answer call lights promptly, both to give quality care every day and to discover an emergency situation early. Most resident calls are not emergencies, but you never know what's behind the door until you check. It could be a fire starting in a waste can, someone choking, or a resident having severe chest pain.

Cardiac Arrest

Each facility has its own protocol for what to do if a resident has a cardiac arrest. Become familiar with the procedure where you work. Not all residents will receive cardiopulmonary resuscitation (CPR). Some residents have signed a living will or advance directive stating they do not wish to be resuscitated. Sometimes the family and physician decide this if a resident cannot make his or her wishes known.

If you find a resident who is not breathing and has no pulse, get help from a nurse immediately. Every second counts. The nurse knows who should receive CPR and who should not.

You may assist with CPR, depending on the facility's policy. If so, you need special training and certification. Talk with the charge nurse, head nurse, or staff development nurse for more information. If your facility does not offer CPR training, you can take a CPR course from your local American Red Cross, American Heart Association, or even your community hospital.

Aid for a Choking Resident

Many people die of choking every year, most often when food or another object gets stuck in the throat. Residents are at a great risk for choking on food. Many have difficulty swallowing or try to swallow food that is not adequately moistened by saliva. The signs of choking are:
▶ A resident cannot breathe
▶ A resident cannot talk
▶ A resident is turning blue

You must act quickly, as usually you have only 4-8 minutes to save the person's life by dislodging the food or object using the Heimlich maneuver. You need formal training and practice with this procedure before trying to use it. When a person is choking:
1. First, call for a nurse immediately. Never leave a resident. This is a life-threatening situation.
2. If a nurse is not available, you need to help now with the Heimlich maneuver to get the food out of the airway.
3. If the person can speak or is coughing, do not do the Heimlich maneuver. Coughing is the body's way of clearing the airway by itself.

How to Perform the Heimlich Maneuver

If the resident is sitting or standing:
1. Stand behind the person.
2. Wrap your arms around the waist.
3. Put your fist on the resident's stomach below the rib cage and a little above the naval. Keep your thumb on the stomach and place your other hand over your fist (Fig. 18-29).
4. Sharply thrust your fist inward and upward. This causes a burst of air from the lungs to dislodge the food or object.
5. Repeat the thrusts up to 10 times or until the airway is clear.

If a resident is standing and then becomes unconscious, gently lower him or her to the floor. Once the resident is lying down:
1. Place the resident on his or her back, face up.

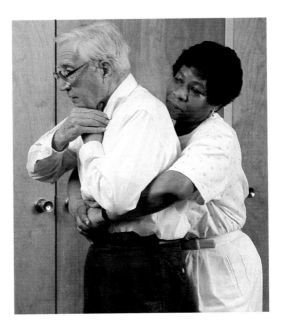

Fig. 18-29. Performing the Heimlich maneuver on a resident who is standing.

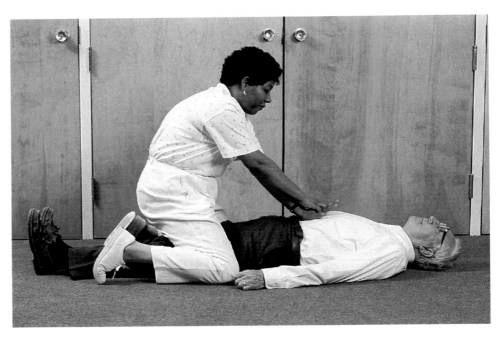

Fig. 18-30. Performing the Heimlich maneuver on a resident who is lying down.

2. Get on your knees and straddle the resident across the hips.
3. Place the heel of one hand on the stomach, below the rib cage, a little above the naval. Place your other hand on top of your first hand (Fig. 18-30). Interlace your fingers and point them upward off of the abdomen.
4. Push inward and thrust upward suddenly. This should dislodge the food or object.
5. Repeat up to 10 times or until the airway becomes clear.

Seizure

You may care for a resident with a seizure disorder. Seizures are often called convulsions. Most people with seizure disorders take medications to help prevent seizures. There are many types of seizures, ranging from a blacking out (petit mal) period for a few seconds to a hard convulsion (grand mal) that can last quite a while. The grand mal type is more of an emergency. It is characterized by generalized jerking movements of the body that the person cannot control.

Sometimes a resident can tell you he or she feels a seizure coming. Many people who have seizures feel an aura before an attack. The aura is an unusual sensation in smell, taste, sight, or sound. This can occur immediately or even hours before a seizure. Follow these safety guidelines if a resident feels a seizure coming:

▶ Since a resident may fall during a seizure, protect him or her from injury. Help ease him or her to the floor using the method described in Chapter 13.

▶ Remove objects the person may strike against because of the jerking movements.

▶ Never try to restrain or hold down a person during a seizure. This could result in an injury.

▶ Oxygen may be needed and should be available.

What to Do if a Resident Has a Grand Mal Seizure

▶ Call for help from the charge nurse.

▶ Remove any objects in the person's way that could cause injury during the seizure.

▶ If possible, turn the head to one side. This helps the person breathe by letting saliva drain out and by preventing the tongue from blocking the airway.

▶ Loosen belts, ties, or other clothing to help the person breathe better.

▶ Help the nurse by noting:
a. Parts of the body involved
b. Strength of the activity
c. Whether bowel and bladder functions stayed controlled
d. Resident's mental state after the seizure and how long the seizure lasted (this can be of help to the physician)

▶ Remain with this resident until the seizure is over. Reassure and comfort the person to the best of your ability. He or she may be confused, disoriented, frightened, and even embarrassed.

Residents Who Wander from the Facility

A resident who wanders away is an emergency in every facility. A confused resident may go out of a door and become lost. This resident may not be familiar with the outside surroundings and could become frightened and more confused. Residents who wander should be identified so that all staff know who they are and can watch them more closely. Chapter 19 explains alternatives for caring for wandering residents.

When a resident is announced missing, all staff who can be spared without compromising others' safety should help search for the person. The nurse may call the police with a description of a resident who is not found by the staff within a few minutes. Find out what the protocol or procedure is in your facility.

IN THIS CHAPTER YOU LEARNED TO:

▶ provide general information on admission, discharge, and transfer

▶ demonstrate the following skills: vital signs, specimen collection, use of nonsterile bandages and dressings, use of support hose and elastic stockings, application of topical preparations, hot and cold applications, and ostomy care

▶ state what to do in the event of cardiac arrest, seizure, or choking, and describe how to find a wandering resident

19

ALTERNATIVES TO THE USE OF RESTRAINTS

Imagine sitting in a chair or lying in a bed, unable to move freely, for hours at a time, day after day. Imagine having your hand movements restricted so you cannot scratch your nose when it itches or drink a glass of water when you are thirsty. Imagine not being able to turn over in bed because you are restricted to one position and not being able to go to the bathroom when you want to. How would this make you feel? Wouldn't you spend your time trying to be free so you could move?

In your facility some of your residents may fall, some cannot sit straight, some wander, some pull out the tubes that keep them alive, and some act out. Some of these may be restrained, and to them being restrained is like being tied up. The intention of the restraints is to prevent residents from harming themselves, but often the restraints and residents' endless efforts to get free actually cause more injury.

This chapter discusses how you can provide good care without using restraints. You will learn what a restraint is, the problems they cause, why restraints should be used only after everything else has been tried, and legal implications of using restraints. You will also learn the main reasons why restraints have sometimes been used and alternative approaches for these residents. Finally, you will learn about the exceptional cases when restraints are appropriate on a temporary basis.

WHAT IS A RESTRAINT?

A physical restraint is anything used to restrict a resident's movement or ability to reach a part of the body. Restraints prevent residents from moving freely. Restraints include waist or pelvic restraints, seat belts, vests, mittens, straps, siderails, or trays fastened to the chair (Fig. 19-1):

▶ Waist, pelvic, seat belt, and Velcro strap restraints are used to prevent residents from getting out of bed or up from a chair. These restraints are attached to the bed or chair and strapped across a resident's waist or pelvis.

▶ Vests or jacket restraints are also used to restrict residents from getting out of bed or a chair. These restraints are like a sleeveless jacket that crisscrosses in front of a resident and is attached to the bed or chair.

▶ A tray fastened to a chair restricts a resident from getting up from a chair. It crosses over the person's lap and locks into the side of a chair.

▶ Mitt restraints restrict the movement of the fingers. The mitt is placed over the person's hand and wrist.

▶ Siderails are placed on the sides of a resident's bed and restrict a resident's ability to get out of bed. The rails are pulled up and locked in place.

COMMON REASONS FOR RESTRAINT USE

Restraints are generally used for six kinds of problems of residents in long term care facilities. The following problems create safety concerns for residents, and thus necessitate the use of restraints:

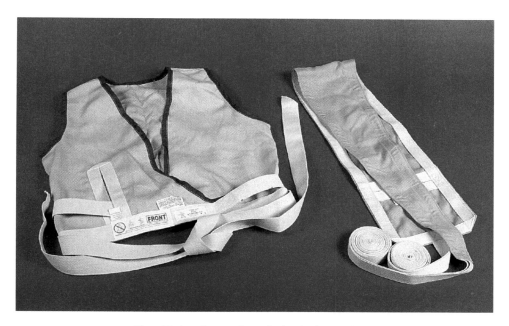

Fig. 19-1.   Examples of physical restraints.

Walking and Falling Problems

Walking and falling problems occur when residents are unsteady on their feet. For many different reasons, a resident may lose his or her balance while standing or walking or may have trouble transferring from a sitting position to standing, from one seat to another, or from lying to sitting to standing.

Positioning Problems

Some residents cannot sit safely or comfortably because of positioning problems. The person may fall or slide to the floor, lean forward, or lean to one side. These problems may be due to weakness, arthritis, or another chronic illness or condition. Muscle and bone deformities and the restlessness caused by discomfort are also sometimes classified as positioning problems.

Agitated Behavior

Residents who behave in an agitated way are sometimes restless or combative. Some wave their arms around; some kick, bite, and scratch; and some talk and act angrily. Some residents behave like this often, others only at certain times.

Wandering

Wandering is the restless roaming of a resident. Residents may wander in a wheelchair or on foot.

Life Support Equipment Problems

Some sick residents are confused and agitated and try to pull out the tubes that help keep them alive (Fig. 19-2). For example, they may pull out a feeding tube, an IV providing medicine, or a catheter. They may also pull off bandages. Often they do not realize what they are doing. Other residents may pull out tubes because they are depressed or for other reasons. Some may have decided to reject a treatment.

Stress of Admission

Moving into a facility is stressful for new residents and those returning from a hospital. Under stress, residents may behave in ways they would not normally behave, such as wandering and acting out.

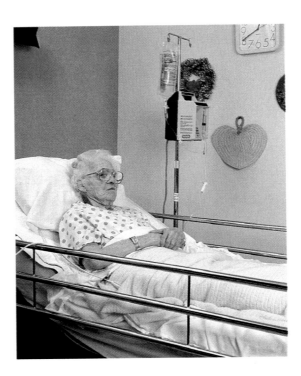

Fig. 19-2. Sometimes a resident may be confused or agitated and try to pull out the tubes that keep them alive.

SOLUTIONS

Although the six kinds of problems described above are often cited as reasons for putting a resident in restraints, there are usually other solutions that do not involve using restraints. Staff can work to create individual plans of care for certain behaviors and prevent the use of restraints. For example, an individual who falls may need a particular kind of muscle exercise to strengthen a weak muscle. A resident who wanders at night may have been a night watchman and needs a solution based on his lifelong habits. Coming up with solutions and creating individual plans of care takes the whole team. You must work closely with the charge nurse and other staff. Here are some solutions you can individualize for residents you assist.

Solutions for Falling and Positioning Problems

For any resident at risk for falls, ask why the person is getting up unassisted. Is he or she hungry, uncomfortable, in pain, needing to use the toilet? If so, you must intervene; for example, providing snacks and offering comfort measures like pillow changes and back rubs will ease hunger and discomfort. A change in toileting or other schedules can prevent getting up in the night. Work with other staff and discuss potential problems in the environment—such as poor lighting, uneven or slippery floor surfaces, poorly designed bathrooms, incorrect bed height, inadequate storage, clutter, and inappropriate chairs—that can contribute to falling problems. Consider the following:

▶ A chair alarm, consisting of a cord attached to the person's clothing at one end and an alarm device at the other, is sometimes a solution. The alarm sounds when the person starts to stand and the cord pulls on the alarm, summoning help before he or she can fall. Alarms are good for residents who are recently out of restraints because they help staff, family, and resident alike feel more secure.

▶ Change the chair residents sit in. Most residents do better if they sit in different chairs throughout the day, such as a lounge chair, a reclining chair, a dining chair, or a beanbag chair. Residents cannot easily stand up from chairs, reclining lounge chairs, and soft-seated chairs. These chairs can provide greater safety for some residents, and maintain good seating position.

▷ For a resident who falls or slides to the floor because of positioning problems, correct positioning can increase comfort and decrease agitation, often reducing or eliminating the need for restraints. A physical therapist or a rehabilitation nurse does the assessment and makes recommendations for residents with positioning problems.

▷ A resident who uses a wheelchair should have his or her own that is individually adjusted for comfort and ease of use. For example, for residents who spend most of the day in a wheelchair, the chair probably needs a special cushion to take up the slack caused by the sling effect. A cushion with a rounded bottom and a flat sitting surface is called a solid-seat insert. A cushion with a rounded bottom higher at the front than the back is called a wedge cushion, used for residents who lean forward or who tend to slide out of the chair. Both kinds of cushions should be attached to the chair with Velcro or a similar fastening (Fig. 19-3).

▷ Residents who tend to lean toward one side and have trouble sitting straight can be helped by specially shaped lateral supports. Lateral supports can be purchased or made from firm foam. Wheelchair anti-tippers are devices attached to wheelchair wheels that make it almost impossible for a wheelchair to tip, even if the person leans off center. Leg rests provide comfort and help to correctly position the legs. A rehabilitation nurse or therapist can decide exactly what equipment is appropriate.

Solutions for Agitated Behavior

Agitated behavior sometimes results from an illness requiring medical attention. Report any changes in behavior to the charge nurse. Work closely with this resident and other staff to find a pattern or cause of his or her agitated behavior. Is he or she hungry? Does it happen at a certain time each day? You may observe when the restless agitated behavior occurs. If you can find the cause, you can often prevent the behavior and thus the need for restraints. Consider the following:

▷ If a resident is agitated or expressing distress, check for discomfort, pain, and toileting needs. Does the toileting schedule need adjusting? Is his or her clothing comfortable and well fitting? Is the chair or bed the correct size and type so he or she can get comfortable? If you can identify the specific problem, you and the team should discuss what to do to solve the problem.

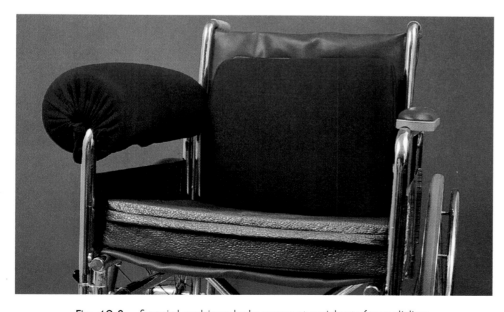

Fig. 19-3. Special cushions help prevent residents from sliding.

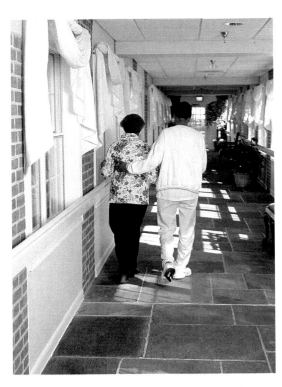

Fig. 19-4. Walk with a wandering resident to see if it gives you clues about why they wander.

▷ Work to communicate clearly with agitated residents. Make sure residents wear their glasses, teeth, hearing aids, and any other assistive devices they may have. Use simple sentences, be aware of your body language, and use gestures to reinforce your message. Like someone who speaks another language, confused residents often cannot understand the words but will understand gestures. Never argue with an agitated resident, but be as calm and patient as possible.

▷ Sometimes residents are overcome by stress. In this case, try using simple relaxation exercises, giving a gentle shoulder and neck rub. If you think a resident is stressed by noise, reduce or remove the noise. Ragged nerves can be soothed by music through headphones.

▷ Encourage family and friends to visit often. Involving each resident and family members in as much decision making as possible helps them feel in control. Put yourself in their position: what would you want to know and decide?

Solutions for Wandering

Many of the techniques for residents with behavioral symptoms also work for residents who wander. Remember, wandering is OK as long as a resident is in a protected environment. Consider the following:

▷ Maintain familiar routines and regular exercise schedules. Follow a wandering resident to see where he or she goes, and you may discover why a resident is wandering (Fig. 19-4).

▷ Some residents wander because they are bored, so you need to find activities they will enjoy.

▷ Others need a safe place, such as a courtyard or locked area, to wander. Use hidden door locks or alarms on doors so that wandering residents do not go beyond the safe space.

▷ In the unit, use large signs and pictures to help residents find their room, bathroom, dayroom, etc.

▷ A wandering resident should wear a name band for identification in case he or she slips away and gets lost. This situation is considered a facility emergency.

▷ Frequently check on a wandering resident's whereabouts.

Life Support Equipment Problems

A resident on life support equipment who is moving lines or tubes may be feeling irritation and discomfort where the tube, line, or catheter enters the body. Consider the following:

▷ Keep the tape clean and free of irritation. Report to the nurse if the tape needs to be changed or repositioned.

▷ If a resident is bothered by an IV line or feeding tube, maybe exploring other ways he or she can safely take food and liquids by mouth is a solution.

▷ Keep tubes out of sight and out of the person's reach. This may mean putting clothing over the tubes such as long sleeves, jumpsuits, and clothing with an opening at the back where it is hard to reach.

▷ Make sure there are no dangling ends on tubes or IVs a resident is tempted to pull on.

Solutions for the Stress of Admission

The stress of the change due to the admission may be more than a resident can handle. Consider the following:

▷ Adopt a routine similar to the one the person had at home.

▷ Be patient and help the person get used to the new environment.

▷ All staff should learn as much as possible about new residents from these residents themselves and their families and friends. When a new resident is admitted to a restraint-free unit, the interdisciplinary team should evaluate him or her for strengths and needs.

▷ Orient this resident and family to the floor plan and procedures. Be sure to give them time to absorb new information. And be patient, repeating yourself as often as necessary and being reassuring often.

Case Studies

The following two cases show how to use possible solutions for residents as alternatives to using restraints.

Mrs. Brown

Mrs. Brown is 79 years old and for many years has had osteoarthritis in both knees and Parkinson's disease (Fig. 19-5). She has poor balance and needs help with moving and positioning. Her husband is 84 years old and usually visits once a week. He became ill about a month ago and has not visited since then. Two days ago, a nurse found Mrs. Brown on the floor next to her bed. She said that she fell as she was trying to go to the bathroom. She said that she felt dizzy when she stood up, and then she fell. The nursing staff were afraid that Mrs. Brown would fall again, so they worked out the following plan of care:

1. The nursing staff discussed the situation with Mrs. Brown's physician so she could be evaluated for medical problems.
2. They checked that her shoes fit well and were comfortable, and had a firm, rigid, nonskid sole. They decided the floor surface was slippery and added nonslip strips by the bed.
3. They checked whether she had been tired at the time of the incident.
4. They ensured her bed was adjusted to the right height so that she could rest her feet on the floor to stand. They checked that the bed wheels were and stayed locked.
5. They created a regular toileting schedule for Mrs. Brown.

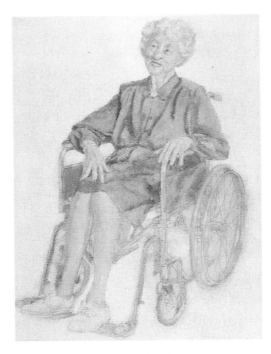

Fig. 19-5. Mrs. Brown.

6. Because Mrs. Brown worried about her husband's health, staff decided she could benefit from talking to the social worker.
7. They assisted or supervised Mrs. Brown when transferring from bed to chair or chair to bed.
8. Mrs. Brown's wheelchair was adjusted for ease of use and comfort.

Miss Schwartz

Until recently, Miss Schwartz, age 76, lived with her sister. Miss Schwartz is a retired journalist who never married (Fig. 19-6). Over the years her memory has grown worse, and last year she was diagnosed with Alzheimer's disease. At home Miss Schwartz wandered, and twice she left the house and got lost. Miss Schwartz can still perform most activities of daily living—eating, toileting, and dressing—but she needed help with household tasks. When she needed 24-hour supervision, concerns for her safety led to admission to the facility.

Miss Schwartz rarely stays in her room. She wanders throughout the facility and is often found on different floors in other residents' rooms. For the next two weeks, she became increasingly agitated, telling staff, "I have a deadline to meet. Get the phone!" She also insisted on taking daily "walks through the neighborhood." Her gait was unsteady, and she tended to shuffle rather than walk. Staff were afraid that she would hurt herself, so they worked out the following plan of care:

1. By closely monitoring Miss Schwartz, they established that she became agitated only at two times in the day: in the morning when she used to leave for work or the library and later in the afternoon when she would leave work. She was, in fact, reliving her earlier work routine. (The technique for tracking a resident's behavior to determine a routine is sometimes called *behavior mapping*.) (Fig. 19-7).
2. Like many other confused residents, Miss Schwartz found it reassuring to have personal items and pictures in her room. Miss Schwartz responded well to the photos and other personal items that her sister brought in.
3. The staff also encouraged family and friends to visit often, particularly at the times when she became agitated.

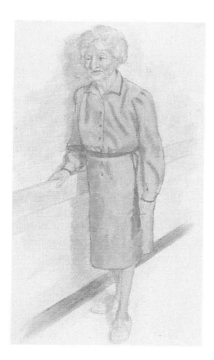

Fig. 19-6.   Ms. Schwartz.

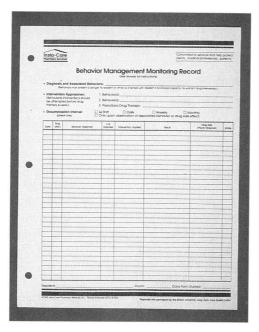

Fig. 19-7.   Behavior mapping helps to determine a resident's routine. (Courtesy of Insta-Care Pharmacy Services.)

4. When no family or friends were visiting, in the morning, staff encouraged Miss Schwartz to spend time with her books and papers in the part of the dayroom they called the library. In the afternoon if she again became restless, a nurse assistant walked with Miss Schwartz to an enclosed patio garden where she could walk about safely.

CONSEQUENCES OF RESTRAINTS

Finding a balance between the use of restraints for safety reasons and resident's rights to be free from restraints is a major challenge. Many health care workers feel restraints can prevent residents from falling and hurting themselves. Experience shows this is not true: residents continue to fall, and often their injuries are just as serious. Imagine what could have happened if Mrs. Brown had struggled hard to stand up while restrained in a wheelchair. The wheelchair might have fallen on top of her, almost certainly causing an even greater injury.

Residents who are restrained for a long time are also more likely to develop medical and psychological conditions. Restraints can cause bowel and bladder problems because residents cannot access the bathroom freely. Such problems are uncomfortable, medically unsafe, and potentially dangerous, and they may require treatment. Lack of movement can negatively affect circulation and skin condition. People who are restrained for long periods often have swollen legs because of the immobility and impaired circulation. Skin breakdown many develop due to prolonged pressure and lack of mobility. Some restrained residents develop muscle contractures, rigid joints, loss of muscle mass, tone, and strength, and loss of bone density. All of these reduce functioning and well-being.

One possible reason why Mrs. Brown fell is that her blood pressure may have dropped because she was confined to her bed. When she stood up, she felt faint and then fell. Restraining Mrs. Brown in one place would not prevent more episodes. Residents like Mrs. Brown need to be as active as possible.

Think how you would feel if you were restrained. Some restrained residents feel humiliated and angry, and then are labeled as behavior problems if they express their feelings. Others feel sad and ashamed, feeling they are being punished. Restrained residents often get less attention than unrestrained residents. This lack of attention can lead to a loss of interest in life, dependence on others, depression, and confusion.

As you can see, there are many reasons not to use restraints. It is better not to restrain a resident unless there are absolutely no other alternatives.

ADVANTAGES OF RESTRAINT-FREE CARE

There are many advantages for residents, staff, and families in not using restraints. Residents will be stronger, more independent, and healthier. They will feel better about themselves, about living at the facility, and about life generally. Happier residents often mean happier families and happier staff. Communication among staff members, residents, and family members improves as everyone gets involved in learning more about the person and providing the best possible care.

Each of the residents you care for, even those with the most severe impairments, has the right to be free of restraints. Many residents are calmer and can do more for themselves when the restraints are removed. Staff feel better about their work and having their opinions about alternatives valued.

The concept of restraint-free care is based on the fact that each resident is a special human being. Care must be individualized. Staff should adapt to the needs of residents, rather than making residents adapt to the needs of staff. To treat each resident in the best possible way, you and other staff must assess each resident carefully and individually. Get to know the residents by gathering information about their habits, routines, preferences, strengths, and weaknesses. This information helps you come up with more effective alternatives to restraints. In the long run, your job will also become easier, more fun, and not as physically demanding.

The Nurse Assistant's Role in Keeping Residents Restraint-Free

Since you provide the most care, you know residents better than other staff members. You spend more time with residents and are in the best position to monitor their routines. You can improve the quality of care.

For example, you know what a resident likes and dislikes. You know what, when, and how he or she likes to eat. You know if a resident is a "night" or a "morning person." And you know if there are certain times, day or night, when a resident tends to become tired or unsafe.

To keep your residents restraint-free, communicate what you know about residents to other team members. This helps the team provide individualized care to avoid restraints. Be careful to distinguish between what you see (objective observation) and what you read into a situation (subjective interpretation). For example, the statement "Mrs. Brown was found lying on the floor beside her bed" is objective because it is factual. To say "Mrs. Brown slipped because she was impatient to get to the bathroom" is a subjective interpretation. At team meetings, give an accurate and objective account of your observations of each resident, to allow an effective plan to be developed. Avoid subjective opinions and interpretations that might be incorrect and could lead to an ineffective care plan (Fig. 19-8).

Many family members know you deliver most of the hands-on care, and because of this they feel comfortable talking with you. Often you are the first staff person with whom families share information about a resident's life-style, likes, and dislikes. You therefore have much to contribute to the team's assessment. Once the team has a good sense of a resident's condition, interests, likes, and dislikes, everyone should work together to come up with a plan of care that avoids using restraints.

Another important responsibility is to ensure that equipment and devices are properly used and that the care plan is carried out. There are right and wrong ways to put cushions and other positioning devices, for example, in the chair. Most positioning aids have a front and a back, and many should be fastened in place with Velcro or a similar fastening. With alarms, be sure that the batteries are good, that the alarm is turned on, and that the ends are properly attached. Be sure to ask for assistance if you do not know how to use any device.

Keeping a resident free of restraints may require following a napping or toileting schedule closely. Notify the charge nurse if you do not understand the schedule, if you cannot keep to the schedule, or if you have an idea about a better schedule.

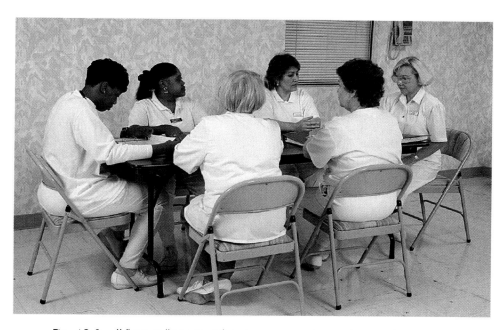

Fig. 19-8. When talking to other team members, always give an accurate and objective account of your observations and interactions with the resident.

WHEN RESTRAINTS ARE NECESSARY

While restraints are undesirable and a last resort, occasionally a resident must be restrained on an emergency or temporary basis. A resident may need restraint because he or she is delirious, and the agitated behavior could dislodge a life support device such as an IV line, feeding or drainage tube, catheter, or dressing or bandage.

Other residents sometimes restrained are those with severe deformities or involuntary movements. Restraints may provide safe and comfortable positioning for these residents. Finally, some residents may need restraints because they are dangerous to themselves or others, such as residents who are violently agitated and must be temporarily restrained for safety until the cause is found and solved.

1. Restraints must be ordered by a doctor. They must be the least restrictive possible. They should be secure enough to protect a resident but not completely restrict movement. You must be able to slide your fingers comfortably between the person and the restraint (Fig, 19-9).

2. If you have to apply restraints, think of how you'd feel in the person's position or how you would want your own mother, father, or grandparents to be treated. Make sure the restraint is not too tight, and check often to make sure the person is as safe and comfortable as possible. Also check the condition of the skin around the restraint for chafing, redness, or bruising. Check the circulation by checking their pulse and watching for any swelling. Never tie the restraint to a moveable object, such as a bed rail or furniture that can be moved. Always use a quick release knot when restraining a resident, such as a knot used for tying shoe laces or a square knot. Remove the restraint at least every 2 hours for toileting and walking. Your facility may require documentation of release of restraints. You should become familiar with all policies and procedures.

3. Regardless of the type of restraint, the above principles hold true. The following is the procedure to follow if using a waist restraint while sitting in a chair.

   ▶ Assist this resident into the sitting position desired, using skills described in Chapter 13.

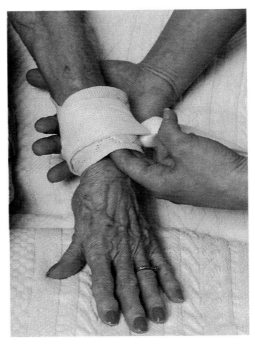

Fig. 19-9. Restraints need to be secure but not to the point that they completely restrict movement.

- Place the restraint around the resident's waist, bringing the ties around the back of the chair.
- Place the ties through the slots.
- Secure the ties, using a bow tie knot or a square knot.
- Be sure the waist restraint is not too tight by placing your hand between the person and the restraint.

4. Remember that residents have the right to refuse any treatment or intervention, including doctor-ordered restraints. Restraints should be used for the shortest possible period and never only for the convenience of staff. The decision to restrain should be a team decision, and the family or resident representative must be notified.

5. When restraints are used, all staff members should continue seeking alternatives. For most residents, restraints should be only a temporary measure. Tell the charge nurse any time you think restraints could safely be untied (such as at mealtimes) and speak up in team meetings.

BEYOND RESTRAINTS

Taking restraints off is the first major step: keeping restraints off is a continuing challenge. Involve residents in structured activities at the facility. Focus on residents' interests and assist in creating a safe environment. Keeping the restraints off requires that everyone be alert and continue to work as a team. Once in a while, a particularly challenging resident may tempt the team to seek a restraint order. Always ask yourself, "Would I like someone to do this to me? Is there anything else I could do that would take care of the problem?"

Residents need activities to build on their restraint-free status and to enhance the quality of their lives. Because you work closely with residents, you play an important role in helping residents live with dignity and satisfaction.

IN THIS CHAPTER YOU
LEARNED TO:

- list various restraint devices, the reason for their use, and alternative solutions
- state the advantages of restraint-free care
- define the nurse assistant's role in ensuring a restraint-free environment
- list the "rules of use" when restraints are necessary

RESTORATIVE ACTIVITIES

Have you ever watched a very young boy trying to get dressed by himself? After three or four tries he manages to get his pants on without both feet in the same pant leg. For a long time he can't seem to get all his toes into the socks. You offer to help but he pushes you away, saying he'll do it by himself. Finally the socks are on but he can't get the shoes on the right feet. Still he rejects your offers to help. This is the stage of a typical 2-year-old craving independence.

Watching a child getting dressed can seem humorous because to us, these simple tasks are so easy we take them for granted. By age 30 we've put on socks over 10,000 times—almost never even thinking about it, much less having trouble doing it.

Think of other activities in your daily life you take for granted. Getting out of bed in the morning, walking to the bathroom, brushing your teeth, showering, getting dressed—and hundreds more things every day. We take for granted our ability to get to the bathroom, to raise the toothbrush to our mouths, and so on. But many residents do not have these same abilities because illness, disease, or disabilities have limited capability for movement. A resident may not be able to reach his or her feet to put on socks or get out of bed to the wheelchair by himself or herself.

Imagine what it must feel like, after decades of taking such actions for granted, to not be able to do these things by yourself or to have to learn to do them in a different way. Imagine how frustrating it can be to have to ask and rely on someone else for help in the activities of daily living.

This chapter is about you becoming a teacher, and residents learning or relearning information and skills that can help them regain or maintain their level of independent functioning. You will learn how to work with residents in restorative activities and how to help residents use special equipment and devices to function independently. With your mindful attention to residents' physical and emotional needs and your knowledge of how to provide care, you can help much to promote their independent functioning and thus improve their quality of life (Fig. 20-1).

The word "function" is used often in this chapter. Restorative activities are designed to help residents be as independent and functional as possible. Function may involve how well a particular part of the body works or how well the whole person can perform an activity. The more residents can do for themselves safely, the more functional they are.

What is Rehabilitation?

You may hear the terms "rehabilitation" (rehab) or "retraining." These words describe the process by which residents improve their functional abilities, such as walking, getting up, moving, dressing, and bathing. Rehabilitation is an approach to care that focuses on restoring and retraining. A resident in rehabilitation is developing new skills or working on old ones to live as independently as possible (Fig. 20-2). Although rehabilitation seems to focus on physical well-being, the goal is psychological well-being and independence. You can help in the rehabilitation process by using restorative activities in your nursing care. You use all the information you have about how to care for residents and teach, prompt, and encourage them to care for themselves. You work with residents in those activities that benefit them most.

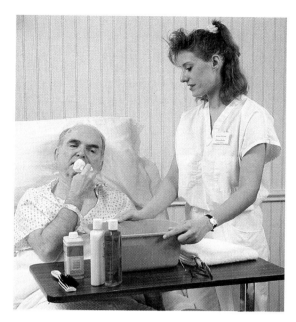

Fig. 20-1. Being attentive to the physical and emotional needs of the residents, will help promote their independence.

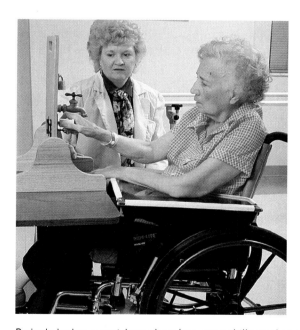

Fig. 20-2. Rehab helps a resident develop new skills and work on old skills.

WHAT ARE RESTORATIVE ACTIVITIES?

With restorative activities you have the opportunity to help residents regain or maintain the ability to care for themselves. Everything you do with a resident must have a restorative theme. Ask yourself when assisting a resident, "What can I do to help this person regain or maintain his or her independence?"

Restorative activities promote independence in areas of feeding, bathing, dressing, toileting, continence, and moving and positioning. These are called the activities of daily living. The goal is to achieve the optimal or best level of functioning.

Restorative activities are any activities done in a way to restore function. How you interact with a resident is important for optimizing a resident's function. How you ask residents to do something, how patient you are with their capabilities, and how you encourage and prompt them make all the difference in their ability to do a task. These activities can be simple everyday routine activities such as teaching a resident how to get out of bed, get dressed, use a walker or wheel themselves in a wheelchair, or they can be special activities added to the normal routine such as exercise. Following are some examples:

Mr. Ellis can sit up by himself. It is better for him if you ask him to sit up and give him the time to do so while you stand by to assist if needed, than if you say you would like him to get up and then lift him to a sitting position.

Mrs. Weiss uses a walker to walk to the dining room with help from a nurse. It is better for her if you walk with her to the dining room using her walker and your help, than if you wheel her in a wheelchair to the dining room.

Mr. White cannot move at all by himself, yet is alert and can converse. It is better for him if you do his range of motion (ROM) exercises and talk to him about what you are doing and why, asking how he feels or if anything hurts as he does the exercise, than if you move his arms and legs for him without involving him at all in what you are doing.

Mrs. Wong is confused and hard of hearing. She can walk by herself yet forgets to at times. It is better for her if you face her and clearly ask her to get up and walk to the bathroom, than if you remind her to walk to the bathroom by speaking with your back to her.

What did you notice in each example? Which technique is most helpful to that resident and why? In these examples, the promotion of the resident's independence is shown. The importance of each resident's success is the primary focus instead of the nurse assistant doing the task.

Helping Residents in the Restorative Process

Consider four primary areas when working with a resident:
1. Establishment of short and long term goals
2. Cuing, prompting and encouragement
3. Identifying assistive devices
4. Strengthening exercises

Establishment of Short and Long Term Goals

To improve ourselves, we often set goals, short term and long term, that we can strive to accomplish. When helping residents optimize their independence, be aware of their problems and the goals set by the members of the health care team. As a vital part of this team, your input is necessary in establishing these goals because you spend the most time with residents each day. Once you know a resident's goals, desires, and preferences, use your creativity to find ways to help the person accomplish these goals and to feel good about his or her progress.

For example, a resident has a goal of learning to use a walker safely to transfer to a chair and walk short distances. You might start to help him or her to achieve this goal by first determining his or her current ability to use the walker. Work closely with a resident and discuss the established goal as you find the starting point. Then observe the person firsthand and learn his or her capabilities. Now you are ready to assist in accomplishing his or her goals.

For example, a resident can get out of bed with some cuing from you, and requires a little help to stand up, but has great fears about letting go of your arm and using the walker. In this example, your short-term goal may be to help this resident feel comfortable using the walker to stand and transfer to the chair. Your long term goal would be to assist him or her to walk with the walker. To establish the long term goal, you must first tackle the short term goal. The following are some ideas:

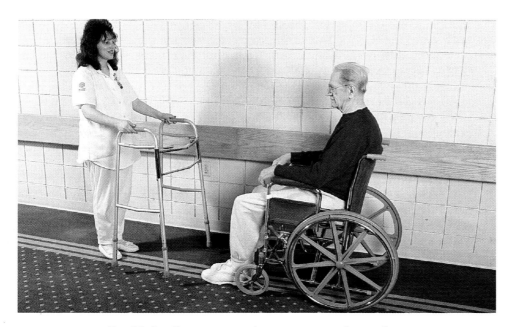

Fig. 20-3. Demonstrate the correct use of a walker.

▷ Demonstrate the use of the walker (Fig. 20-3). Show how to use it when trying to stand up.

▷ Reinforce the safety of the walker. Show the rubber stoppers on the bottom that prevent slipping.

▷ Tell the person you will stay close by. Ask him or her where you should stand.

▷ Encourage and support a resident's efforts.

Once the short term goal is accomplished, you can establish the next. Always keep in mind the long term goal—the person will walk with a walker.

Your goals should compliment the care plan and be realistic for a resident to attain. Always discuss these goals with the nurse for further input before trying with a resident in case you need additional information.

Cuing, Prompting, and Encouragement

In your role as the daily caregiver, you need to use restorative activities throughout a resident's care. Take the time to offer residents the cuing or prompting and encouragement that may help them to do the task more independently. Cuing means that you prompt a resident by telling him or her part or all of the steps in a task.

In the chapter on mobility and positioning, you learned how to move and position a resident in bed, transfer him or her, and position him or her in a chair. How can these activities become restorative? When helping a resident to do an activity, you use common sense and your personal knowledge of how to do the skill steps to teach him or her. Here are some suggestions on how to teach residents while doing activities with them:

▷ Explain to residents what you would like to help them do. If they do not understand what you are saying, try to say it in a different way. If a resident is hard of hearing, try to speak louder or more clearly while facing him or her. Try speaking on the side of a resident's better ear. Write it down if necessary.

▷ Always give a resident time to respond to a request. Often a resident may be trying to move but just has trouble getting started and moves slowly.

▷ If residents look puzzled or you think they might be confused by what you said, try to break down the activity into simple steps. For example, you would like a resident to get up out of bed, yet he or she seems to be having trouble responding. You might say, "I would like you to get out of bed now. First, please roll toward me. Good. Now bring your legs over the edge of the bed. Good. Now push your upper body up to sitting." Or even more simply, you can say "Please sit up. Now stand up. Now let me help you get into the chair."

▶ If a resident is still having trouble, you may need to also show him or her what to do or even start each step for him or her. This is called cuing. For example, you want a resident to brush his or her teeth, but the person is having trouble getting started. You might place the toothbrush in a resident's dominant hand and hand him or her the toothpaste (Fig. 20-4). If he or she still does not understand, try to put the toothpaste on the toothbrush and help him or her to hold the toothbrush while brushing.

▶ If a resident does not want to participate in care, try gently encouraging him or her to participate before you do it for him or her. Explain to the person, in terms he or she can understand, how important it is for them to try to do as much for themselves as possible.

Residents' Equipment: Identifying Proper Assistive Devices

Often a resident has equipment in his or her room, such as braces, walking devices, splints, trapeze, and dressing aides. These pieces of equipment most of the time have been given to a resident by the therapist at some point in their rehabilitation to help him or her be more independent. It is extremely important to the restorative (rehabilitation) process and the resident's functioning to become familiar with each piece of equipment, how it is used, and why it is used. Then you can guide residents in using their equipment if they need help. Residents may also forget to use equipment or resist using something that helps keep them safe from injury. You must talk with the charge nurse about a resident's abilities to help identify equipment to improve functioning. For example, you may identify a problem, such as a resident having difficulty using a fork. You tell the charge nurse and together with the therapy department find an assistive device. A simple change in eating utensils may dramatically improve a resident's nutritional status. The following devices can be used to improve a resident's function:

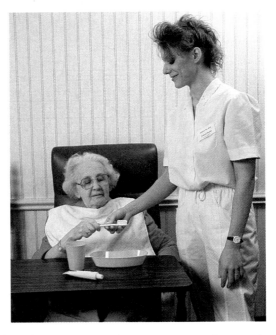

Fig. 20-4. Residents may need assistance or to be cued when beginning the task of brushing their teeth.

Assistive Devices. Assistive devices are equipment that enable a resident to transfer or walk more independently and safely. Generally, they provide support or assistance, depending on the support needed. Following are examples of assistive devices, arranged from those that provide the most support to those that provide the least.

A *walker* is used when a resident needs the most support from an assistive device. It is used by moving the walker first, then the weaker leg, then the stronger leg. If a resident's legs are equally strong, the person just moves the walker forward and then steps with one leg and then the other.

A *rolling walker* is used for a good amount of support. Because it has two wheels in front, it allows a resident to push it instead of lift it up while walking. It is used by residents who may lose balance lifting a walker off the floor (Fig. 20-5).

Both types of walkers should always remain in front of the body while walking. The height of the walker should be at his or her hips so that he or she is not bending forward during walking.

Crutches are not often used in long term care facilities because of the balance and flexibility required. There are two types of crutches: axillary (under the arm) crutches and forearm (also called Canadian or Lofstrand) crutches. Crutches are used to keep weight off a leg while walking or to provide support for a resident who needs less support than a walker (Fig. 20-6).

Canes are used when a resident needs less support than a walker or crutches. A cane can be used to support a weaker leg or just to provide support for a slight balance problem. If the cane is used to support a weak leg, it should be in the hand opposite the weak leg. If it is used for balance, it can be used in either hand, although a right-handed person usually prefers the right hand, and vice versa. The height of the cane should be at the level of the person's hip so that he or she is not bending forward when using it.

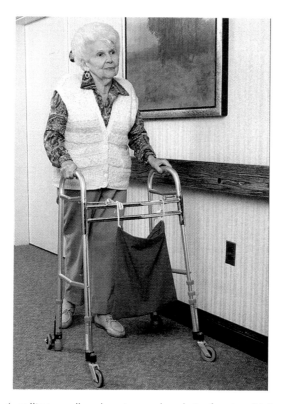

Fig. 20-5. A rolling walker has two wheels in front, which allows the resident to push the walker instead of lifting it.

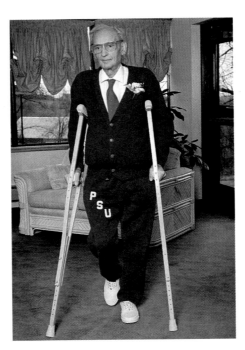

Fig. 20-6. Auxillary crutches support from under the arm and are used for residents who need less support than a walker.

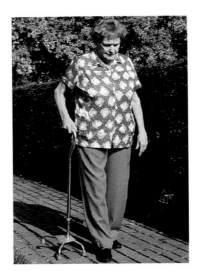

Fig. 20-7. Canes are used when a resident needs less support than a walker or crutches. A quad cane can have either a large or small base with three or four prongs.

There are two types of canes:

▶ A quad cane has a large or small base, usually with three or four prongs. The end of the handle faces backward and the flat side of the base stays at the person's side (Fig. 20-7).

▶ Straight cane (also called cane or J cane): This is the typical cane made of either wood or metal.

An assistive device, as the name implies, is used to assist residents in moving. Always keep the assistive device next to a resident and use it when transferring or walking. Its use is essential in optimizing residents' functional independence.

Prosthetic and Orthotic Devices. Prosthetic devices are equipment specially made for a resident such as artificial limbs, hearing aids, and glasses, that improve the function of a body part that is missing or not fully functioning. (A prosthetic device may also be referred to as a prosthesis.)

Orthotic devices are equipment specially made for a resident, like braces, splints, or shoe inserts to improve or help restore the function of a limb or body part during functional activities. (An orthotic device may also be referred to as an orthosis.)

You need to use a resident's prosthetic or orthotic devices in all functional activities or other activities as intended. Always check with the charge nurse if you have any questions.

There are many kinds of *artificial limbs*, but the most common among residents are artificial legs (Fig. 20-8). A resident may need your help in putting the artificial leg onto the leg stump. Use the necessary stump socks and prosthesis liners to protect a resident's skin at the end of the stump. If you notice a resident's stump is red or bruised when you take off the artificial leg, notify the charge nurse.

Leg, neck, and back *braces* are common with long term care residents. Braces are designed to do what the name implies, brace a body part during transfers and walking when that part of the body does not have the strength to support the body weight by itself. Braces may be used permanently by someone for an injured, chronically painful, or weak joint; or temporarily during a recovery from a stroke, injury, or surgery. Usually the firmer the brace material, the weaker or more severely injured that body part is. Some braces are worn only when a resident is out of bed, and others are worn all the time. You must learn how to put each brace on correctly and know when it should be worn. You may see several typical types of braces:

▶ A knee brace is made of either elastic, for less support, or other materials. Metal strips are located on either side of the knee for more support.

▶ An ankle foot orthosis (AFO) is either a shoe with metal uprights attached to a calf band or a plastic shoe insert that usually covers from the back of the calf to the bottom of the foot (Fig. 20-9). If a resident has lost use of the leg above the knee, you may also see a knee-ankle foot orthoses (KAFO), which supports both the knee and the ankle.

▶ A back brace may be a corset type elastic brace that closes in front with either Velcro or straps. Harder materials are used to support any part of the back. Usually braces support the lower back, but occasionally after a surgery or spinal cord injury, you may also see a body jacket. This type of back brace extends from the lower back to under the arms. If a resident is to wear this type of brace, it usually means that the back problem is very severe.

▶ Residents may wear soft or hard neck collars to support the neck (Fig. 20-10). Some residents use these devices just in bed, some only when up, and others all the time.

Splints are used to immobilize a joint or body part, or to restrict its motion in a certain way (Fig. 20-11). You most commonly see them on a hand, wrist, knee, or foot. Usually a resident's splint was given to them by their therapist. The therapist will tell you when and how it should be worn.

Positioning/Seating Devices. These are cushions, supportive chairs, pillows, towel rolls, splints, and heel and elbow protectors used to position a resident who has limited independent movement, in the best functional position while lying or sitting. As you learned in Chapter 14, these also help prevent other problems such as skin breakdown and contractures (arms or legs becoming stuck in a certain position).

Heel and elbow protectors are cloth sleeves that cover the elbow and heels to protect against pressure sores.

Splints keep a joint in a good position or restrict certain undesirable motions that may cause tightness, pain, or injury. Splints include finger, hand, wrist, knee, and ankle splints. A resting splint keeps a body part at rest in the splint, whereas a

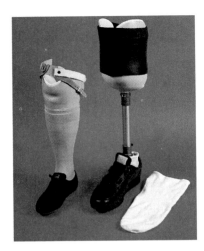

Fig. 20-8. Artificial legs are the most common type of artificial limbs. Use special care when assisting a resident with putting on an artificial limb.

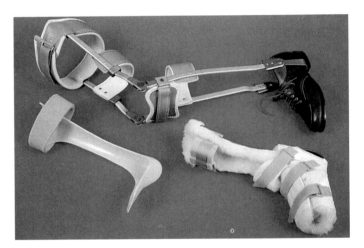

Fig. 20-9. An ankle foot orthosis is used when the ankle needs help in supporting body weight.

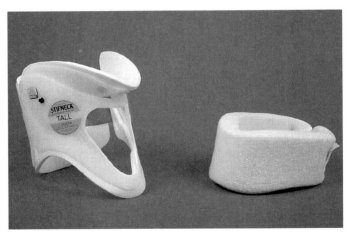

Fig. 20-10. Soft and hard neck collars are a type of brace used to support the neck.

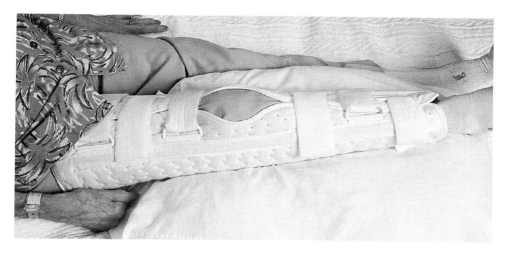

Fig. 20-11. Splints are used to restrict movement of a joint or a body part.

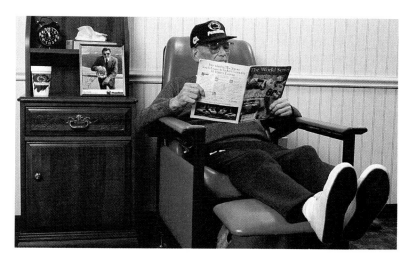

Fig. 20-12. Reclining chairs are best for residents who sit for long periods or who tend to tip when seated in wheelchairs.

dynamic splint allows some motion of the body part while restricting undesirable motions.

Reclining Chairs. These are also called gerichairs, recliners, or cardiac chairs. They are generally larger chairs with more padding on the seat and back. They can be positioned in the upright sitting position or reclined at different angles. These chairs are used for residents who are unable to move, who sit for long periods throughout the day, or who tend to tip over regular wheelchairs (Fig. 20-12).

Wheelchairs. There are many types of and features on wheelchairs: high backs versus regular backs, lightweight versus regular weight, reclinable versus standard upright position, removable arm and leg rests versus stationary arm and leg rests, swing away leg rests, swing up arm rests. If a resident you are working with has his or her own wheelchair, learn about the features on that chair and how they work before using it. If a resident does not use the same wheelchair every day, try to use a wheelchair that will accommodate that resident's needs. Generally, residents who need to be in a chair and can move themselves in that chair safely should be in a wheelchair instead of a recliner. Wheelchairs give residents the ability to get around by themselves.

You need to become familiar with the different parts of wheelchairs and how to adjust them (Fig. 20-13). The brakes are located below the arm rests on both sides in front of each wheel. The leg rests are attached to the front of the chair under the seat on each side of the chair. They may or may not be removable, swing away, or elevate. Leg rests should have foot pedals and calf pads on each side that can be swung out of the way. Learn how to elevate and remove leg rests as needed.

The arm rests are on either side of the seat. They may or may not be removable. You might want to remove them, for example, to do a sliding board transfer.

Aids for the Activities of Daily Living. These aids help a resident perform the activities of daily living (ADLs) such as dressing, bathing, eating, writing, toileting, etc. Much equipment is available to help residents in daily activities. The more commonly used devices are described below. If you have any questions regarding how to use these or other equipment, just ask the therapist. Once you know what is available, you can contact the therapist if you notice that a resident has difficulty with a task.

Dressing sticks, long-handled shoe horns, long-handled sponges, and reachers allow residents to reach further during dressing and bathing without having to bend down as far (Fig. 20-14). Many residents are not supposed to bend down because of a hip surgery, because they become dizzy or lose their balance, or because they are just unable to bend down very far. Sock donners, for example, are devices that fit around the lower leg with a rope that allows the sock to be pulled over the foot without the resident having to bend down.

A raised toilet seat is higher than the average toilet. This can either be fixed to the floor or temporarily placed over the toilet. This is used for residents who have difficulty bending down to sit on a toilet or difficulty getting off of a regular height toilet. It is used by a resident who is recovering from a hip fracture or any leg surgery or who has had a total hip replacement.

Grab bars are metal bars on the walls of bathrooms, tubs, and showers to give residents something to hold onto when transferring onto a toilet, into a tub or shower, or just standing during bathing (Fig. 20-15).

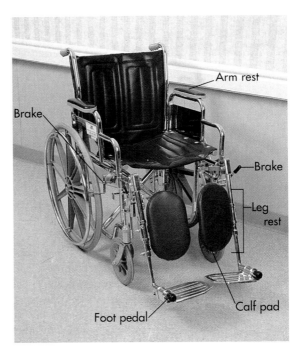

Fig. 20-13. Become familiar with wheelchairs and the operation of different parts.

Built-up grips are raised grips on any piece of equipment to help a resident with a weak grip hold onto it better. For example, these can be placed on eating or writing utensils or even a toothbrush. The grip may also have a strap that can be wrapped around the hand for more support.

Most of this equipment is given to a resident by the therapist or nurse to help them improve their independence. Try to make the equipment available for residents for their ADLs. If you notice a resident having difficulty with a certain activity, contact the therapist so that together you can come up with a solution to help that resident function better.

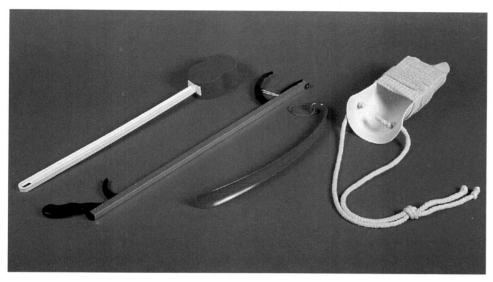

Fig. 20-14. ADL devices, such as a dressing stick, long handled shoe horn, and long handled sponge and reachers, are used by residents who cannot bend far.

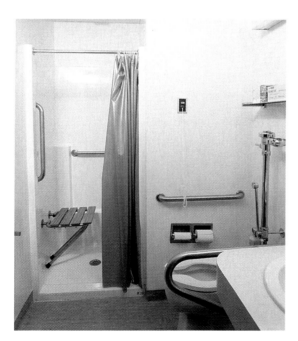

96% of accident happen in bathroom

Fig. 20-15. Grab bars give the resident something to hold onto when moving onto a toilet or into a tub.

Dicehem = grip it.

Preventing Injury to Residents During Functional Activities

Most resident injuries during functional activities are caused either by improper use of equipment or faulty equipment. You can help prevent both types.

Improper Use of Equipment. Help to prevent unnecessary injuries to residents by:

▶ Noticing when a resident is using a piece of equipment improperly or unsafely

▶ Assisting residents to a safe position until the problem is resolved

▶ Reporting a problem to your supervisor and/or notifying the therapist involved with a resident's care.

Following are examples of using these guidelines:

1. You see a resident pushing a walker too far in front of him or her. You explain how he or she can best use the walker (Fig. 20-16). You should always notify your supervisor and/or the therapist of the problem as well.

2. You notice that a walker a resident is using is too short. First check to see if he or she is using his or her own walker. If so and it is the wrong height, call the therapist so that the height of the walker can be assessed.

3. You see a resident using crutches unsafely. Try to have him or her sit down safely and notify the nurse or therapist.

4. You see a resident who is not supposed to put weight on a leg, using a cane or a rolling walker. But using either of these still puts weight on the leg. You explain this to the person and notify your supervisor or the therapist as soon as possible. This is important because a resident who is on a restricted weight bearing status has an injured leg that will heal best if no weight is put on it (Fig. 20-17).

Faulty Equipment. Another way to help prevent injury when using equipment is to watch for any equipment that is broken or faulty. If you notice that any equipment has broken, missing, or wobbly parts, notify the therapy or maintenance department to fix or replace the device. All staff must try to correct these minor problems quickly before a resident falls and is injured by a faulty piece of equipment.

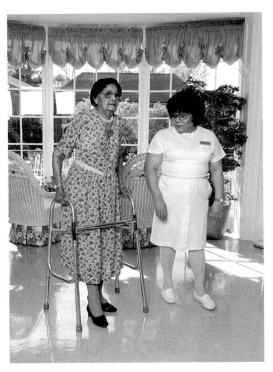

Fig. 20-16.   Improper use of equipment can result in injury, so explain to a resident using a walker how to use it properly.

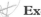

Exercise

Restorative activities involve making everyday activities restorative and interacting with a resident in a restorative way. Exercise is an additional restorative activity to add to a residents' routine. All residents benefit from exercise. You can be a tremendous asset in a resident's rehabilitation process by incorporating a prescribed exercise routine in your nursing care activities. The two basic types of exercise are range of motion exercises and walking.

Range of Motion Exercises

Range of motion (abbreviated ROM) exercises are exercises that move each body part through its own range of motion. ROM exercises may be active (abbreviated AROM, where the person moves the body part using his or her own muscle power), active assisted (where you help the person to move the body part), or passive (abbreviated PROM, where you move the body part for the person).

A resident's physician along with the physical therapist and nurse determines which type of ROM exercise a resident should do, depending on each resident's capabilities and motivation.

Active Exercise. Exercise is active when a resident can do it independently. How can you help with this type of exercise? You help residents based on their needs. A resident may need someone to just remind him or her to do the exercises. He or she may need you to read the exercise program aloud as he or she is doing it. Or he or she may need you to cue how to move each body part correctly.

Active Assisted Exercise. Some residents need you to assist them physically through each exercise because they have an injury to a certain body part that is healing and doing active exercise would be too strenuous, or because they need your help to move that part of their body.

Passive Exercise. Passive exercise means that you do the exercise for a resident, usually because he or she is unable to move that part of the body at all or enough to help with the exercise. However, some residents may be recovering from an injury or surgery and although they can move a body part, they should not, so that this part of their body can heal better. Always ask the charge nurse.

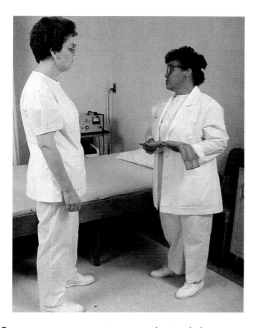

Fig. 20-17. Report to a supervisor or physical therapist to prevent injury if you see a resident who is not using recommended restorative equipment.

Different types of ROM exercises can be performed with the same resident. Residents may be able to move some parts of their body better than others or may not be able to move some parts of their body at all. For example, you may need to help a resident to move the right arm (active assisted ROM exercises), yet he or she may be able to move the left arm independently (active ROM exercises). Yet the person may be unable to move the legs at all (passive ROM exercises).

Guidelines for ROM Exercises

Following are general guidelines for doing ROM exercises with a resident:

▶ You should be familiar with what type of exercise a resident needs for each part of his or her body, the positions he or she should be in during each exercise, and the amount of assistance required during each exercise. If the therapist has written out the exercise program, use this for reference.

▶ Remove any obstacles that may be in the way of a motion. Move the pillows, bed sheets, and blankets out of the way. Accidentally banging a frail elderly resident's body part can cause bruising, skin tears, or even more severe injury.

▶ Explain to the person what you would like to do and why.

▶ Use your knowledge of moving and positioning a resident to move him or her to get into the appropriate position for each exercise.

▶ Remember your body mechanics and pay attention to your body position. Experiment with different standing positions, hand placements, and bed heights until you have found the best position for you to keep your back safe while giving residents the help that they may need. Sometimes it may help to put one knee up on the bed while standing on the other. Always ask the person if this is OK before lifting your leg onto the bed.

▶ Keep both hands on the person's extremity if possible during each exercise to provide the best support and guidance.

▶ When you are ranging a specific joint, have one hand above and the other hand below the joint. Generally, the hand above the joint stabilizes the extremity (holds it in place) and the hand below the joint does the range of motion. For example, if you are ranging the elbow joint, use one hand to stabilize the upper arm (above the joint) and the other to move the forearm up and down (below the joint)

▶ While ranging an extremity, be gentle and never force the joint because you can cause severe damage if you push or pull too hard. This can rupture a tendon, pull a muscle, tear skin, break a bone, or just cause pain or swelling. Many residents have osteoporosis or other conditions that cause weakened bones; weakened muscles, tendons, or ligaments; fragile skin; or unstable joints. The most easily damaged joints are in the neck, hands, wrists, and feet.

▶ During the exercise, frequently ask the person how he or she is doing, if he or she has any pain with a particular motion or part of a motion, or if your hand pressure on the extremity (arm or leg) is OK. Watch the person's facial expression and response because a resident may not always be able to tell you that he or she is uncomfortable.

▶ The full exercise routine should be done at least once a day. Try to encourage activities using the arms and legs throughout the day as well. If a resident has an exercise program from the therapist and can do the exercises independently, also figure out ways to motivate him or her to do these throughout the day by reminders, setting him or her up to do the exercises, or cuing him or her during the exercises. You may even take your break in the resident's room to keep him or her company during the exercise routine.

Which Joints to Exercise

A resident may have specific exercises designed by a therapist for certain problem areas. Follow these exercises and ask the therapist about any others for this resident.

If a resident is not actively seeing a therapist, he or she will usually benefit from a general ROM exercise program on a daily basis. A general ROM program works on each joint of the body. The joints that you should include in your ROM program are the shoulder, elbow, wrist, hand (fingers), hip, knee, ankle, and foot (toes).

Ask your supervisor or the therapist if the resident has any restricted joints. If there are no restrictions, move each joint through its full available motion at least once a day. Based on a resident's ability to help you, you may be doing some joints actively, some with active assistance and some passively, or all joints the same way. Let the person do as much as possible and help them with the rest. Give residents time to respond to what you are asking them to do.

How Joints Move

Each joint moves in different types of motions based on the structure of the joint. The box below lists the specific motions of each joint for a general ROM exercise program.

Starting a ROM Program

You can do an entire ROM exercise program with a resident in about 15 minutes when you have a system. Here's some things to consider to get you started:

▶ Think about each motion and see if you can think of any nursing care activities that use these motions. For example, when bathing under the arm of a resident, use shoulder flexion or abduction. If you lift each shoulder up a few times or have a resident do it while bathing, this can be part of the daily exercise rou-

---

Motions of Major Joints

SHOULDER

Flexion: bringing the arm up toward the head in front of the body
Extension: bringing the arm straight back to the bed
Abduction: moving the arm away from the body out to the side
Adduction: bringing the arm back toward the side
Internal rotation: turning the shoulder in
External rotation: turning the shoulder out

ELBOW

Flexion: bending the elbow
Extension: straightening the elbow
Supination: turning the palm up
Pronation: turning the palm down

WRIST

Flexion: bending the wrist up
Extension: bending the wrist back
Ulnar deviation: with the hand held at the same level as the forearm, moving the hand toward the pinkie finger side
Radial deviation: with the hand as above, moving the hand toward the thumb side

HAND

Finger abduction/adduction: fingers spread apart and then together
Finger flexion: bending the fingers at each of finger joints

(3 on each finger, 2 on the thumb)
Finger extension: straightening the fingers out at the finger joints
Opposition: touching each finger tip to the thumb

HIP

Flexion: bending the knee toward the chest
Extension: bringing the hip behind the body
Abduction: bringing the hip out to the side
Adduction: bringing the hip back toward the side
Internal rotation: turning the hip inward
External rotation: turning the hip outward

KNEE

Flexion: bending the knee
Extension: straightening the knee

ANKLE

Dorsiflexion: bending the top of the foot up toward the face
Plantarflexion: pointing the foot down like stepping on a gas pedal
Inversion: turning the bottom of the foot inward
Eversion: turning the bottom of the foot outward

FOOT

Toe flexion: bending the toes down
Toe extension: straightening the toes back up

tine. Still keep the separate exercise program, but you can include some of the exercises during your nursing care.

▶ Figure out a system to use every joint in an exercise routine. Then once you have a system, use the same exercise order for each resident. You may have to change the specifics based on each resident's needs.

Range-of-Motion Exercises

▶ Resident preference
▶ Common preparation steps
▶ Equipment and supplies needed
▶ Environment preparation
▶ Resident preparation

Note: Do each exercise 5-10 times, depending on a resident's tolerance with each extremity.

The Arm

Start with the shoulder and work your way down to the hand. During each exercise, help the person move the extremity or move it yourself, depending on how much he or she can do independently.

The Shoulder

Place one hand just above the shoulder and the other hand below the shoulder on the mid arm above the elbow. Allow the forearm to rest on your body as you move the arm. If the person is on his or her back, you should stand close to the side of the arm you are moving.

1. Help the resident to lift his or her arm up toward the head of the bed with the elbow straight (flexion) (Fig. 20-18).
2. Bring the arm back down to the bed (extension) (Fig. 20-19).
3. Help the resident to lift his or her arm out to the side with the elbow straight (abduction) (Fig. 20-20).
4. Bring the arm back toward the side (adduction) (Fig. 20-21).
5. Help the resident to lift his or her arm halfway out to the side and with the elbow bent, rotate the arm down (internal rotation) and up (external rotation) (Figs. 20-22 and 20-23).

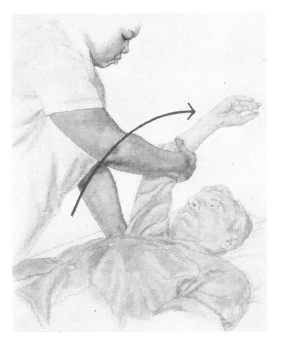

Fig. 20-18. Help the resident to lift the arm up with the elbow straight (flexion).

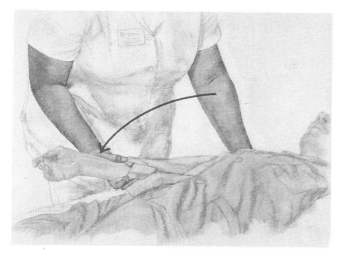

Fig. 20-19.   Bring the arm back down to the bed (extension).

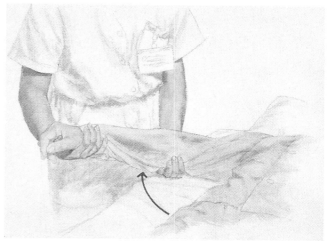

Fig. 20-20.   Help the resident lift the arm out to the side with the elbow straight (abduction).

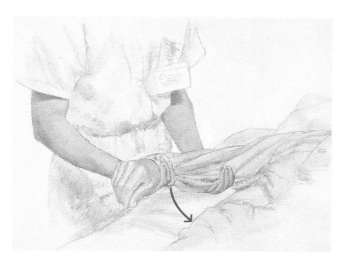

Fig. 20-21.   Bring the arm back toward the side (adduction).

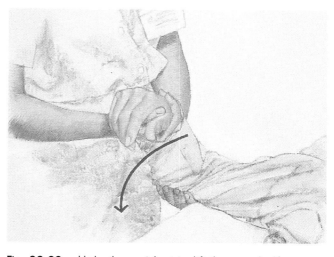

Fig. 20-22.   Help the resident to lift the arm halfway out to the side and with the elbow bent, rotate the arm down (internal rotation).

(Bedbath)

Best time bath time
for ROM Am.

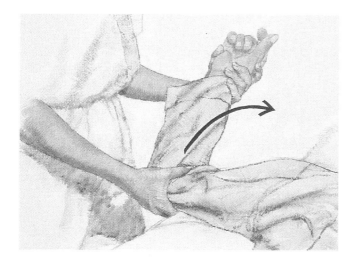

Fig. 20-23.   Help the resident to lift the arm halfway out to the side and with the elbow bent, rotate the arm up (external rotation).

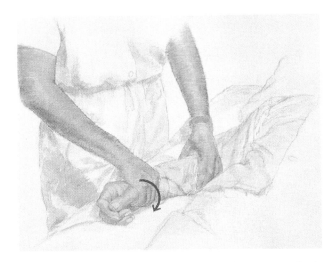

Fig. 20-24. Help the resident to turn the palm over with the elbow fairly straight and the wrist in neutral position (pronation).

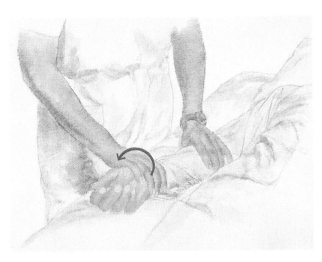

Fig. 20-25. Help the resident to turn the palm back up with the elbow fairly straight and the wrist in neutral position (supination).

The Elbow

Place one hand above the elbow and the other below on the forearm across the wrist to the hand. The wrist should be in neutral, not bent forward or backward.

1. Help the resident to bend the elbow by bringing the hand toward the upper arm with the palm facing up (flexion).
2. Help the resident to straighten the elbow by bringing the hand down toward the bed until the elbow is as straight as possible (extension).
3. Help the resident to turn his or her palm over with the elbow fairly straight and the wrist in neutral (pronation) (Fig. 20-24).
4. Help the resident to turn his or her palm back up with the elbow fairly straight and the wrist in neutral (supination) (Fig. 20-25).

The Wrist

Place one hand around the forearm just above the person's wrist and the other hand in his or her hand.

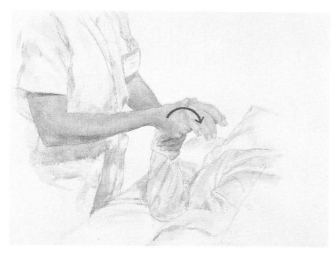

Fig. 20-26.   Help the resident to bend the wrist down (flexion).

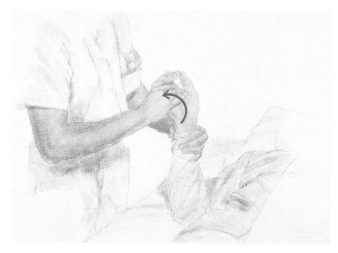

Fig. 20-27.   Help the resident to straighten the wrist and then to bend the wrist back (extension, hyperextension).

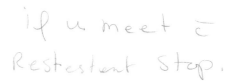

1. Help the resident to bend his or her wrist down (flexion) (Fig. 20-26).
2. Help the resident to bend his or her wrist back (extension) (Fig. 20-27).
3. Help the resident to move his or her hand toward the pinkie side of the wrist (ulnar deviation) (Fig. 20-28).
4. Help the resident to move his or her hand toward the thumb side of the wrist (radial deviation) (Fig. 20-29).

The Hand

Use your fingers to help the person move his or her fingers one by one.
1. Bend and straighten each finger at each of the creases (joints of the fingers). Then, curl the hand into a fist and straighten the fingers back out (flexion and extension) (Figs. 20-30 and 20-31).
2. Spread the fingers away from the third finger (abduction) and then toward it (adduction) (Figs. 20-32 and 20-33).
3. Bring each finger across the palm to the thumb and back out (opposition) (Fig 20-34).

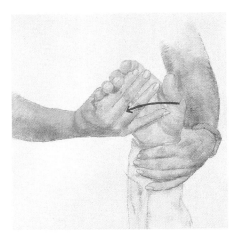

Fig. 20-28. Help the resident to move the hand toward the pinkie side of the wrist (ulnar deviation).

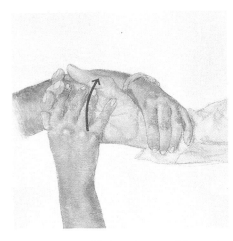

Fig. 20-29. Help the resident to move the hand toward the thumb side of the wrist (radial deviation).

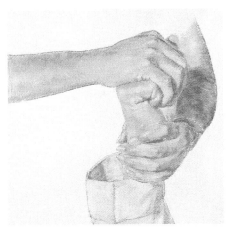

Fig. 20-30. Curl the hand into a fist (flexion).

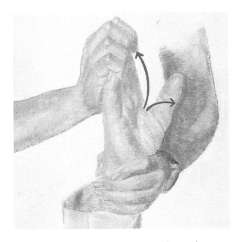

Fig. 20-31. Straighten the fingers back out (extension).

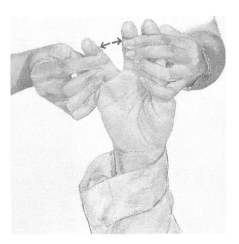

Fig. 20-32. Spread the fingers away from each other, one at a time (abduction).

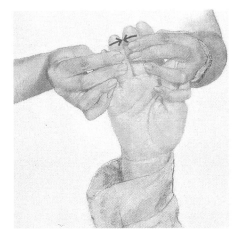

Fig. 20-33. Bring the fingers together, one at a time (adduction).

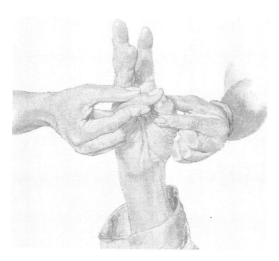

Fig. 20-34. Bring each finger across the palm to the thumb and back out (opposition).

The Leg

Start with the hip and work your way down to the foot.

The Hip

Place one hand under the thigh and the other hand below the knee around the calf. You may have to adjust your hand placement, depending on what feels comfortable to both you and the resident.

1. Help the resident to bring his or her hip up toward the chest with the knee bent (flexion) (Fig. 20-35).
2. Bring his or her leg back down toward the bed (extension) (Fig. 20-36).
3. Help the resident to bring his or her leg out to the side (abduction) (Fig. 20-37).
4. Bring his or her leg back toward the other leg (adduction) (Fig. 20-38).
5. Help the resident to bring the leg partly up toward the chest with the knee bent. Now gently turn the leg in (internal rotation) and out (external rotation) (Figs. 20-39 and 20-40).

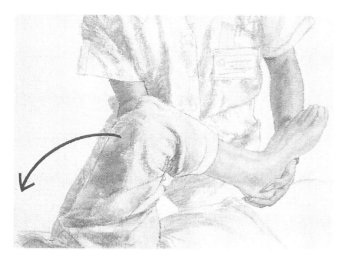

Fig. 20-35. Help the resident to bring the hip up toward the chest with the knee bent (flexion).

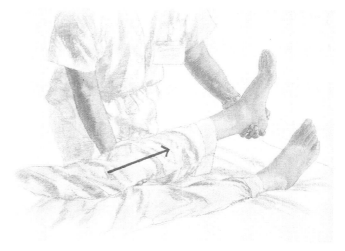

Fig. 20-36. Bring the leg back down toward the bed (extension).

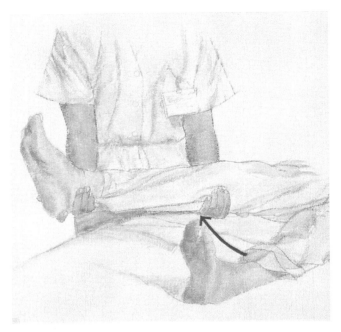

Fig. 20-37. Help the resident to bring the leg out to the side (abduction).

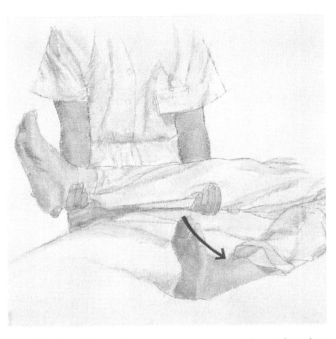

Fig. 20-38. Bring the leg back toward the other leg (adduction).

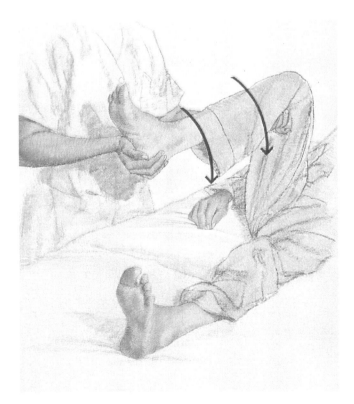

Fig. 20-39. Help the resident to bring the leg partly up toward the chest with the knee bent and gently turn the leg in (internal rotation).

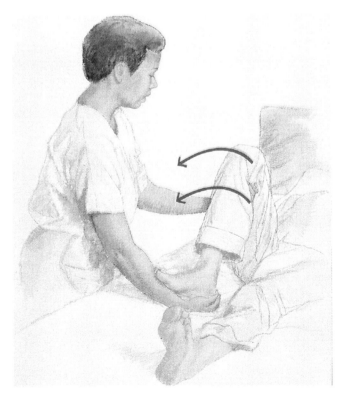

Fig. 20-40. Help the resident to bring the leg partly up toward the chest with the knee bent and gently turn the leg out (external rotation).

The Knee

Place one hand above the knee under or on the thigh and one hand below the knee around the calf.

1. Help the resident to bend the leg up toward the chest slightly. From this position, help him or her bend the knee (flexion) (Fig. 20-41).
2. With the hip in the same position as described above, help the resident straighten the knee (extension) (Fig. 20-42).

The Ankle

Place one hand above the ankle around the lower part of the calf and the other hand around the bottom of the foot.

1. Help the resident to bend the foot up toward the head while the knee is held straight (dorsiflexion) and then point the foot downward (plantarflexion) (Figs. 20-43 and 20-44).
2. Help the resident turn the bottom of the foot outward (eversion) and then inward (inversion) (Figs. 20-45 and 20-46).

The Foot

As with the hand, place your fingers around each toe and gently bend (flexion) (Fig. 20-47) and straighten each toe at each of the joints (extension) (Fig. 20-48). You can also bend and straighten all the toes at once (extension).

Remember:

▶ Meet resident needs
▶ Common completion steps
▶ Clean and put away equipment and supplies
▶ Environment completion (Is it safe? Is it clean?)

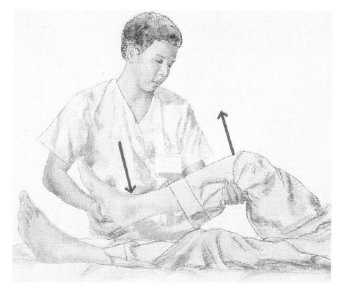

Fig. 20-41. Help the resident to bend the leg up toward the chest, then bend the knee (flexion).

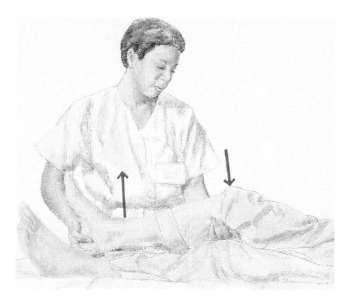

Fig. 20-42. With the resident's leg bent, straighten the knee (extension).

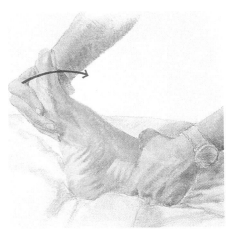

Fig. 20-43. Help the resident to bend the foot up toward the head with the knee held straight (dorsiflexion).

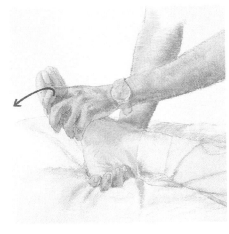

Fig. 20-44. Help the resident to point the foot downward (plantarflexion).

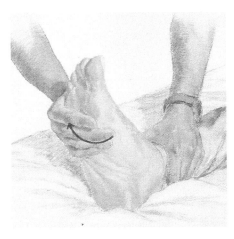

Fig. 20-45. Help the resident turn the bottom of the foot outward (eversion).

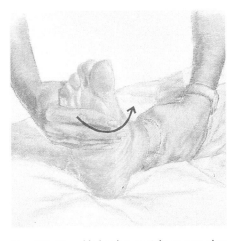

Fig. 20-46. Help the resident turn the bottom of the foot inward (inversion).

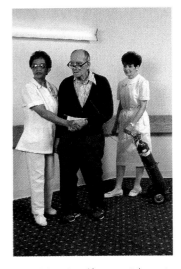

Fig. 20-49. If a resident is on oxygen, he or she may need two people to assist when walking.

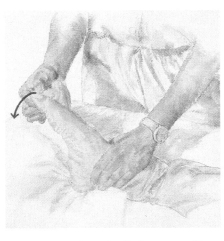

Fig. 20-47. Bend all the toes (flexion).

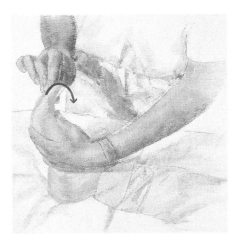

Fig. 20-48. Straighten all the toes (extension).

Walking with a Resident

Once you have assessed a resident's abilities and the situation, prepare for walking. Then follow these principles:

1. Put the guard belt on the resident.
2. If the resident walks without an assistive device, stand to his or her side so that you can watch his or her face as you hold onto the belt from behind. If the resident uses a walker or cane, stand to his or her side with one hand on the back of the belt and the other on the walker (or cane if the resident needs help with the cane). Most residents who have a cane can hold it, which means you can stand on the opposite side. Make sure that the cane is in the correct hand.
3. Walk with the resident. Have him or her take small steps and slowly progress to larger ones. When walking in the hallways, encourage the resident to use the safety bars for added support. Always stand on the other side of the resident so he or she may use the bars. *Note:* Try to use short walks during other activities such as getting out of bed, coming back from the bathroom, going to meals, going to activities, etc. For residents who can walk on their own, encourage them to do so throughout the day. For example, a resident has just finished using the toilet and needs to get back into the chair. If this resident can walk a fair distance before becoming tired, place the chair outside of the room or down the hall instead of next to the bathroom and have him or her walk to the chair.

Certain situations may occur when assisting residents with walking. Following are four common situations and actions you can take:

1. A resident questions why he or she has to walk. You can encourage walking by explaining that walking will help him or her get stronger or stay strong.
2. A resident generally walks a lot during the day yet does not feel well or you know he or she is sick that day. Respect the person's right not to walk that day and try again when he or she feels better.
3. The resident is on oxygen. Ask the nurse or therapist if it is OK to walk this person. Find out if and how much oxygen is needed when he or she walks. If so, see if the nurse can put this resident on a portable tank for the walk. You may need another staff person to walk a resident with oxygen if he or she needs much help to walk. One person pulls the oxygen tank and chair while you walk holding onto the guard belt and walker if using one (Fig. 20-49).
4. A resident tends to act unpredictably when walking, such as his or her legs get tired and give out easily, or the person is confused and tends to sit without telling you. In this case, have another person follow you with the chair as you walk with him or her. This way the chair is ready to be placed under him or her if he or she needs to sit suddenly.

Walking

Walking is an important part of moving as well as an excellent way for a resident to exercise and maintain optimal function. Walking is also called ambulation. Gait refers to the way someone walks. If a resident needs help to walk, either physical help or supervision, you need to know the following:

- What assistive device they use, if any?
- What amount of help they need to walk, if any?
- How much cuing do they require for safety reasons?
- Do they need any braces, prostheses, or other equipment?
- How far can they walk safely?
- Will you need another staff person to help?
- How much body weight can they place on the legs while walking?

Remember:

- Resident preference
- Common preparation steps
- Equipment and supplies needed
- Environment preparation
- Resident preparation

Remember:

- Meet resident needs
- Common completion steps
- Clean and put away equipment and supplies
- Environment completion (Is it safe? Is it clean?)

IN THIS CHAPTER YOU LEARNED TO:

- define the nurse assistant's role in promoting independence
- list various kinds of equipment for use in promoting independence
- demonstrate range-of-motion exercises and assist with walking

21

THE DYING PROCESS

Death is a natural stage in life, but most people do not like to talk about it. When we face the death of another person, we are reminded that we too will die some day. Many people fear death because of a fear of the unknown. One also will have no more chances to do the things one wanted to do. Often at this time people ask themselves, "What is the meaning of life? What have I done that has made a difference or will be remembered after I am gone?" These fears and thoughts lead to issues that you as a nurse assistant can help residents with.

DEATH AS A NATURAL PROCESS

Although residents do not come to facilities to die, many are older and debilitated and thus more likely to die sooner than younger, healthier persons. Elderly people often have faced the death of loved ones, and because of this they may think more about life and death (Fig. 21-1). The need for spirituality becomes more important as people do a life review. Feelings about impending death may vary greatly among different individuals, depending on their life experiences and spiritual beliefs. Cultural background also plays a role in what a person believes and how he or she responds to dying. Some welcome death as release from pain and suffering. Many have positive expectations based on their religious beliefs. Following are some common beliefs:

▶ There is a life after death free of pain and hardship.
▶ One will be reunited with loved ones who have already died.
▶ One is reincarnated into another body or form.

To support a resident through the dying process, you must first understand what he or she believes. For example, some dying residents fear dying alone, even when they accept death as positive or freeing. If a resident seems fearful about being alone, develop a plan to be with him or her as needed. Give the person a bell to ring when afraid and be sure to respond. Many also fear pain as a part of dying. Ask the charge nurse to discuss pain management with the person. Residents may also have fears related to how they have lived their lives:

▶ Residents may feel they have unfinished business, such as an unresolved argument with a family member, or a disabled child who needs lifelong care.
▶ Residents may not feel good about how they lived their lives or may feel they failed to achieve all they wanted.
▶ They may feel guilty about something they did or did not do, such as not being supportive enough of a family member.

The process of life review is very important. Be supportive, open, nonjudgmental and always listen to the person (Fig. 21-2). Think about basic human needs as you care for the dying residents, and try to meet as many needs as possible.

THE STAGES OF DYING

Regardless of individual attitudes and spiritual beliefs, most dying people experience common stages of feelings. Dr. Elisabeth Kubler-Ross, a psychiatrist who worked extensively with dying patients, described the five stages. Her descriptions

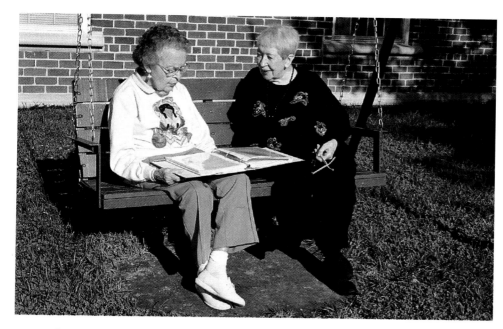

Fig. 21-1. Some elderly people, may spend more time thinking about life and death than younger, healthier people.

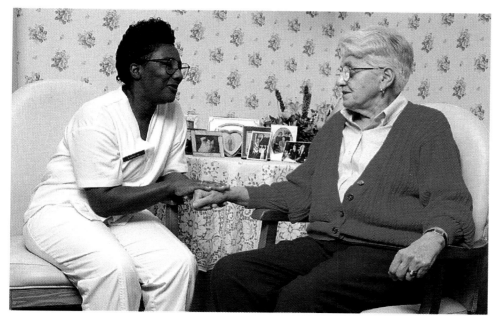

Fig. 21-2. Be sympathetic and nonjudgmental with residents. Listen and meet as many of their needs as possible.

apply to reactions to any kind of loss. These stages of feelings are now commonly known as the stages of grief:

1. For most people, the first stage when they learn that they are dying is denial, or the "not me" reaction. The individual may refuse to talk about death or to acknowledge physical evidence that he or she is dying.

2. The second stage is anger, when the individual asks "Why me?" He or she may lash out at family members, caregivers, or even God, looking for someone to blame.

3. The third stage is called bargaining, when the individual seems to be saying, "OK, maybe it's going to happen soon, but before it does I want to. . . ." The person often tries to bargain to gain time to complete unfinished business.

4. The fourth stage is depression, which occurs when the individual acknowledges that death is coming. Now the person is getting in touch with his or her sadness and begins the process of mourning the loss of self.

5. The fifth and final stage is acceptance, when the dying person has worked through most of the earlier feelings and has reached a calm or peacefulness.

Reaching the last stage does not mean a resident has decided to stop living because he or she is dying. Typically, a person who has reached acceptance is more able to focus on living each day to its fullest. You may even see a dying resident helping friends and family work through their feelings of grief and loss over his or her impending death.

As with the hierarchy of basic human needs, people do not necessarily move through the five stages of grief in one smooth movement. Often a person may move back and forth. For example, someone who has accepted his or her death may go back to bargaining, to try for more time "just to see my son graduate." Not everyone goes through all the stages. Someone with a strong spiritual belief in an afterlife, for example, may move more quickly to the stage of acceptance. Someone else may never get beyond the stage of anger.

Almost everyone who is terminally ill knows death is inevitable. You may pick up clues from a resident who asks questions such as, "Am I going to get any better?" You may have heard family or staff talk about a resident who hasn't been told about his or her impending death. This does not mean that he or she does not know. It usually only means that the person cannot yet talk freely with loved ones about his or her fears and feelings. You may need to let family members and other staff know about clues you pick up that he or she does know. Encourage them to listen carefully to what the person says. Use your communication skills to let a resident know that it is all right to talk to you about his or her feelings. Some residents may even ask you to help their loved ones accept that they are dying.

HELPING DYING RESIDENTS COPE WITH THEIR FEELINGS

Death can occur very quickly or be a long process. This chapter focuses on dying that is approaching within a matter of days.

Use the communication techniques you have already learned to help residents cope with their feelings. Listening is still the best thing you can do for most people. If you listen carefully, they will tell you what they need. Your physical presence will provide reassurance that they are not dying alone.

Use the technique of reflection to encourage residents to talk about their fears and feelings, saying something like, "It must be hard to talk about these things with anyone." Ask open-ended questions such as," What are you most worried about?" If a resident is worried about his or her care, ask what he or she would like to have done. Assure residents they will be made as comfortable as possible, and they will not be left alone. Whenever possible, take time to sit with a dying resident, holding hands or touching. You do not have to say anything.

When a resident's behavior shows that he or she is denying the impending death, do not try to force a resident to "face reality." The person is not ready to deal with these feelings, and you can do more harm than good by forcing the issue. Accept that a resident will move at his or her own pace in adjusting.

Residents in the stage of anger often blame caregivers for not doing enough treatment or keeping them comfortable. They may be short-tempered with everyone around, including other residents and even the most devoted family members. Don't take personally any anger directed your way. Do not try to talk a resident out of being angry by saying things such as, "You shouldn't feel that way" or "You shouldn't talk to your wife that way." Acknowledge the person's feelings with statements like, "What you're going through is really hard, isn't it?"

A resident in the stage of bargaining may say things such as, "I just want to be able to hold my grandson one more time." Relay these wishes to the family, and help any way you can to meet the request for "one more. . . ." Often the bargaining involves what the person considers unfinished business. If the person can complete it, he or she may be able to move more easily to the stage of acceptance.

The stage of depression may be marked by withdrawal from social contacts, crying, or a lack of interest in anything outside oneself (Fig. 21-3). Your role is again supportive: be there, and accept a resident's need to go through these feelings. You might try to express the feelings you see, such as by saying, "You seem very sad," or "You're having a really hard time today." Even if you do not get a verbal response, you have communicated your concern and your presence as a listener.

When residents reach the stage of acceptance, you usually see a much calmer attitude. Residents can more easily talk about dying. They often want to talk about what they would like to have done with their belongings, how they would like to be cared for at death, and even funeral arrangements. In this culture, people often avoid talking about these things openly and directly with a dying person. Family members often refuse to talk about death with a dying loved one. You and other staff may be the only ones residents can talk to openly and without fear of upsetting the family. Keep listening.

THE SIGNS OF DEATH APPROACHING

These are the physical signs that death is impending: You may see these signs a matter of minutes or hours before the person dies.

- Decreased blood circulation causes the resident's hands and feet to feel cold to the touch, and his or her face becomes pale or gray and mottled. The person looks spotted.
- The resident's eyes may stare blankly into space, with no eye movement, even when you pass your hand in front of his or her face.
- Breathing becomes irregular, sometimes rapid and shallow, at other times slow and heavy.
- Heavy perspiration is common.

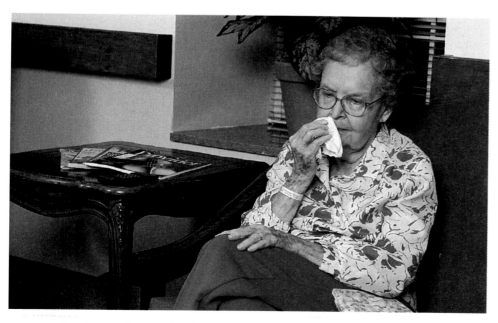

Fig. 21-3. Facing death may cause a resident to withdraw or cry.

▶ Loss of muscle tone causes the body to seem limp; the jaw may drop with the mouth staying partly open.
▶ What is sometimes called the "death rattle" results from mucus in the throat affecting breathing.
▶ The resident's pulse becomes rapid, weak, and irregular.
▶ Respiration stops and the pulse gets very weak.

When you recognize the signs of impending death, be sure to notify the nurse. The family should be contacted. If you had enough advance knowledge of death coming, you should already have talked with the person or the family about any final wishes. Make every effort to meet the resident and family's requests for the last hours of life. Surviving family members will remember for a long time their last interaction with their loved one, and this will have lasting effects on their emotional health.

YOUR ROLE THROUGH THE DYING PROCESS

Your role for the time a resident is dying includes comfort measures for him or her and helping family members and other residents cope with their feelings. Remember the length of time varies from resident to resident. You may also need to manage your own feelings. The following sections discuss these issues.

Comfort Measures for the Dying Resident

You demonstrate caring by doing everything you can to ensure the dying resident is comfortable. Continue to incorporate the themes of care in your activities with this resident. Continue to provide for his or her privacy. Follow these guidelines:

▶ Keep the room well lighted and well ventilated.
▶ Identify yourself frequently, and explain everything that you are doing, even if the person is not responsive.
▶ Offer food and fluids as tolerated.
▶ Change the resident's position often, and change clothing and bedding when soiled by perspiration, urine, or feces.
▶ Give skin care to prevent or reduce breakdown.
▶ Because the dying resident often breathes through the mouth, frequent mouth and lip care is necessary.
▶ Take the resident's vital signs as often as directed by the charge nurse, and notify the nurse of any change.
▶ Spend time talking, reminiscing, and listening to the person.

Helping the Family During the Process of Dying

Family members go through the same stages of grief as the dying person. They do not necessarily move through the stages at the same time, however, and you may have to assist the communication between family members and resident because of this difference. Some families do not pass beyond the denial stage at all while their loved one is still alive. They may refuse to talk with the person about his or her wishes for care or funeral arrangements, saying, "No, you're not going to die." You may have an opportunity to tell family members a resident is trying to talk about things that really need to be said.

Some family members deal with their anger and guilt by insisting on providing all the care to their loved one, or being very critical of the care you give. Others may withdraw and not visit the person, unable to express their feelings directly.

Encourage family members to participate as much as they can. You may have to encourage them to take time out to rest and to take care of their own health. Reassure them that their loved one will be well cared for in their absence and that you will call them if there is any change. Do not take personally any criticisms or complaints the family makes during this time. Give them time to talk, and listen, listen, listen (Fig. 21-4). Be sure to communicate to all staff the wishes of a family member to be notified about any change in the person's condition.

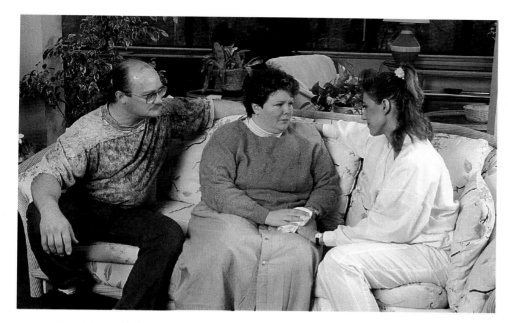

Fig. 21-4. Offer your support and comfort to the family of a resident who has died.

When a resident dies, offer the family time alone with the body. Offer to sit with them. Pray with them, if they request and you feel comfortable doing so. Give them privacy, and offer to call a clergyman.

Religious and Cultural Practices

Hopefully, you will have had a chance to learn from residents and family members what their religious beliefs and practices are, along with their wishes for rituals at the time of death. Many residents want religious symbols, medals, statues, or pictures at hand. You may be asked to read from the Bible or another religious book, or to pray with them. A rabbi, priest, and minister may visit this resident and family regularly, and their presence is often requested at the time of death. Often religious residents want to talk with their clergyman or make a confession, when they know death is near (Fig. 21-5). During such visits, be sure to provide privacy.

Take care to understand the concerns of family members at the time of death. A family member may insist on staying with the body. Although in some cases this may show difficulty accepting the death, usually it involves traditional religious or cultural practices for care of the body after death. Family members often want assurance the body will be treated with respect. Reassure them by explaining what will happen with the body. If the family wants to bathe the body or perform another ritual cleansing, let them assist in preparing the body if the request is appropriate and within facility policy. Their participation is often important for their emotional healing.

Helping Other Residents Cope with Their Loss

A resident's death affects all residents. For some, it is a reminder that their own death is not far away. For others, the death means the loss of a good friend. Residents should always be informed of the death. Encourage them to talk about their sadness, loss, anger, fear, and other personal feelings. Reminisce with them about the resident who died. A memorial service held in the facility is a good way to give residents and staff a chance to talk about their feelings of loss and to remember the good things about the person who died.

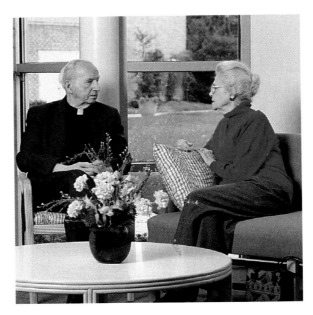

Fig. 21-5. Provide privacy when a resident requests to see a member of the clergy.

Often other residents want to know about how the person died. Was he or she in pain? Was someone there? These questions often arise from a concern for how they will be treated "when my time comes." Answer their questions as much as you can without violating confidentiality.

Managing Your Own Feelings

You often develop close relationships with residents. When they die, or as they are dying, you too may experience the same feelings as the family and other residents. You are trying to help the dying resident, the family, and other residents deal with their feelings. Who will help you deal with yours? If you are really listening, however, you can learn much from the dying resident. He or she may be offering support in various ways to everyone involved. If you have helped the person to a peaceful death, you can take comfort from that knowledge.

Talking with other staff is another good way to manage your feelings. Knowing what your feelings are is the first step in resolving them. Knowing that others too feel this way also helps, and you will probably find that other staff members have similar feelings. Realize too it's OK to cry sometimes.

THE PHYSICAL CARE OF THE BODY

Every facility has specific procedures for caring for the body after death. Typically these are written in a policy titled "Post-Mortem Care." The box on page 357 lists common practices.

Your facility may include other procedures in postmortem care. Be sure to read and follow the facility policy.

LIVING WILLS

A living will is a document a resident may use to communicate his or her wishes about care in the event he or she becomes incapacitated and cannot make decisions (Fig. 21-6). This is a legal document called an "advance directive." The Patient Self-Determination Act, a federal law passed in 1991, requires that health care facilities inform residents of their right to have such a directive and explain the pro-

Caring for the Body after Death

1. Treat the body gently and with respect.
2. If the resident has a roommate who is aware of his or her surroundings, arrange for the roommate to be somewhere else until the body is removed.
3. Close the door or pull the curtain for privacy.
4. Remove any tubes and dressings.
5. Put the body in a flat position with the limbs straight. Place one pillow under the head to prevent the face and neck from becoming discolored.
6. Put the hands on the chest.
7. Put in false teeth.
8. Wash the body as you would when giving a bed bath. Place a fresh dressing over any open or draining wounds.
9. Comb the hair.
10. Cover the perineal area with a pad to absorb any drainage.
11. Put a clean gown on the body.

cedures for using one. Different states have different forms that must be used, but they are similar in meaning. The most powerful type of advance directive is the durable power of attorney for health care.

A living will must be written while the individual is mentally competent, and the person can revoke it at any time by verbal notice or simply tearing up the document. A living will states the person's wishes about withdrawing or withholding life-sustaining procedures if he or she becomes terminally ill. The durable power of attorney for health care is not limited to conditions of terminal illness. It designates someone, usually a family member or an attorney, to make health care decisions for the person if he or she becomes incapacitated. The document also spells out which treatments the person would accept or reject. Not all types of advance directives are living wills, as there are some important legal differences. You need not know those differences, but your facility will handle them differently. Read your facility's policy. You should know which residents you care for have advance directives.

IN THIS CHAPTER YOU LEARNED TO:

▶ describe why death is a natural process

▶ list the stages of dying

▶ list specific measures the nurse assistant can do during the dying process

▶ describe the care of the body after death

▶ describe a living will

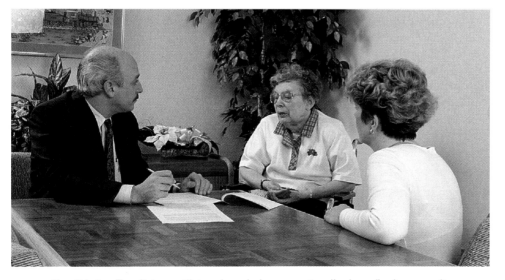

Fig. 21-6. The living will is a legal document called an "advance directive." It is used when a resident can no longer make his or her own decisions.

CARE OF A RESIDENT WHO IS COGNITIVELY IMPAIRED

Think about your first day at a new job. Wasn't it exhausting? You encountered what seemed like a million new things and new people. You tried to process and remember all of it at once, and most of the time you felt overwhelmed and wondered how you'd make it through the day. For cognitively impaired residents, each moment is a new experience, like the first day of a new job.

In this chapter you will learn about cognitive impairment, dementia, and other mental disorders. A large percentage of residents in facilities are cognitively impaired. You will learn about residents with cognitive impairment and dementia behaviors, abilities, and disabilities, as well as how best to care for these residents. You will learn specific techniques for helping these residents accomplish the activities of daily living.

UNDERSTANDING COGNITIVE IMPAIRMENT

Cognitive impairment is an illness of the mind that causes temporary or permanent altered thinking. With normal thought processes, you can learn and remember because of your cognitive abilities. You can take this course, for example. Your cognitive abilities let you live a productive life. When a person is cognitively impaired, more than just memory loss may result. Other abilities affected may include language comprehension and expression (the abilities to understand others and to speak to others), attention span, judgment, and the recognition and proper use of common objects (Fig. 22-1).

Cognitive impairment can be caused by a number of things. Temporary causes may include stress, medications, depression, vitamin deficiency, thyroid disease, alcohol, and head trauma. Permanent causes include severe head trauma, illness, brain disease, and brain damage at birth. In long term care facilities, most cognitive impairments are caused by brain disease. Alzheimer's disease is the most common incurable dementia-causing illness and is the fourth leading cause of death in adults older than age 65. No one yet knows exactly what causes brain deterioration. Nurse assistants play an important role in compassionately caring for people who have Alzheimer's and other dementia-causing illnesses. Your role is to give assistance and direction to help a resident with cognitive impairment get through each new day.

Stages of Cognitive Impairment

Cognitive impairment may not be obvious in early stages, although you may see clues in the person's behavior. A person who is cognitively impaired moves through different stages of decline. Dr. Barry Reisberg has defined seven stages of cognitive decline in the Global Deterioration Scale. Early stages include forgetfulness and confusion. Later stages are more severe and include dementia, a state in which a person cannot live without assistance.

In Stage 1 the person has only mild forgetfulness and occasional confusion. The condition is still so mild that neither the person nor most others around the person will view this as anything more serious than forgetfulness.

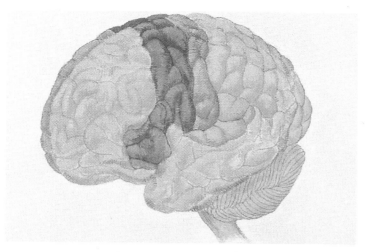

Fig. 22-1. Cognitive impairment can affect different areas of the brain.

In the forgetful stage, Stage 2, a person forgets simple things like familiar names and where he or she put things. But the person can still hold a job and has no apparent change or difficulty. These residents may become fearful and frustrated as they realize they are losing their mental abilities.

In Stages 3 and 4, the confusional stages, in addition to forgetfulness, residents become disoriented about the date and time, where they are, and who they and others are. They may lose things of value or become lost when traveling to unfamiliar places. They have trouble remembering familiar family and friends. Others begin to notice that something is wrong. The primary behaviors for Stage 3 include anxiety and agitation. In Stage 4, depression is the primary behavior.

Behavioral symptoms for Stages 2, 3, and 4 include tearfulness, agitation, depression, and anxiety. Affected residents realize they are becoming forgetful and confused. It is frightening to them and often depressing. An individual may try to cover up his or her losses. Residents need patience and nonjudgmental interaction during these phases.

Residents moving into Stage 5 are now moving into dementia. Stage 5 is early dementia. These persons still look "normal," wear their clothes correctly, speak relatively well, and retain fairly good social skills. They still understand concepts of the past, present, and future. They can still form a thought, plan an action, and follow through with it, although their reality is based on inaccurate perceptions; they believe they still have responsibilities and they don't believe they need help. The primary behaviors for Stage 5 may include purposeless activities like fidgeting and pacing, suspiciousness and paranoia, and sleep disturbances.

Stage 6 is middle dementia. These persons seem "not-quite-right." They are less concerned for their appearance and may not want to change their clothing. They may begin to stand and walk differently and lose their social graces. They may have noticeable speech problems and obvious trouble recognizing or using common objects. They no longer understand the "future" and have trouble keeping a thought. Finally, they are unconcerned about their whereabouts (Fig. 22-2). Primary behaviors for Stage 6 include purposeless activity, agitation, and the fear of being alone.

In late dementia, Stage 7, residents are generally lost in their own world. They look "abnormal." They wear clothes oddly, have lost all social graces, have lost the ability to walk, sit up, hold their head up, and swallow, and have obvious speech problems. They have tremendous difficulty recognizing and using common objects. It is hard to get and keep their attention.

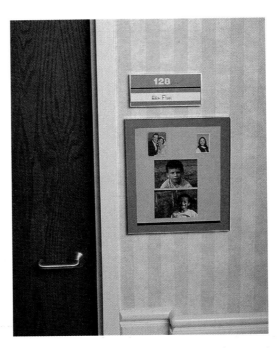

Fig. 22-2. Visual cues are used to help cognitively impaired residents recognize their whereabouts.

Stage 7 behavior includes agitation. This behavior dominates in Stages 6 and 7 because it is the only way this resident can communicate needs or feelings, like a young child.

Dementia

Dementia is a severe state of cognitive impairment. A person can be cognitively impaired (in earlier stages) but not have dementia. All persons with dementia share the same cognitive losses, which are called universal deficits. These deficits are in three areas:

▶ Memory (initially short term memory loss about information learned, later long term information about their life)

▶ Judgment (abstract thinking), such as when a resident has difficulty following directions

▶ Orientation (residents can be confused about day and night, where they are, and who they are—a person with dementia is disoriented in at least two of these areas)

These deficits lead to loss of ability in five other areas:

1. Self-care (eating, bathing, dressing, etc.)
2. Attention
3. Language (verbal and comprehension)
4. Recognition
5. Motor planning (balance, walking, posture)

With these types of losses, you can see why a demented person can no longer live without assistance.

YOUR ROLE CARING FOR A RESIDENT WITH COGNITIVE IMPAIRMENT OR DEMENTIA

Your role in caring for a resident who is cognitively impaired is different than your role with other residents. You must adjust your focus from the promotion of independence and regaining loss of function to meeting changing basic needs. The problems caused by a resident's brain-damaging disease cannot be reversed. The disease cannot be cured. Your role is to support the person and limit agitation and fear. You can meet many of their needs and work closely with family to lend support. In the following sections, you will learn the six major roles you will take on in caring for cognitively impaired residents.

Provide Guidance and Direction

Your first role is to gently guide and direct residents through the day (without becoming bossy), helping them focus on the task they are trying to accomplish. Treat them as you would a visitor in a foreign land. Every day they awake to a new world they do not understand and must attempt to cope with (Fig. 22-3).

Think again of that first day at a new job when everything is new and you are trying to process everything at once. By late afternoon, you feel you cannot deal with anything else that day. You are worn out and maybe irritable. This is how a cognitively impaired resident feels. By late afternoon or early evening, their coping abilities are weakening. You may see a change in their behavior. They may become irritable or combative or tearful and withdrawn. This is called sundowning. This is why your gentle direction helps get them through each new day.

Discover and Use Residents' Abilities

As residents move through the stages of cognitive decline, they are losing many of their abilities. Instead of focusing on what they cannot do, your role is to "discover" what they can do and try to incorporate these abilities into your caregiving. Whenever possible you should do "with," not "for" or "to," a resident. This means that you involve residents in any way they can in their care and assist only as needed. For example, encourage a resident to put soap on the washcloth before you wash his or her face. Or suggest a resident hold the wash items before you start washing. Later in this chapter you will learn techniques to enable residents to understand what you are doing and your expectations of them.

As you notice a resident's abilities declining, share these observations with the charge nurse. Try to avoid situations that "showcase" residents' disabilities and doom them to failure. For example, a resident with cognitive impairment should not get the same dietary tray as a cognitively intact resident. He or she may improperly use silverware and condiments, licking the butter pats, sucking the sugar out of sugar packets, and drinking the coffee cream. Besides frustrating a resident, you make your job harder as you now have to go back and fix things.

Instead, cognitively impaired residents' meals should be ready to eat as soon as the food is served (Fig. 22-4). This means that the meat is cut, the cream is in the

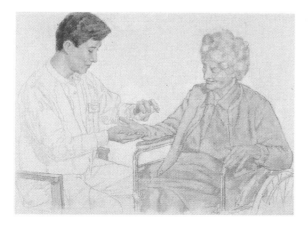

Fig. 22-3. Gently guide and direct cognitively impaired residents through daily tasks.

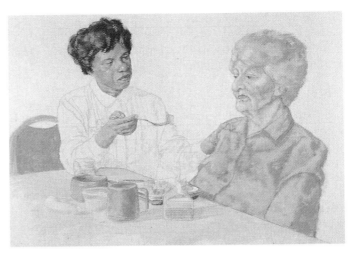

Fig. 22-4. Cognitively impaired residents' meals, should be ready to eat as soon as the food is served.

coffee, the butter is on the roll, etc. Now this resident is in a situation to succeed while using his or her remaining abilities.

In every situation, think of yourself as the person's champion and rescuer in this foreign land. You are "rescuing" him or her from the disabilities by optimizing his or her abilities.

Promote Each Resident's Dignity

Another important role is to promote their dignity. Each person has a different idea of what dignity means and what is embarrassing or undignified. You can tell if you are compromising a resident's dignity by his or her reaction to your care. If a resident gets upset when you do something, then stop and ask yourself if you are compromising his or her dignity. Remember to be gentle with your assistance and do not offend.

Be especially careful not to assume that a resident does not understand what is happening or being said. Cognitively impaired persons sometimes experience windows of clarity or lucidity when their brain functions well for a moment or two and allows them to clearly understand what is happening. Always treating residents with respect and dignity avoids hurtful situations.

Comfort and Reassure Each Resident

Your role is also to give comfort and reassure these residents (Fig. 22-5). They are literally losing their mind and abilities. Distress often results. Help them find physical, emotional, or spiritual support throughout the day. Do this by anticipating needs, providing gentle touches, sitting with them, reading from familiar books, and asking clergy to visit.

Anticipate Basic Needs

Anticipate and meet the basic needs of a resident with cognitive impairment. In every situation, especially if a resident is resisting care, you should first ask yourself, have this resident's most immediate basic needs been met? Think about Maslow's hierarchy of needs. For example, if a resident does not want to sit down to eat, he or she may need to go to the bathroom first. Ask yourself, when was the last time this person ate, had a drink of water, or was taken to the bathroom?

Always address these basic needs first in your caregiving. The hierarchy of needs helps you remember the priorities for meeting these five levels of common needs (see Chapter 2).

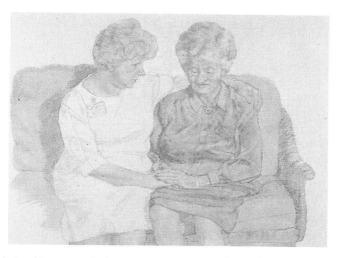

Fig. 22-5. Your comfort and support throughout the day is very important to a cognitively impaired resident.

Enjoy Residents and Help Them Enjoy Life

Your final role is to enjoy residents and help them enjoy life moment to moment. Residents can enjoy life when they feel successful and secure. You can help them feel this way when you are gentle and guiding, when you optimize their abilities, when you promote their dignity, when you give them comfort, and when you satisfy their basic needs. Your job will also go smoother and you will be able to appreciate and enjoy your residents. When residents with dementia can no longer use their minds, they still respond to emotions. A pleasant expression and sensitive use of laughter often bring a positive response (Fig. 22-6).

TECHNIQUES FOR RESPONDING TO BEHAVIORAL SYMPTOMS

Cognitively impaired residents often misinterpret what is going on around them. They may not understand what you are asking them to do or why. They may become frustrated, upset, or agitated and, because of this, resist the care you are giving.

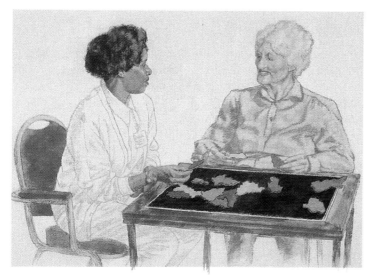

Fig. 22-6. A pleasant expression and sensitive use of laughter often bring a positive response.

Remember, behavioral symptoms such as verbal outbursts and tearfulness are common signs that a person with dementia is in distress. Recognizing what causes this distress is an important part of providing good care. This also makes your job easier and your interactions with these residents more enjoyable. So pay close attention to residents, see if you can identify a time of day they get upset, what tasks are pleasurable, which ones are not. Share information with other staff. Maybe together you can discover what brings happiness to residents.

The following sections describe techniques to better understand and work with these residents. Some of the techniques are for certain stages and others can be used throughout all stages. Apply the techniques not to a stage but as needed for an individual resident. The stages of dementia are continuous. A resident goes back and forth along the continuum many times each day. These stages are only a guideline.

Enter a Resident's Reality

Reality orientation is a common practice in long term facilities, based on the belief that residents benefit from knowing current information or reality. Reality orientation does not work with residents who are demented because they no longer can understand reality. Trying to convince them of something they are incapable of understanding only frustrates and agitates residents and sets up resistance to caregiving situations.

A positive care practice is validation therapy. With this approach you try to understand their feelings (enter their world) and then comfort their feeling (validate their perception of the world). By doing this, you are reassuring and comforting them while making your job easier. For example, if a resident tells you she would like to dress up because her husband is coming. You should accept this and help her dress up even though you know the person's husband is dead. Remember that a resident with dementia is a visitor in a foreign land and the foreign land is in their mind, not yours. You are helping to guide them through this new, strange foreign land of theirs.

Always remember that there is more than one way to view things. You may not feel that the behavior of a resident with dementia is normal, but for that resident it is. The behaviors of each dementia stage are normal for that person at that stage. When you understand how they view the world, you can see their behaviors in a whole new light. The world can be viewed in many different ways. Your goal is to find out how the dementia resident views the world so that you can enter that world and care for him or her.

Know Your Resident

To care for your residents, you need to know what makes them tick. How do they like things done? How did they used to do things? Gather as much information as possible to help understand residents. Ask questions of a resident, other staff members, and family members and friends (Fig. 22-7). Be mindful and discover his or her routine. Consider these questions:

- What did they do for a living?
- What is their religious affiliation?
- Did they have any hobbies?
- What social background do they come from?
- What did they take pride in?
- What made them feel sad?
- Did they experience major losses?
- What were they afraid of?
- How did they handle stress?
- What was a typical day like for them before their illness?
- What behavior symptoms do they have? What stage are they on the Global Deterioration Scale?

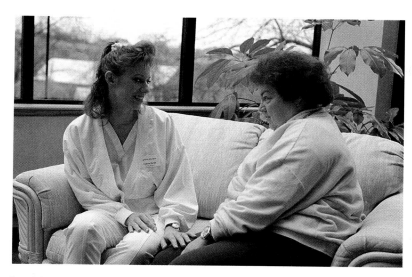

Fig. 22-7. Find out as much as you can about residents from their families and loved ones.

This information can help you enter their reality and make your caregiving easier. Residents often exhibit what is called "agenda behavior." This means that they feel they have a certain agenda to follow of things to do during the day. This "agenda" is often based on a past routine a resident still tries to follow. Disrupting this agenda may be stressful for him or her. Once again, knowing the "agenda" and trying to honor it as much as possible will ease your caregiving.

Know Your Resources

Besides knowing your residents, know what available resources can assist you with your caregiving tasks. This includes facility equipment and department resources. Does the nursing or dietary department have things or procedures to make your job easier? Have you read each resident's latest care plan? Does the activity department have special items a resident enjoys using? Can you offer sweets to a resident to make a bath a more pleasant experience? Make sure you are aware of any such resources. They will make your job easier.

Communicating with a Resident Who Has Dementia

The most important skill you can learn is to communicate with cognitively impaired residents and learn how residents communicate with you. As dementia progresses, residents do not always communicate their needs in an obvious manner, and they eventually lose the ability to speak and understand. Be aware of the signals residents send you to communicate their needs. Also be aware of the signals you send them. Chapter 6 covered the basic principles of communication. This section covers specific communication techniques for residents with cognitive impairment.

Body Language

Being aware of residents' body language will help you anticipate their needs. When a resident wraps his or her arms around the chest and is rocking back and forth, you can see that he or she is having trouble accepting what is going on. This resident needs comfort and reassurance, not someone insisting on care at that moment. Be careful of what your body language says. Try to send positive messages to residents.

Facial Expressions

As dementia progresses you will notice that residents "mirror" or copy your facial expressions, voice tones, and sometimes body language. We all know that a smiling, welcoming face is much more appealing than frowning. Residents take their cues from us on how to respond, and your facial expression affects how you communicate with a resident who has dementia.

Tone of Voice

Tone of voice often communicates more than words. Your gentle, patient tone tells residents they can feel safe with you and trust you. Residents' tone can also help you understand what they need even when their words do not make sense. Is their tone angry or desperate? Is it light-hearted or concerned?

Stage-Specific Communication Techniques

At each stage of cognitive decline, dementia residents have different communication skills and needs. Change your communication techniques as a resident's disease progresses (Fig. 22-8). Stage 5 residents can communicate fairly well verbally and generally understand simple, one-step commands. They generally state needs simply, such as saying "My lips are dry" instead of asking outright for help. They commonly have problems finding the right word ("tip of the tongue" syndrome), especially nouns and names. They may use inappropriate words, ramble, or talk around the point. They may also stutter mildly.

Stage 6 residents begin to have problems forming full sentences or understanding simple sentences. They may stop speaking unless spoken to and have more trouble finding the right word. Their responses may be limited to a few words, and they have difficulty staying on the topic. Residents who speak English as a second language will return to their first language.

Stage 7 residents lose all but the most basic verbal and comprehension abilities and the ability to feel. They communicate mainly through body language. They may also let out infrequent moans or screams.

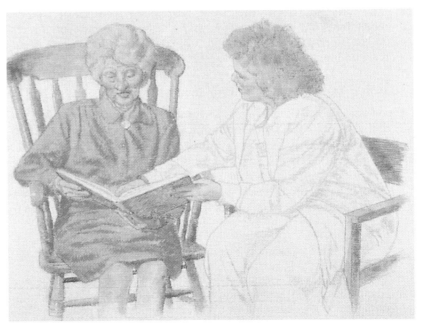

Fig. 22-8. Communication skills and needs will change as the resident's disease progresses.

Use the following techniques to communicate with a resident with dementia:

▷ Speak slowly and clearly using simple one-step commands, allowing residents time to process and respond to the information. You may have to give a resident 5-10 minutes; you can go away and come back. In interactions with Stage 6 residents, limit choices to two things, stating each choice simply. Allow time to respond to the first choice before offering the second. With Stage 7 residents, use only the simplest verbal interaction and communicate through gentle, pleasant tones of voice, facial expressions, and gentle touch. Meet residents' need for simplistic instruction without treating them like children. Remember they are adults and their feelings are still intact.

▷ Listen for a resident's verbal "cues" (simple statements like "Do me" or "My mouth is dry").

▷ Validate a resident's perception of reality whenever possible and then try to distract him or her from any problematic or troubling thoughts. Do not try to force a resident to do anything that is upsetting (see the later section on resistance to care).

▷ Avoid testing a resident, as this may set him or her up for failure. For example, avoid asking questions that will force him or her to use nouns or names, such as "Who came to visit today?" or "What is my name?" or "What is this called?" Try to phrase interactions simply so that the person will be able to respond with a "yes" or "no" whenever possible. Say something like, "How nice, your wife came today," or "Did you have a nice visit with your wife?"

▷ When giving direction, use one-to-one word directions and nonverbal cues whenever possible. As a resident's communication skills decline, send nonverbal cues to as many different senses as you can. For example, at bath time, first show him or her the towel, then soap and shampoo, then run water in the sink and let him or her feel the wet washrag. While doing this, never stop talking: "There is the towel for your bath, and here is the soap. Do you want your hair washed? I am turning on the water now. . . ." The person will understand your tone, if not the words.

▷ Observe a resident's body language for any signs of physical discomfort or unmet basic needs. Try to meet these needs before continuing.

Motivate Residents with Dementia

Besides being aware of how to communicate more effectively with residents with dementia, be aware of what you are communicating. People only do what they want to do. When someone asks you to do something, you may consider why you should do what the person wants or what's in it for you. Residents with dementia are motivated in the same way. When you learn what motivates them to want the care they need, you avoid unpleasant behavior that leads to difficult caregiving.

What motivates a resident with dementia? Residents want to do things that feel good, physically and emotionally. A warm washcloth is more inviting than a cold one. Emotionally, strange people, unfamiliar places, and equipment make people feel threatened. The care setting should be familiar to a resident. Expecting or insisting someone do more than he or she can is also emotionally threatening. Even residents with dementia like to feel successful.

Residents are often motivated by something funny (a silly hat or clown nose) or anything new, interesting, or unexpected. Curiosity is a big motivator. These techniques are also distractions that allow you to do care.

Another key to motivation is catching someone at the right time. Is the person ready to do something? Does it meet his or her needs at that time? For example, residents who are hungry and thirsty concentrate only on those needs until they are met. If you are trying to coax them into changing their clothes, they are not very motivated to go along with you. Meet basic needs first and other motivators will be easier.

Residents, like everyone, are motivated by things and people that are pleasant and inviting. Is the environment inviting, and pleasant for residents? Are you inviting to residents, someone they want to be with or go with? Does the person like you, feel safe and secure with you, find comfort being with you?

Finally, almost no one is motivated by something perceived as work. So don't make it work—make it fun! If you are setting out to bathe, groom, and dress Mrs. Mancino, tell her she has won "Queen for the Day" and your job is to pamper, bathe, groom, dress, and spoil her all day long.

Stop When a Resident Resists Your Care

As you work with a resident, communicating properly and offering motivators, keep assessing the results of your approach. If you accomplish your task and this resident is happy, you have developed a successful technique. Look for verbal and nonverbal signs whether a resident is enjoying the activity or becoming tired or agitated. When residents resist your care, this is your signal that they are becoming distressed.

Resistance to care is a resident's way of telling you he or she is stressed. When confronted with this situation, cease caregiving immediately! A resident with dementia cannot resist if you do not insist. Next, assess the person or situation for a possible cause of the resistance. Take care of this first and then try to continue care. If you avoid confrontation then you were successful. The box below describes common factors that may cause resistance to care.

Factors that Cause Resistance to Care

MEDICAL/EMOTIONAL FACTORS

A resident has an unmet basic need (pain, hunger, thirst, or elimination need). Do not try time-consuming care like bathing and dressing before meals with Stage 6 and 7 residents because hunger will make them unable to cooperate.

COMMUNICATION FACTORS

A resident may be responding to negative body language, tone of voice, or facial expressions.

ENVIRONMENTAL FACTORS

The room is uncomfortable or upsetting to a resident (too cold, too large, too much equipment, etc.).

NATURE OF THE TASK

A resident does not understand the care procedure. This includes not knowing what is expected of him or her, not knowing what is being done, not understanding the need for the care or when the care will end, and not knowing you. You might give Stage 7 residents something sweet to eat or hold during the procedure since they may be initially resistive to care for these reasons. Often you can use alternative care that will work with a particular resident. For instance, a resident who is frightened of a tub bath can have a bed bath or shower.

STAGE OF DISEASE

A resident's needs and abilities change as the dementia increases, and care procedures need to be simplified to match his or her new needs and abilities.

Finally, if routine care must be given to a resistive resident because the situation could become life-compromising otherwise, you should validate the person's distress and try to provide comfort through and after the care. Offering a drink of juice on completion of a care procedure is a good approach.

SPECIFIC TECHNIQUES FOR ACTIVITIES OF DAILY LIVING

Residents with cognitive impairment and dementia have unique needs that must be met to accomplish basic routine care and the activities of daily living. You will be challenged to find caregiving approaches that do not cause a resident distress. Tailor caregiving techniques to each dementia stage to help residents accomplish these activities easier and with dignity. Keep in mind the person's approximate mental age for needs and abilities according to the dementia stages, as shown in Table 22-1. Use this table as a general guide, but always individualize your care based on each resident's needs.

As you can see from the table, within any stage a resident's abilities can fluctuate. By the time people have dementia, they have become child-like because of their brain damage. But they are not *childish*. Childish implies that a mature person is acting immaturely. In residents with dementia, the disease process shuts their brain down in a reverse of how it develops, and thus they no longer have a mature intellect. As the brain shuts down, thinking and functioning become similar to young children, driven by their immediate bodily needs. For example, Stage 6 and 7 residents (whose thinking and functioning are like a child 1-5 years old) are hungry when they wake in the morning. This is their immediate need, and they cannot wait for bathing and dressing to meet that need. The challenge is to use the same kind of patience and understanding you would with a child, while honoring and respecting them as the adult they are.

Toileting

Residents with dementia all eventually lose control of their bladder and bowels. This can happen sooner if residents have difficulty locating restrooms or communicating their need to toilet. Once again, verbal and nonverbal cues help you to know when a resident needs to go to the bathroom. For example, Mrs. Morgan may not ask you directly where the bathroom is or say, "I need to use the restroom." She may be pacing around agitated and may seem to be trying to take off her skirt. Be aware of these cues. You can prevent residents from becoming prematurely incontinent and make your own job easier.

TABLE 22-1. The Global Deterioration Scale

Stage	Characteristics	Mental Age
5	Requires assistance choosing proper attire	5-7 years
6	Requires assistance dressing	5 years
	Requires assistance for proper bathing	4 years
	Requires assistance with mechanics of toileting	2 years
	Incontinent of bladder	36-54 months
	Incontinent of bowel	24-36 months
7	Speech limited to about six intelligible words	15 months
	Intelligible speech limited to one word	12 months
	Cannot walk	12 months
	Cannot sit up	24-40 weeks
	Cannot smile	8-16 weeks
	Cannot hold head up	4-12 weeks

Adapted from Reisberg, B. (1986). Geriatrics, 41(4): 30—46.

Stage 5 residents have control of their bowel and bladder when they receive assistance in locating bathrooms and reminders to toilet. Stage 6 residents begin to have episodic incontinence, times when they cannot control their bowel and bladder. They also require your help in the mechanics of toileting, such as wiping, flushing, and pulling down and up their underwear. Stage 7 residents are completely incontinent. They may not hear or understand reminders to use the toilet and may resist your help in changing incontinent products.

Follow these guidelines to help a resident remain continent as long as possible and to make toileting easier for both of you.

▶ Always be ready to help in finding bathrooms or in toileting.
▶ Be aware of residents' individualized toileting schedules so that you know when they may need your help. This also helps you to recognize cues that a resident needs to use the bathroom. As a general rule, a resident often needs to use the bathroom 1/2 to 1 hour after meals or snacks.
▶ Help a resident with incontinent products when the need arises. One way to ease the transition into using incontinent products is to place underwear over them.
▶ Always communicate slowly and gently with a resident while toileting, and allow extra time to process information.
▶ Remember that providing a distraction may help when a resident does not accept your help in toileting. One pleasant way to distract is with something sweet to eat.

Finally, remember that toileting is a personal matter. The wearing and use of incontinent products can be embarrassing and upsetting. Put yourself in the person's position and think how you would like to be treated. Remember respect and dignity.

Hydration

One of the basic needs is to replace body fluids. This is called hydration. Water is the primary source of hydration. Often, you may not understand why a resident is thirsty when a bedside water pitcher and water fountains are within easy reach. But think a moment; do you have a water fountain in your home or water pitcher by the side of your bed? Neither did most residents. These now unfamiliar objects go unnoticed or unrecognized by dementia residents. Thus, a resident may go thirsty without your help in locating or providing water.

Because dementia residents have difficulty telling you what they need, you must watch for both verbal and nonverbal cues that help you anticipate their needs. For example, a person may say "My mouth is so dry" or display other signs of thirst like agitation, dry mouth, or seemingly aimless searching. As the dementia progresses, residents' needs change. Residents in Stages 5 and 6 can usually drink independently, but they may not be able to find water fountains or water pitchers and may not ask you for something to drink when they are thirsty. In the last stage of dementia, Stage 7, residents cannot do any of these things. They will need help holding a glass to their mouths to drink and may have trouble swallowing (Fig. 22-9).

Follow these basic techniques to ensure that residents with dementia are not going thirsty:

▶ Offer residents hydration according to each resident's individual needs. For Stage 5 residents, encourage them to participate as "hosts" or "hostesses." This can be both fun and useful for you and residents. For Stage 7 residents, offer fluids more often in smaller amounts. If a resident has trouble swallowing, inform the nurse immediately.
▶ Offer fluids when a resident gives spoken "cues" of thirst (like "My mouth is so dry").
▶ Offer fluids when a resident shows nonverbal signs of thirst (like dry mouth, agitation, tongue hanging out, seemingly aimless rummaging or searching behavior).

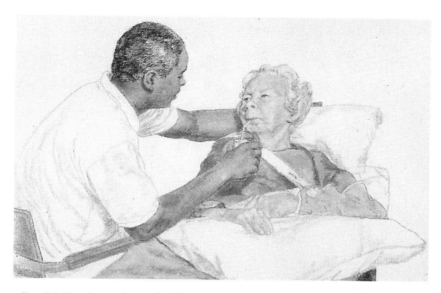

Fig. 22-9. A resident who has cognitive impairment may need assistance with drinking.

Eating

All residents with dementia need assistance finding the dining area and eating. Many techniques, unique to each dementia stage, can ease the dining experience for both of you. Be sure to inform the nurse of any changes in residents' abilities to ensure that dietary tray set-ups and food choices are appropriate for the abilities of each resident at each dementia stage.

Stage 5 residents can eat independently, but be careful that they continue to use their knife properly. Stage 6 residents begin to lose eating skills such as using knives, forks, and straws and may have problems with positioning and swallowing. Techniques you should follow for Stages 5 and 6 include:

▶ Prompting and providing cues to continue eating, chewing, and swallowing when necessary.

▶ Allow more time to eat.

▶ Precut, preseason, and debone their food. The food should be ready to eat when the tray is placed in front of them.

▶ Watch for misuse of utensils and provide only a fork and spoon to those who cannot use a knife properly (Fig. 22-10).

▶ There is no reason why residents cannot use their fingers.

▶ Watch for things like the person ignoring one side of his or her plate, which may result from a visual problem; not being able to handle food and drinks served at the same time; not eating other food if dessert is served with the meal; and difficulties with swallowing and positioning.

Stage 7 residents have completely lost their eating skills. Techniques that you should add to the techniques used in Stages 5 and 6 include:

▶ Ensure proper body positioning.

▶ Move slowly to allow the person more time to understand.

▶ Peel all fruit.

▶ Watch for pouring of drink into his or her plate. If a resident does this, do not give food and drink at the same time.

▶ Add sweetener to increase the appeal of food if necessary.

▶ If a resident cannot use a fork appropriately, provide only a spoon. If unable to use a spoon appropriately, the person needs to transition into eating only finger foods.

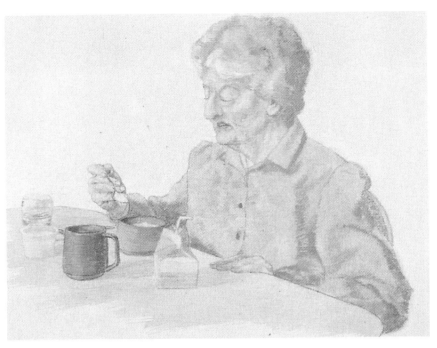

Fig. 22-10. Give residents a fork and spoon if they can no longer use a knife properly.

Dressing

As you have seen with other ADLs, the ability of a resident with dementia to dress varies as the disease progresses.

Stage 5 residents can dress themselves independently with limited supervision. Your assistance may be needed only to choose things to wear that are appropriate for the season or occasion. Some Stage 5 residents may need coaxing to change their clothes or remove their clothes at night. Others may try to change their clothes repeatedly throughout the day.

Some Stage 6 residents may also need only limited supervision, while others need a lot more help. They need help putting their clothes on properly, like putting shoes on the right feet and tying laces. They also may begin to have problems wearing their glasses, dentures, and hearing aids for the entire day. They may resist your efforts to help them change clothes.

Stage 7 residents need total assistance in dressing and cannot wear supportive appliances. They may begin taking their shoes and socks off, along with clothes that fasten in the front. They may fiddle constantly with buttons, zippers, or hems. They may not only resist changing their clothes but may resist wearing underclothes.

Follow these procedures to make dressing more simple and enjoyable for you and residents with dementia:

▶ Always be ready to assist residents in any stage when you see that your help is needed.

▶ Simplify dressing according to the needs of each stage of dementia. In Stage 5, offer no more than two outfits to wear and ask the person to select one. In Stage 6, select clothing for the person to wear. Simplify dressing by laying clothes out in the order they are put on. You may also need to place their arms, legs, and head in clothing openings and fasten any buttons, snaps, etc. (Fig. 22-11). In Stage 7, dress residents in clothing that can be easily taken on and off. For example, use over-the-head dresses and shirts, elastic waistbands, no front closures (like buttons and snaps), and no belts or ties.

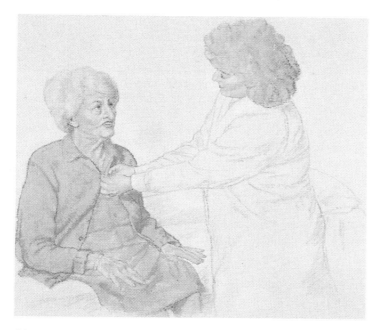

Fig. 22-11. You may need to assist residents in dressing themselves properly.

▷ If residents become resistive to your efforts to dress or undress them, they may need friendly coaxing. If this is not enough, take these steps:

  ▷ If resistance is in the morning, do not try dressing until after the person has eaten breakfast.

  ▷ If resistance is at night, encourage the family to bring in clothing that can be worn day or night, like jogging suits, housecoats, or muu-muus. This will limit clothing changes to once a day, in the morning.

  ▷ If resistance is to nonessential clothing like bras, slips, or nylons, do not force the person to wear them.

▷ Remember to always be gentle and patient. Use words and gestures to communicate and move slowly to give a resident time to understand what is happening.

▷ Residents who begin walking with one shoe off and one shoe on may need to be assessed for foot problems, or their shoes checked for fit and condition. If neither is a problem, he or she may need to wear slipper socks with nonslip soles instead of shoes. Inform the nurse of such a change.

Bathing

Bathing is often a traumatic experience for dementia residents, but it need not be. With your help, bathing can be done smoothly and in a manner least upsetting to a resident. Showers are often stressful in all stages, so bathtubs are generally preferable. Consider each resident's needs and the actions you can take to meet these needs.

Early dementia, Stage 5, residents rely completely on you to tell them when they need to bathe and need help finding bathrooms and bathing supplies, like soap, washcloth, towel, and shampoo. They may need very little or quite a lot of help in actually bathing themselves, getting into and out of the shower or bath, adjusting the water, and washing and drying themselves. Take these actions to help a Stage 5 resident:

▷ Assist with any activities to help get ready for bathing like getting undressed, finding the bathroom, etc. You do not always have to help, but you should be ready to help if you see that a resident is struggling.

▷ Assist with hair washing if a resident needs help.

▷ Give direction (talking a resident through it or using body language) during washing and drying to make sure a resident does a good job.

Stage 6 residents need much more help in bathing. These residents are experiencing many more physical and cognitive difficulties. In bathing, their abilities may be limited to washing and drying their hands and face. Even when it seems very little, you should encourage any action a resident can do independently. Stage 6 residents may develop a fear of water from the shower head or in the tub. They may resist your efforts to help them bathe. Help a Stage 6 resident this way:

▷ Assist with undressing, getting into and out of the shower or bath, and washing and drying.

▷ Encourage residents to bathe themselves in easy to reach areas like the face, chest, and thighs. How you communicate with residents will make this easier. Use simple one-step commands ("Rinse your arm . . . now rinse your shoulder") and hand-over-hand demonstrations to show residents how to wash their arm or dry their leg, etc.

▷ Try to avoid doing things that may make residents fearful of bathing. Do not wet a resident's face directly with the shower spray. Sponge bathe as needed to avoid putting a resident completely in the water. Think about the things you would not like done to you if you had a fear of water.

Late dementia, or Stage 7, residents need total assistance. They may resist your efforts to help them bathe because they do not understand the bathing process and may have a fear of water. Often it is better to sponge bathe or bed bathe. Take these actions to help a Stage 7 resident:

▷ Communicate gently during the entire bathing process. Remember to communicate both verbally and nonverbally.

▷ Move slowly to allow the person more time to understand what you are communicating or doing.

▷ When working with resistive residents, you may want to distract them with something sweet to eat and offer a drink after bathing. You can make bathing more comfortable by warming the bathroom before bathing and less fearsome by wetting their feet first, not spraying water right in their face, or sponge bathing. Keep in mind that your role is to help residents feel less fear. Remember you are trying to coax someone into doing something he or she doesn't want to do.

Grooming

Proper grooming is important to preserve the dignity of a resident. Often, improper or incomplete grooming leads to family complaints. Grooming includes combing the hair, washing the face, brushing the teeth, removing and reinserting dentures, shaving, and applying make-up, and cologne or lotion. Meeting the grooming needs of residents with dementia is not difficult.

Stage 5 residents can groom independently with your encouragement and supervision. As residents decline into Stage 6, their grooming needs may involve just your supervision, or they could need extensive assistance. Stage 6 residents may begin to resist having their hair washed and stop using glasses, hearing aids, and dentures. Stage 7 residents completely depend on you for their grooming. They also resist shaving and do not use supportive appliances.

Use these techniques to make grooming an easy and more pleasant activity for both you and residents:

▷ Be ready to provide help with the mechanics and tasks of grooming and locating bathrooms whenever necessary (Fig. 22-12).

▷ Simplify the tasks of grooming as needed to encourage self-grooming, and "press the starter button" to initiate an activity. For example, you may put the toothpaste on the toothbrush for residents.

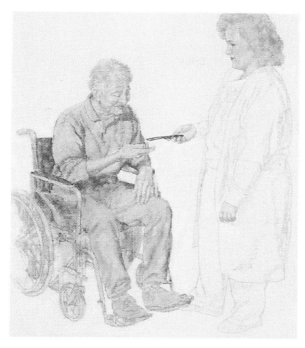

Fig. 22-12.   Be ready to assist the resident with grooming.

▷ Encourage a resident to attend the morning grooming program in your facility to apply any "finishing touches" like cologne and make-up. This promotes a positive self-image and good self-esteem.

▷ When a resident stops wearing supportive appliances, give them to him or her when it is most beneficial. For example, dentures are required at meals but are not absolutely necessary at other times.

▷ Always gently communicate with resident while grooming using sensory cues (like warm washcloth on face and warm shaving cream applied with a shaving brush) to encourage grooming. As always, move slowly to give more time to understand.

▷ If resistance to shaving occurs, assess for physical pain, like oral problems and ear aches, or discomfort from other unmet needs. If resistance continues, do not force shaving at that time. Try later using more sensory cues. If resistance still continues, try every day but do not force care. Be sure to advise family that this is a normal behavior for Stage 7 and that you will resume shaving when this behavior diminishes and the person stops resisting.

To accomplish the activities of daily living, you must consider a dementia resident's particular needs for each dementia stage and adapt your care accordingly. Keep in mind the general principles of preparing yourself, using good communication and motivation skills, and assessing the situation for resistance. If things become confusing, remember that the simpler you keep what you are asking of them, the easier it will be on everyone.

Be sure to discuss with the charge nurse any concerns you have about caring for a resident with cognitive impairment. Share your ideas of adapting care with other team members. Use your philosophy of mindful caregiving and the themes of care. A resident with cognitive impairment will challenge you, but you will find your successful caregiving rewarding.

Other Mental Impairments

Other disorders too can severely affect a person's ability to think, reason, and learn, such as mental retardation, depression, anxiety, suspiciousness, paranoia, delusion, and schizophrenia. These conditions are cognitive impairments in general, but they are unlike other conditions such as Alzheimer's in that usually they do not progress to dementia.

Mental Retardation

With mental retardation, a child's brain development is slowed or stopped so that the child never mentally matures. The most common causes of mental retardation are difficult birth, Down's syndrome, and high fever in infancy or childhood.

Depression

Many things can cause residents to be depressed or not feel good about themselves or others in their life. This can result from being sick for some time, losing persons or things we care deeply about, or being kept from doing what we want to do. If we aren't able to adapt, these feelings may make us angry and resentful. The longer this lasts, the more depressed we become. Many nursing facility residents suffer from depression for these reasons. Symptoms of severe depression include:

▶ Weight problems (loss of appetite and weight or overeating and weight gain)
▶ Tiredness and not being able to sleep
▶ Crying spells
▶ Complaining of not feeling good all the time
▶ Being negative and unable to work with staff
▶ Loss of will to do anything
▶ Thoughts of suicide or death

As you can see, severe depression has many of the symptoms of dementia. This may be considered a "pseudo dementia," a false dementia. But when you respond to these symptoms with supportive care and antidepressant therapy, the "dementia" ends.

Anxiety

Anxiety is a vague uneasy feeling that can lead to feelings of nervousness, fear, and high blood pressure. In extreme cases, the person loses the ability to think about anything else. This can lead to panic. Anxiety can be caused by chemical imbalances in the brain. Prolonged anxiety can prevent the ability to function and affect quality of life. Severe cases require medical intervention.

Suspiciousness, Paranoia, Delusion, and Schizophrenia

Suspiciousness is the distrust of others. Paranoia is a feeling of being mistreated (persecution). Delusion is a false belief or idea not supported by reality. When a person has all three of these conditions and is frightened by his or her thoughts, that person is said to have schizophrenia. This condition requires medical treatment.

23

Additional Infection Prevention and Control Procedures

IN THIS CHAPTER YOU WILL LEARN TO:

▶ state how the body responds to infection

▶ define the nurse assistant's role in identifying signs, symptoms, and clues of infection

▶ explain the facility's policy and procedures relating to isolation precautions

How do you define a challenge? Most of us think of a challenge as something that is difficult but important and gives us a feeling of satisfaction when we accomplish it.

Infection control is often a challenge in long term care facilities—both caring for residents with an infection and preventing the spread of infection to other residents. Residents who are elderly and may be frail or weakened by other illness are more susceptible to infection and can be seriously affected by infections that may not be as serious in younger, healthier adults. This makes your challenge even greater.

As you learned in Chapter 7, you play a very important role in prevention and control of infections in residents. You can do many things to prevent the transmission of microorganisms.

You can also learn to identify infection when it first appears. You are often the first person to notice a change in a resident's normal behavior or condition. Sometimes this change is a "clue" that a resident is developing an infection. If you tell the nurse about this change so that this resident can be evaluated promptly, the doctor can often start treatment before the infection becomes serious (Fig. 23-1). Treatment with antibiotics that destroy microorganisms works much better early in an infection than after a resident becomes seriously ill.

In this chapter you will learn to identify signs and symptoms of skin infections, urinary tract infections, and respiratory tract infections. By recognizing early clues to infections, you can help improve the quality of life for residents.

Some residents admitted to nursing facilities already have infections, and others develop infections in the facility. Some facilities use special infection prevention and control measures for these residents, often called "isolation precautions." Isolation precautions mean using barriers for certain care activities and assigning residents with certain types of infections to private rooms.

In this chapter you will learn about the different types of isolation precautions used when caring for a resident diagnosed or suspected of having an infection. This care includes helping residents in isolation meet their psychosocial needs.

HOW THE BODY RESPONDS TO INFECTION

When microorganisms cause infection, a person's body responds in many different ways. The response depends on the severity of the infection. There are three general types of responses: localized, whole body, and silent.

Localized Responses

Some kinds of infections can be seen by looking carefully at a resident's skin. For example, if a resident has a skin tear that becomes infected, the area around the tear becomes warm and red, and there may be yellowish pus in the wound. This is called

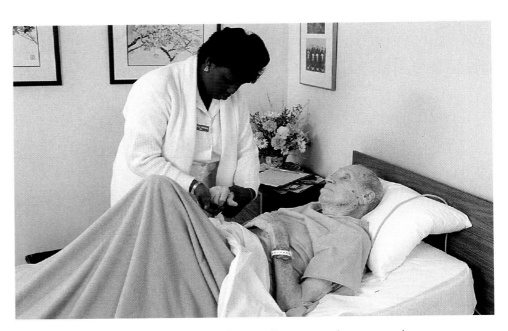

Fig. 23-1. Look for signs of infection. Reporting changes early on can prevent a serious infection.

a localized response because it affects only one isolated area. Other parts of the body are not affected.

Whole Body Responses

Pneumonia is an example of infection that affects the entire body. When this happens, the body usually responds in many ways, including becoming warm with fever. Other signs and symptoms may occur, such as respiratory distress, achiness, pain, cough, sputum production, and possibly a change in mental status—the whole body is affected. However, fever is probably the primary sign. In older people the temperature usually doesn't get as high as it does in children and younger adults. A temperature a little over 100° F. in a person 80 years old may be as serious as a temperature of 102° F. in a small child. When a resident doesn't feel well, a fever may be an early clue that he or she is coming down with an infection.

Silent Responses

Some infections are called silent because they cause no symptoms and are found only with lab tests. For example, most people infected with the human immuno-deficiency virus (HIV) (the virus that causes AIDS) have silent infections and can be identified only with special blood tests.

Some microorganisms that cause infections in childhood can stay in the body silently for many years. An example is the chicken pox virus. As some people get older and the immune system weakens, the chicken pox virus wakes up and causes painful blisters called shingles. If you have never had chicken pox, you can catch the virus from a resident with shingles, and you can then become ill with chicken pox. (To avoid this, you should wear gloves when caring for a resident with draining shingles and wash your hands well.) However, if you have already had chicken pox, you cannot catch it again.

IDENTIFYING CLUES TO SIGNS AND SYMPTOMS OF COMMON INFECTIONS

Because the body responds to infections in certain ways, you can learn to identify the clues of common infections.

Key Terms

You have already learned signs and symptoms of infection. A *symptom* of infection is something that happens in a person's body when microorganisms cause disease. Symptoms often are not visible to another person but are felt by the infected individual and must be described by him or her. For example, a fever blister on the lip causes burning or tingling of the skin before the fever blister breaks out. If a resident cannot describe this symptom, you cannot know that a fever blister is about to erupt.

A *sign* of infection is apparent to someone else. Some signs of infection are visible, such as redness and drainage caused by an eye infection. Other signs of infection are identified by lab tests (Fig. 23-2). For example, a complete blood count can identify a high number of white cells in the blood, which is a sign of infection.

Other signs of infection are measured with special instruments. For example, a thermometer is used to measure elevated temperature, a sign of fever, and X-rays can identify signs of pneumonia in the chest.

We use the term *clue* for those signs and symptoms of infection that you as a nurse assistant can observe in your daily care of residents. When you put several clues together, you form a picture of more specific symptoms or signs of infection, even if residents can't tell you where they hurt or how they feel. When you put clues together well and report these to the nurse promptly, you improve the quality of life for residents.

Signs, Symptoms, and Clues to Infection in Older Adults

Signs, symptoms, and clues for infections are not as clear in older adults as they are in younger people. As well, a resident with cognitive impairment may not be able to tell you when he or she feels symptoms, so you will have to use your senses to identify changes. You can also look at factors that may be influencing the sign or symptoms. Using the information about the aging process in Chapter 3, you can identify signs and symptoms and put clues together. Some clues to infection that you can observe during daily care include drainage from a wound, dark and smelly urine, and greenish thick sputum.

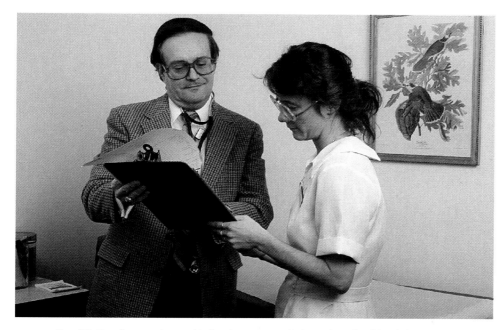

Fig. 23-2.   Some signs of infection can only be identified by laboratory tests.

Signs, Symptoms, and Clues for Common Infections
Fever

A common sign of infections affecting the whole body is fever, an elevated temperature measured with a thermometer. But you might not think to take a resident's temperature unless you have some clues that a resident may have a fever (Fig. 23-3), since taking temperatures is a daily routine at most facilities. You can take a temperature whenever you suspect a resident may have an infection without being told by the nurse.

Pneumonia

A symptom of pneumonia is chest pain, but you can't see chest pain in someone else directly. A clue to chest pain is a resident's pained facial expression or holding the chest when coughing. Other clues to pneumonia are shortness of breath or more coughing than is normal for a resident, and coughing up thick sputum that is white, yellow, or any other color. Since many older adults with pneumonia do not have the energy or muscle tone to cough up sputum, you may not see this clue. Be sure to report any clues for pneumonia promptly to the nurse so that this resident can be evaluated further (Fig. 23-4).

Urinary Tract Infection

Some symptoms of urinary tract infection include difficulty voiding, burning while voiding, increased frequency, and some back aches. Fever is sometimes but not always present. Signs that you can observe include cloudy, bloody, or smelly urine. For residents whose habits you know well, you may see clues such as residents asking to void more frequently than is normal or being incontinent when they usually can hold their urine until they get to the toilet. When you identify signs or clues to possible urinary tract infection, report them promptly to the nurse.

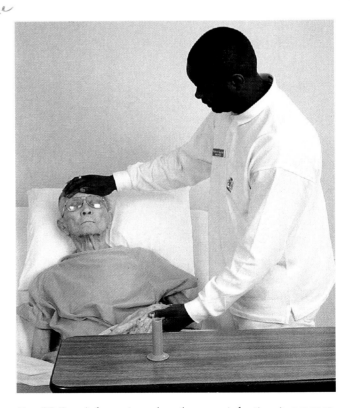

Fig. 23-3.   A fever is a clue than an infection is present.

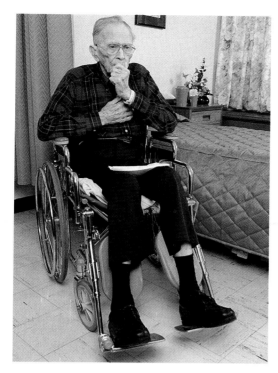

Fig. 23-4. Watch for symptoms of pneumonia and report them to the nurse immediately.

Describe your observations as specifically as possible. The nurse can then use your information to evaluate this resident further before talking with the doctor (Fig. 23-5).

Skin Infections

As people age, the skin becomes thinner, less elastic, and easier to damage. Skin tears are common in older people and can let microorganisms from the skin or from

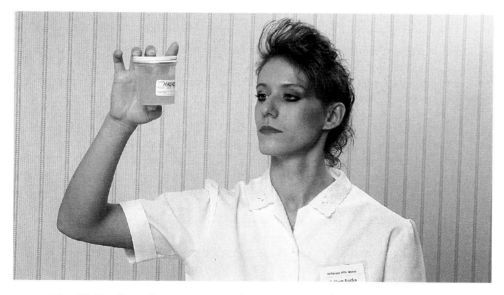

Fig. 23-5. Describe symptoms of urinary tract infections as specifically as possible.

your hands enter the body. Sometimes skin tears become infected. When you provide daily care to residents with skin tears, look for infection clues such as redness, swelling, or bad-smelling darkened tissue in the wound. A clear sign of infection is pus at the site.

Scabies Infestations

Scabies outbreaks are common in long term care facilities. Scabies is caused by a mite transmitted by skin-to-skin contact. Unfortunately, it takes 2-6 weeks for someone newly infested with scabies to develop symptoms of itching, so early scabies infestations are silent. The first clue may be scratches you notice on a resident's skin.

In the evaluation for scabies, mites are often found in the finger webs, at the wrists and elbows, under the breasts, and at the belt line. In people with weakened immune systems, the whole body may be affected.

To prevent outbreaks of scabies, all newly admitted residents should have a complete head-to-toe skin assessment by a nurse. Any suspicious rashes must be evaluated carefully. You can help the nurse by looking at a resident's skin during your daily care activities and reporting any rashes or scratches.

Treatment for scabies requires the use of special baths or skin medications. When an outbreak of scabies occurs in a facility, other residents and employees are usually treated also to stop the outbreak.

Putting Clues Together

When you identify clues to a possible infection, you need to put them together in a meaningful way. You know residents better than anyone else in the facility, and you know when a resident looks, acts, or sounds different from usual. These differences from normal may be clues to infection, but you need to put them together and report your observations to the nurse so that action can be taken if needed. Consider the following example:

> Ms. Anderson is usually eager to get out of bed and be active. On Tuesday morning when you go in to get Ms. Anderson ready for breakfast, she tells you she didn't sleep well and was cold all night. She coughs a couple of times, and you notice that her nose is running. She tells you she really doesn't feel like getting out of bed this morning.

The first thing you might want to do is take Ms. Anderson's temperature because this is a sign of infection. However, if Ms. Anderson just has a cold she may not have a fever. The runny nose and cough are other clues you want to report to the nurse so that she can be evaluated further.

Rather than just telling the nurse that Ms. Anderson "has a cold," it would be better to describe the clues you have observed (Fig. 23-6). That is, tell the nurse that Ms. Anderson has a runny nose and cough and doesn't feel like getting out of bed, but that her temperature was only 98.0°F. This gives the nurse specific information for evaluating Ms. Anderson further and talking with the doctor. The nurse should also be pleased that you have already taken Ms. Anderson's temperature. The doctor may prescribe cold medications to make Ms. Anderson more comfortable. For the next few days, stay alert to changes in her condition because a simple cold can sometimes turn into pneumonia.

Putting clues together also helps identify possible urinary tract infections. For example, a common symptom of urinary tract infection is "burning on urination," but a resident who is cognitively impaired may not be able to describe this. You need to watch his or her facial expression and body language to see if pain occurs during voiding. A pained facial expression during voiding may be a clue of a urinary tract

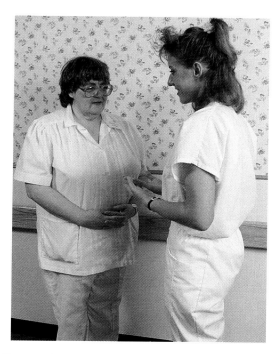

Fig. 23-6. Report detailed clues of a resident's suspected infection to the nurse.

infection, although there could be another reason for the pain. Another more specific clue is dark or smelly urine, or urinary incontinence in a resident who usually can control bladder function. If the same resident has all three clues present at the same time, it is quite likely that he or she has a urinary tract infection. Report this information promptly to the nurse.

ISOLATION PRECAUTIONS

Isolation precautions are the different things a facility does to keep microorganisms from spreading from one resident to others. Isolation precautions are provided in many ways in long term care facilities, and these are usually described in the facility's "Infection Control Manual" or "Isolation Manual." The designated infection control practitioner is responsible for teaching you how to use the isolation precautions system.

State agencies that license long term care facilities have requirements for isolation precautions, which vary from state to state. Guidance for isolation precautions also comes from the Centers for Disease Control and Prevention (CDC). The CDC's "Guideline for Isolation Precautions" provides ways to reduce risks of transmitting organisms from one resident to another, from a resident to a health care worker, and from health care workers to residents.

The Guideline offers facilities three options for a system of isolation precautions: category-specific isolation precautions, disease-specific isolation precautions, or facility-designed isolation precautions. These are described below.

Category-Specific Isolation Precautions

Residents diagnosed or suspected of having an infectious disease or condition are assigned to one of 6 or 7 different categories. Each category includes several different diseases or conditions transmitted in a similar way. A category-specific sign is placed on the door that describes the precautions required for the category. The facility's infection control or isolation manual lists all diseases or conditions in each

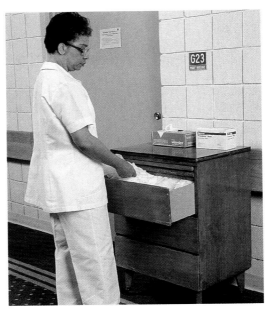

Fig. 23-7. Isolation precautions are used for residents with an infectious disease or condition.

category and details for isolation precautions (such as a need for private room, masks, gloves, gowns) for each category (Fig. 23-7).

Strict Isolation

This category is for a few highly infectious diseases. It requires hand washing before and after caring for a resident and using masks, gowns, and gloves before entering the person's private room. Strict isolation is used for whooping cough, pneumonic plague, chicken pox or shingles all over the body, and certain tropical viral fevers rarely seen in residents.

Contact Isolation

This category is used for many different diseases and conditions listed in the infection control manual. The most common conditions include infection or colonization with multiply resistant bacteria, lice, scabies, certain bacterial pneumonias, and major skin or wound infections. Contact isolation requires hand washing before and after caring for this resident, masks for those who come close to him or her (usually within 3 feet), gowns if soiling is likely, and gloves for touching infective material (wound drainage, pus, sputum).

Respiratory Isolation

This category is used for several diseases, but very few are likely in residents of long term care facilities. A private room is needed, masks are worn by those who come close to the person (within 3 feet), and hand washing before and after care is required; however, gowns and gloves are not necessary.

Acid-Fast Bacillus (AFB) Isolation

This category is used for residents with active pulmonary tuberculosis for as long as they are considered infectious. AFB Isolation requires that this resident stay in a private room with special ventilation and the door remains closed. Gowns and gloves are not needed, but masks are required for room entry. Special masks such as high efficiency filtration masks (also called particulate respirators) are recommended. These masks have two straps to insure a better fit and tighter face seal to protect the airway of the wearer. These masks can also be used for an entire shift (put on and taken off repeatedly and stored in the pocket between wearings) because touch contamination does not transmit tuberculosis organisms.

Enteric Precautions

Diseases requiring enteric precautions include many gastrointestinal infections of residents and health care workers. Enteric precautions require gloves for touching infective material (such as stool), gowns if soiling is likely, and hand washing before and after resident care. Masks are not needed.

Drainage/Secretion Precautions

Diseases requiring drainage/secretion precautions include those with limited or minor production of pus, drainage, or secretions. Residents often have minor or limited infections of the skin, wounds, decubitus ulcers, or abscesses. Drainage/secretion precautions require gloves for touching infective material (such as pus or drainage), hand washing before and after care, and gowns if soiling is likely, but not masks.

Blood/Body Fluid Universal Precautions

In Chapter 7 you learned about blood/body fluid universal precautions, intended primarily to protect health care workers from infection with bloodborne pathogens such as HIV, hepatitis B virus (HBV), and hepatitis C virus (HCV). Universal precautions require gloves for touching blood and body fluids to which universal precautions apply, gowns if soiling is likely, masks and eye protection if splashing of the face or eyes is likely, and hand washing before and after care and after removing gloves. Chapter 7 describes these procedures in detail.

Disease-Specific Isolation Precautions

With disease-specific isolation precautions, only specific precautions to interrupt transmission of the particular disease are recommended. Facilities that use disease-specific isolation precautions list in the infection control manual each disease or condition and requirements for precautions such as private room, masks, gowns, and gloves. The manual also lists specific infective material for each disease or condition and specifies how long precautions should be used. When a resident is diagnosed or suspected of having a specific disease or condition, a special sign is placed on the door that states exactly what precautions should be used (Fig. 23-8).

Facility-Designed Isolation Precautions

Some facilities design their own system of isolation precautions. One of the most popular is called "body substance isolation" (BSI) or "body substance precautions" (BSP).

The BSI system is based on the principle that a resident in a nursing facility always has infectious organisms in some body substances (stool, sputum, oral secretions, wound drainage, vomitus) and may have infectious organisms in their blood and/or urine. However, specific organisms may not be identified unless the person has signs and symptoms of infection or has had lab cultures done. Because all of these body substances can be reservoirs for microorganisms that can cause infection in other residents or health care workers, barriers should be used between the body substance and the care provider to break the chain of infection at the mode of transmission link.

If hand washing and barriers are used correctly (see Chapter 7), then direct and indirect transmission from the reservoir to the susceptible host are interrupted, regardless of whether a resident is diagnosed as having an infection.

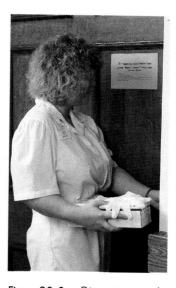

Fig. 23-8. Disease-specific isolation requires a sign be placed on the door stating the precautions that should be used.

Body substance isolation systems also include provisions for diseases such as tuberculosis transmitted by the air. These are the same as those for AFB isolation described above.

APPLYING ISOLATION PRECAUTIONS

You need to know which system of isolation precautions is used by your facility and be consistent in applying it to your resident care activities. The following is an example of an infection and how a facility would handle it.

Tuberculosis is caused by bacteria. When TB bacteria are coughed into the air by a person with pulmonary tuberculosis, some of them remain suspended in the air in very tiny droplets. If you or anyone else inhales enough of these droplets, you can become infected with tuberculosis organisms.

A resident who is diagnosed with active pulmonary tuberculosis is usually transferred to an acute care facility for treatment. But a resident could be returned to the long term care facility while still infectious if the facility can provide adequate care there. This resident needs to be assigned to a private room with special ventilation.

If you are caring for a resident who is still infectious with tuberculosis, you should be sure that the door is closed at all times and wear a mask whenever you go into the room. Teach this resident to cover the nose and mouth with a tissue during coughing, and to discard those tissues in the trash can. Most states no longer consider these tissues regulated waste, since contaminated trash does not transmit tuberculosis microorganisms.

TUBERCULOSIS INFECTION AND TUBERCULOSIS DISEASE

There are two stages in the tuberculosis process. The first stage is "tuberculosis infection" and the second stage is "tuberculosis disease."

Most people who are infected with tuberculosis organisms just have "tuberculosis infection" and are not infectious to others. These people are called tuberculin reactors because they have positive skin tests. They do not have active pulmonary disease and they do not cough up TB organisms. People who have active pulmonary tuberculosis disease are infectious to others. They usually have generalized symptoms of fever, night sweats, and weight loss.

The best way for you to monitor yourself for "tuberculosis infection" is to participate in the facility's skin testing program whenever you are scheduled to have a skin test (Fig. 23-9). This determines if you have become newly infected with tuberculosis organisms and need medical follow-up and treatment to prevent tuberculosis disease.

If you already have a positive skin test, you may have been treated with anti-tuberculosis drugs in the past. The infection control practitioner can help determine if you need additional medical follow-up, depending on your own skin test and past treatment situation.

PSYCHOSOCIAL NEEDS OF RESIDENTS ON ISOLATION PRECAUTIONS

Today, strict isolation is rarely necessary in long term care facilities. Even when a resident is on isolation precautions, that usually does not mean that he or she must be confined to the room without visitors or social stimulation.

Many residents who are not allowed to leave their rooms believe they have done something wrong and are being punished for bad behavior. Help these residents understand about the transmission of microorganisms and prevent fear of the unknown. Consider this example:

> Mrs. Henderson developed an intestinal obstruction in the facility. She is transferred to an acute care hospital for abdominal surgery and develops a postoperative wound infection. The doctor starts treatment with IV antibiotics in the hospital, and her wound infection begins to heal. As she improves, her treatment is changed to oral antibiotics, and she returns to the facility five days after her surgery. Because there is

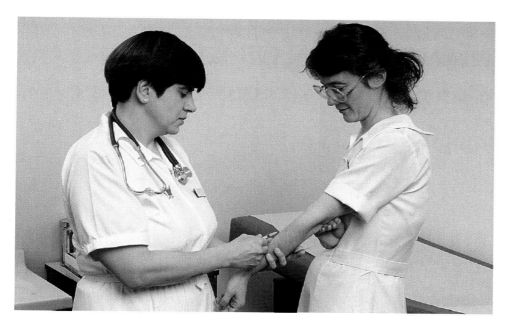

IN THIS CHAPTER YOU LEARNED TO:

▶ state how the body responds to infection

▶ define the nurse assistant's role in identifying signs, symptoms, and clues of infection

▶ explain the facility's policy and procedures relating to isolation precautions

Fig. 23-9. Participate in the facility's skin or blood testing program to monitor yourself for possible tuberculosis infection.

still some drainage from her healing abdominal wound, she is put on isolation precautions when she returns to the facility.

Your facility uses a disease-specific isolation precautions system. For Ms. Henderson's wound infection, this means that caregivers wear gloves during wound care and a gown if soiling of clothing is likely, and wash hands before and after care and when gloves are removed. What kinds of restrictions would Ms. Henderson have?

You are taking care of Ms. Henderson when she has been on oral antibiotics for 3 days, the wound is almost completely healed, and she is feeling much better. She would like to go to the dining room for dinner. Her healing wound is completely covered with a dressing that catches the drainage, and she wants to put on her regular clothing. What would you do? Is there any reason why Ms. Henderson should not be permitted to go to the dining room? At this point you should discuss the situation with the charge nurse. The charge nurse will help you determine if Ms. Henderson presents a risk to anyone in the dining room. Because her wound drainage is completely contained in the dressing and there is no portal of exit for organisms, the charge nurse decides that by eating in the dining room she can visit with other residents and will feel much better. You would help her get dressed and encourage her to eat a good dinner to help her wound continue to heal.

Only in very few situations do long term care facility residents require room confinement and limited visitation. One of those situations is for pulmonary tuberculosis, as described earlier. Confinement can be very disorienting for an elderly person, particularly if he or she is cognitively impaired. Explain to this resident and the family why he or she must stay in the room, how long this will be required, and that this is not punishment. Provide as much mental stimulation as possible during this time through activities a resident enjoys.

MANAGEMENT OF COMMON CHRONIC ILLNESSES, DISEASES, AND PROBLEMS

Have you ever known someone who had many health problems? Maybe you know someone with serious heart problems. Did you ever find yourself calling him "the man with the heart condition," instead of "my neighbor, Mr. Stein"? Doing this labels Mr. Stein: you make illness his most important feature. You tend to think of him as a condition instead of a person just like you.

As a health care professional, take care to avoid labeling residents that way. By referring to a resident as "the woman in 3B with Alzheimer's" or "the blind man," you imply these residents are diseases, not people. If you focus only on what is wrong, you may never see what is right or healthy about them.

Residents with common illnesses, diseases, and problems need the same general care as other residents. Their care just has a different emphasis. In other words, just having a disease does not mean that the person does not receive the same respect and dignity as other, healthier, residents.

This chapter discusses common chronic illnesses, diseases, and problems occurring in different body systems. For each, you will learn its signs and symptoms, your role in the care of residents with the problem, and special care for these residents.

ACUTE AND CHRONIC ILLNESSES, DISEASES, OR PROBLEMS

To understand common health problems, you need to understand the difference between an acute problem and a chronic problem. Acute problems develop rapidly or suddenly. The length of time someone has an acute problem is usually limited and predictable, and then the person usually recovers. A common cold, for example, is an acute problem. It occurs rapidly and lasts 7-10 days, and you recover completely. Infections are also usually acute problems. Identifying an acute problem as soon as possible is important so that it can be treated effectively. Watch for and identify clues to such problems. Clues are signs of infection you observe in your daily care of residents. Some clues, like a skin rash and slight fever, can be specific signs or symptoms of infection, even if residents can't tell you where they hurt or how they feel. The earlier a problem is identified, the quicker the resident's recovery.

Chronic problems are those that last a long time or recur often. Residents with chronic problems usually have days when their signs and symptoms are noticeable and others when they are not (Fig. 24-1). Remember that some residents live with constant pain from chronic illness or disease. Chronic back pain and arthritis are two problems that cause constant, nagging pain. Recognize a resident's efforts to focus on life, however, regardless of the chronic problems he or she may be experiencing.

At times a chronic condition can worsen and need medical intervention. For example, a resident with arthritis on most days wakes up stiff and needs time to get loosened up. But during a flare-up, a resident can have terrible pain. Some joints are swollen, red, and hot to the touch. This is an example of a chronic problem in an acute phase. You must monitor, identify, and report any changes in a resident.

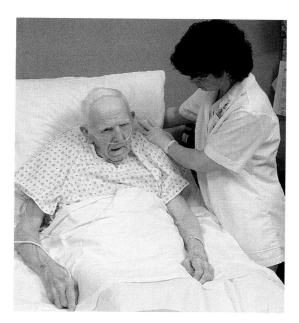

Fig. 24-1. Chronic illness lasts a long time or recurs often.

If you give the charge nurse accurate information about a resident, interventions can be started before the problem gets too serious.

Many common chronic illnesses, diseases, and problems have both acute and chronic phases. A chronic problem can also affect an acute problem. For example, residents with a chronic lung disease have a greater risk of catching the flu than other residents. It also takes longer to recover from the flu because of this chronic illness.

Understanding your residents and their health problems helps you monitor, identify, and report any changes in their condition. Detecting changes in residents is important, such as to assist in identifying early warning signs of cancer.

Cancer

Cancer is a malignant growth of abnormal cells, called a tumor. It grows locally, sometimes rapidly, invading one organ or body system, but also sometimes spreading throughout the body. Health care professionals often talk about the primary site, the first system or organ affected by cancer. For example, a resident's prostate gland (in the reproductive system) may be the primary site of cancer that then spreads to bone (the musculoskeletal system) and the lungs (the respiratory system).

Because of cancer's ability to spread, early detection is important. Report to the charge nurse any cancer warning signs you discover in any resident. The box below lists cancer warning signs.

Cancer Warning Signs

1. Change in bowel or bladder habits
2. A sore that does not heal
3. Unusual bleeding or discharge from a body opening
4. A lump or thickening in the breast or elsewhere on the body
5. Difficulty swallowing or indigestion
6. An obvious change in a wart or mole
7. Nagging cough or hoarseness

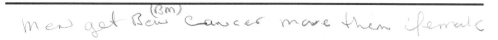
Men get Ben (Bm) Cancer more then female

You do not have to determine what signs and symptoms are a problem and which ones are not. Just communicate the change to the charge nurse.

The treatment of a resident with cancer may include surgery, radiation, chemotherapy, or a combination. Surgery removes the cancer. Often the original organ is removed along with surrounding tissue. Radiation uses X-rays to destroy the cancer cells. Chemotherapy uses drugs that target tumor cells.

Unfortunately, radiation and chemotherapy kill not only abnormal cells but some normal cells also. Residents receiving treatment often experience nausea and vomiting, hair loss, and an increased risk for bleeding and infection. Residents may tell you that they felt better before, with the cancer, than with the treatment. Listen to a resident's concerns and help him or her through the very trying treatment program.

The following sections describe the most common chronic illnesses, diseases, and problems in the nine body systems.

INTEGUMENTARY SYSTEM

The integumentary system is the skin, hair, and nails. It is important to health because it protects the body in two ways:

1. Prevents germs in the environment from entering. The skin is the body's defense against infection.
2. Helps control body temperature.

Common Chronic Illnesses, Diseases, and Problems
Dry Skin

With aging and weather changes, dryness of the skin is a common problem. Dryness may also result from other factors such as irritating wool clothes or rough sheets or linens. Regardless of the cause, dry skin is annoying, but it can easily be handled.

Signs and Symptoms of Dry Skin
- Flaky areas on skin
- Reddened areas
- Complaints of itchiness

Nurse Assistant's Role in Intervention and Management
- Pay attention to a resident's skin when providing care. You may find reddened areas on the skin, or a resident may tell you that his or her skin feels itchy. Dry, itchy skin seems intensified at night.
- Inspect the skin for flaking, redness, or scratch marks. These are signs of a problem.
- Always report any complaints to the charge nurse.

Goals of Care
- Eliminate the dryness and itchiness
- Help the person feel more comfortable
- Prevent problems, like tears in the skin from scratching

Special Intervention or Skills for Care
1. Limit the amount of soap used on the skin.
2. Use moisturizing creams on the affected area. *Note:* Massage moisturizing creams gently into the skin to avoid greasiness. Give residents the option of what cream they would like used on their skin. If resident does not have a preference, any moisturizing skin cream will work.
3. Add bathing oils to bath if resident prefers.
4. Use a therapeutic bath solution as ordered by the physician (see Chapter 13).
5. Increase the amount of fluid resident drinks, especially water if able.

Pressure Sores (Decubitus Ulcers)

Pressure sores are a breakdown of the skin caused by prolonged pressure or friction over any area of the body. The prolonged pressure decreases the flow of the blood carrying nourishment and oxygen to the skin. Skin cells die and an open wound forms. Pressure sores are usually categorized in stages:

▷ *Stage I:* Reddish or blue-grey area over a pressure point that does not go away with gentle massage (Fig. 24-2A).

▷ *Stage II:* Blistering or breakdown of the top layer of the skin (Fig. 24-2B).

▷ *Stage III:* Breakdown of the subcutaneous layers of the skin (Fig. 24-2C).

▷ *Stage IV:* Involvement of muscle and bone (Fig. 24-2D).

Pressure sores occur most commonly over areas where the skin is thin and you can easily feel the bone, such as the elbow, shoulder blades, hips, the base of the back (coccyx), and heels. Other common areas are the ears, under the breasts, between the buttocks, and areas where tubing may be rubbing.

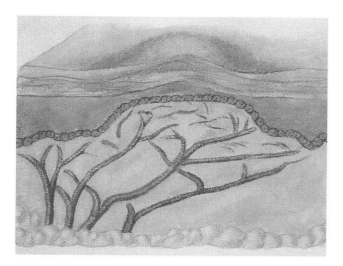

Fig. 24-2. **A,** Pressure sores, stage I.

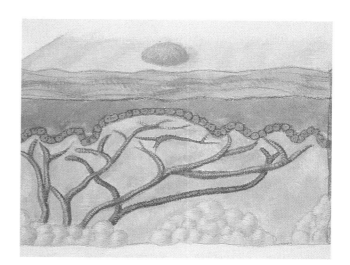

Fig. 24-2. **B,** Pressure sores, stage II.

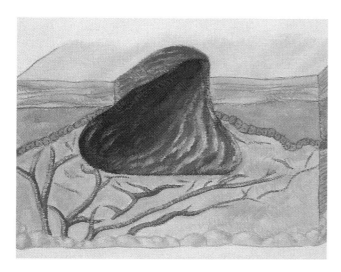

Fig. 24-2. **C,** Pressure sores, stage III.

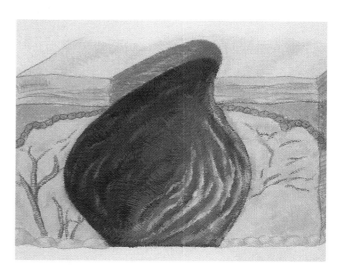

Fig. 24-2. **D,** Pressure sores, stage IV.

Signs and Symptoms of Pressure Sores

▸ Any reddened area of the body that does not return to its original color after repositioning
▸ Any localized skin tear, especially in areas of thin skin
▸ Increased sensitivity and/or pain in early stages

Nurse Assistant's Role in Intervention and Management

1. Promote proper nutrition.
2. Promote exercise: passive or active.
3. Identify any changes in the person's skin.
4. Report any changes to the charge nurse immediately. Identify residents who have had a change in their mobility, appetite, or fluid intake.

Goals of Care

▸ Prevention (It is easier to prevent pressure sores than it is to treat them. Residents who are immobile, seriously ill, poor eaters, poorly hydrated, frail, obese, or incontinent are more likely to get pressure sores.)

Special Intervention or Skills for Care

Constantly monitor the condition of all residents' skin. For high-risk residents, do the following:

▸ Turn residents at least every 2 hours.
▸ Inspect the skin at least every 2 hours.
▸ Perform passive range-of-motion (ROM) exercises at least three times per day.
▸ Use special mattresses and chair and mattress pads such as air mattresses, water mattresses, sheepskins, or flotation pads. These help to distribute weight evenly (Fig. 24-3).
▸ Keep the skin clean and dry.
▸ Avoid friction on a resident's skin. For example, lift him or her in bed instead of pulling him or her up.
▸ Keep beds clean, wrinkle free, and free of objects like crumbs, combs, and glasses.
▸ Minimize skin-to-skin contact by using positioning devices like pillows between knees or under elbows and forearms.

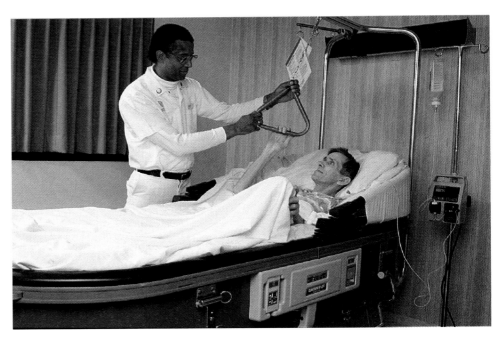

Fig. 24-3. Special mattresses or chair pads help distribute the resident's weight evenly, minimizing the occurrence of pressure sores.

▷ Keep skinfold areas clean and dry. Constant moist contact leads to skin breakdown.

▷ Monitor resident's fluid and food intake closely. Encourage good nutrition.

These steps help prevent pressure sores from developing. If one develops, specific treatments are used along with preventive measures. The facility has treatments for each stage. In addition to these specific actions, keep using the measures used for the previous stages.

Stage I: Pre-sore

▷ Notify the charge nurse immediately. Ask her or him to inspect the area.

▷ Concentrate on preventing pressure on the area. Use all prevention methods.

▷ Gently massage around the reddened area.

Stage II: Blistering of top layer of skin

▷ Cover the blistering area with a dry sterile dressing or a clear plastic bandage.

Note: The charge nurse directs care at this and all later stages. You are responsible for all the preventive measures.

Stage III: Breakdown

▷ Specific treatments with ointments, irrigations, and dressings are used.

▷ Residents are closely watched for infections. Report any signs of infection, such as foul smells, discharge, and increased redness around the area.

▷ Stage IV: Involvement of muscle and bone

▷ Surgical intervention may be needed

▷ Wound care

Contact Dermatitis

Contact dermatitis is a skin reaction resulting from residents contacting things they are allergic to.

Signs and Symptoms of Contact Dermatitis

▷ Rash

▷ Raised, reddened bumps

▷ Complaints of itchiness

Nurse Assistant's Role in Intervention and Management

Identify what changes for resident occurred before the rash developed. For example:

▷ New clothing

▷ New detergents used in laundry

▷ New foods

▷ New medications

▷ New jewelry

Report any rash to the nurse, since it may indicate an infection or an allergic reaction.

Goals of Care

▷ Identify the source of the allergic reaction

▷ Relieve the itchiness

▷ Prevent problems such as skin tears caused by scratching

Special Intervention or Skills for Care

▷ Use over-the-counter topical ointments as recommended by the physician. Such ointments usually have hydrocortisone to relieve the itching.

▷ Cover the area with a dry dressing if the physician orders (Fig. 24-4).

▷ Administer therapeutic bath solutions ordered by the physician (see Chapter 13 on bathing.)

MUSCULOSKELETAL SYSTEM

The musculoskeletal system enables the body to move. Moving and being active are important for overall health.

Common Chronic Illnesses, Diseases, and Problems
Arthritis

Arthritis is a common joint problem that causes pain and limits movement in affected joints. Osteoarthritis is more common, caused by age and a lifetime of "wear and tear" of the joint. The other type, rheumatoid arthritis, can be severely disfiguring and causes much pain.

Signs and Symptoms of Arthritis
▶ Stiffness
▶ Painful joints (Fig. 24-5)
▶ Rheumatoid arthritis joints are painful, red, swollen, and hot

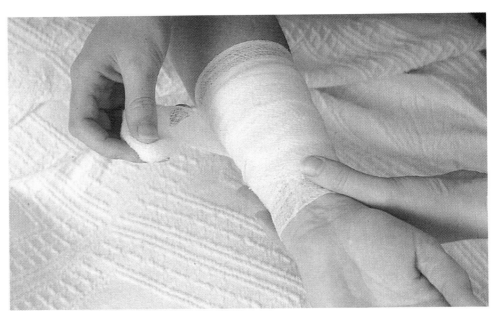

Fig. 24-4. Apply a nonsterile, dry dressing.

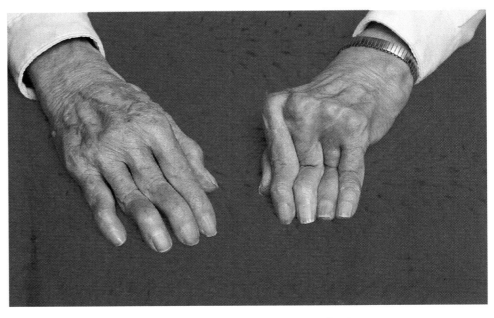

Fig. 24-5. Painful joints are a sign of arthritis.

Nurse Assistant's Role in Intervention and Management

- Identify a resident's capabilities and encourage him or her to do whatever he or she can.
- Plan care around scheduled pain management.
- Support this resident in his or her efforts.

Goals of Care

- Pain management
- Prevention of injury
- Mobility
- ROM exercise to keep joints movable

Special Intervention or Skills for Care

When caring for someone with joint pain, you should:

- Let the residents know you understand and want to help, since residents in constant pain can feel hopeless and depressed
- Plan your schedule for A.M. care and other activities such as ROM exercises to let residents receive pain medication before care. Talk to the charge nurse about this.
- Help this resident with ROM exercises to prevent deformities. However, never move a joint that is very painful, red, or swollen.
- Properly position a resident in bed or a wheelchair. Encourage good posture.
- Assist a resident with putting on splints or braces.
- Plan your schedule to help the person back to bed for rest periods as needed. Don't push a resident to be active when he or she is tired, because this can damage joints.
- Report to the charge nurse any joint problems.
- Encourage a resident to do as much as possible to help maintain independence.

 Osteoporosis wear & tear on bones Shirken

Osteoporosis is caused by a gradual loss of minerals, especially calcium, from the bone. Bones become weak and brittle. Osteoporosis is most common in women after menopause. Often it is not diagnosed until a resident is injured. Other normal aging changes in the musculoskeletal system are exaggerated in a resident with osteoporosis.

Signs and Symptoms of Osteoporosis

- Loss of height
- Falling
- Fractures

Nurse Assistant's Role in Intervention and Management

- Monitor residents who are frail or have a history of falling and previous fractures.
- Anticipate and prevent problems when residents are moving.

Goals of Care

- Promote safety
- Encourage proper nutrition and exercise as tolerated

Special Intervention or Skills for Care

- Always use assistive devices, like guard belts, when moving a resident from bed to chair or chair to bed and when assisting with walking.
- Encourage residents to use canes for support or weight bearing walkers, especially when first starting to move.
- Be sure a resident has a clear path for leaving bed and walking, to prevent injury from bumping into things.
- If a resident starts to fall when you are with him or her, be sure to act as you learned in Chapter 14.

- If you find a resident on the floor, call the charge nurse immediately and follow her or his instructions.
- Encourage residents to eat healthy, balanced meals, especially those rich in calcium.

Fracture

A fracture is a break in a bone, caused most commonly by falls. The one you see most is a fractured hip.

Signs and Symptoms of Fractures

- Swollen, black and blue area at the break site
- Complaints of pain and/or altered sensation
- Inability to put weight on leg or use arm
- Abnormal shape of arm or leg
- History of falls

Nurse Assistant's Role in Intervention and Management

- Report any abnormality you see in a resident's arms or legs.
- Provide a safe environment.
- Promote activities that enhance healing and mobility.

Goals of Care

- Prevent complication of the fracture, such as muscle weakness and contractures
- Help this resident reach the pre-fracture level of mobility

Special Intervention or Skill for Care

- Get the person out of bed as soon as approved by the physician and help with weight bearing
- Do ROM exercises to keep other joints and muscles working.
- Use proper transfer techniques to avoid harmful movement at the fracture site.
- Encourage every resident to do as much as he or she can.
- Support a resident in going to physical therapy for rehabilitation. Prepare him or her well in advance and let him or her know you think it is important.
- Use in the nursing unit what a resident learns to do in physical therapy, such as walking with a walker.
- Recognize that a resident may fear falling and fracturing the bone again and thus avoid activities. Be supportive and offer assistance until the person feels secure.
- Be sure to follow the instructions of the charge nurse and physical therapy staff about positioning a resident properly in bed and in the chair. Improper positioning can lead to improper healing of a fracture.
- Check the wound site if resident has undergone surgery.

RESPIRATORY SYSTEM

The respiratory system takes in oxygen as we breathe and moves it through the lungs to the blood to nourish the body. We breathe out carbon dioxide wastes from the body.

Common Chronic Illnesses, Diseases, and Problems
Cold

The common cold is an upper respiratory infection caused by a virus. Colds sometime accompany the flu, which causes additional symptoms beyond just the upper respiratory complaints.

Signs and Symptoms of a Cold

- Runny nose
- Cough
- Watery eyes
- Stuffiness or a sense of fullness in the face

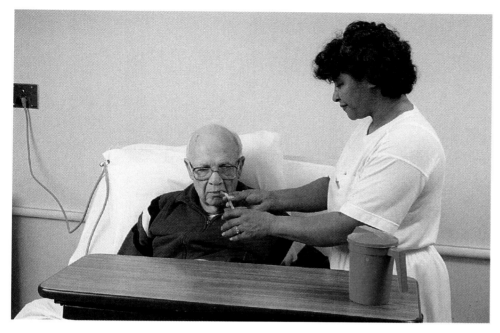

Fig. 24-6. Offer comfort measures to relieve symptoms of a respiratory infection.

Nurse Assistant's Role in Intervention and Management
▷ Identify the symptoms early on to prevent further illness.
▷ Provide care to relieve symptoms (Fig. 24-6).
▷ Practice infection control procedures to prevent spread to other residents and yourself.

Goals of Care
▷ Keep resident comfortable
▷ Monitor symptoms
▷ Prevent spread of infection to self and others

Special Intervention or Skills for Care
▷ Encourage a resident to drink plenty of fluids (unless there are fluid restrictions).
▷ Have him or her rest.
▷ Encourage the person to get out of bed for short periods. If he or she cannot get out of bed, be sure he or she changes position often. Keep the head of the bed elevated to limit respiratory distress.
▷ Remind the person to breathe deeply and cough often to prevent mucus secretions from accumulating in the lungs.
▷ Keep tissues handy.
▷ Provide comfort by fluffing pillows, giving back rubs, etc.
▷ Monitor the resident's vital signs and report any changes.
▷ Monitor his or her symptoms and report even the slightest change to the charge nurse.
▷ Wash your hands before and after contact with a resident.
▷ Dispose of tissue in a proper container, using gloves.

Pneumonia

Pneumonia is a lung infection usually caused by a virus or bacteria. It may follow a cold or bronchitis (an infection in the bronchial tubes).

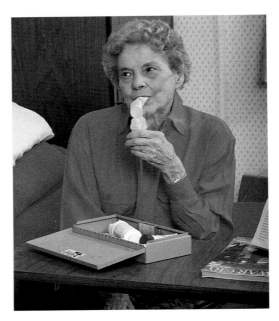

Fig. 24-7. A resident with respiratory impairment, such as pneumonia, usually needs a breathing treatment as part of his or her nursing care to help ease difficult breathing.

Signs and Symptoms of Pneumonia
▶ Difficulty breathing (Fig. 24-7)
▶ Cough, sometimes with increased sputum
▶ Shortness of breath
▶ Complaint of painful breathing

Nurse Assistant's Role in Intervention and Management
▶ Monitor symptoms.
▶ Provide nursing care to relieve symptoms.

Goals of Care
▶ Keep residents comfortable
▶ Relieve symptoms

Special Intervention or Skills for Care
▶ Encourage the resident to drink plenty of fluids (if there are no fluid restrictions).
▶ Have the resident rest.
▶ Encourage the person to get out of bed for short periods. If he or she cannot get out of bed, be sure he or she changes position often. Keep the head of the bed elevated to limit respiratory distress.
▶ Remind the person to breathe deeply and cough often to prevent mucus secretions from accumulating in the lungs.
▶ Keep tissues handy.
▶ Provide comfort by fluffing pillows, giving back rubs, etc.
▶ Monitor the resident's vital signs and report any changes.
▶ Monitor his or her symptoms and report even the slightest change to the charge nurse.
▶ Wash your hands before and after contact with the resident.
▶ Dispose of tissues in the proper container, using gloves.

Chronic Obstructive Pulmonary Disease (COPD)

Chronic obstructive pulmonary disease (COPD) results from many years of problems with the bronchial passageways and lungs. The two most common diseases that cause COPD are bronchitis and emphysema. Chronic inflammation causes narrowing in the bronchioles and alveoli and loss of lung elasticity.

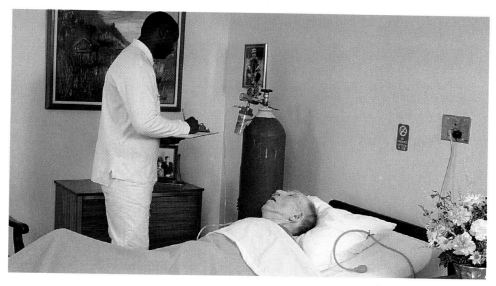

Fig. 24-8. Oxygen can be very drying. Always observe and report nasal passage redness, bleeding, or discomfort.

Signs and Symptoms of Chronic Obstructive Pulmonary Disease (COPD)

▶ Difficulty breathing
▶ Wheezing
▶ Coughing
▶ Cyanosis
▶ Shortness of breath

Bed   HOB ↑

Nurse Assistant's Role in Intervention and Management

▶ Maintain adequate ventilation.
▶ Monitor the resident for secondary conditions such as infection.
▶ Reduce the resident's anxiety.

Goals of Care

▶ Keep the resident breathing comfortably.

Special Intervention or Skills for Care

▶ Encourage a resident if able to take 4-5 deep breaths in and out several times during the day. Deep breathing helps fill the lungs with air to help the chest wall stay flexible.

▶ Encourage the resident to rest between activities such as eating, bathing, exercise, and social activities.

▶ Encourage the resident to breathe slowly and deeply while walking and to rest for a minute frequently during longer walks.

▶ Have the resident when seated lean forward and cross his or her arms in front to make breathing easier.

▶ When assisting with bathing, be careful not to pour water over the head of a resident who is short of breath. This can cause a feeling of suffocating.

▶ Watch for any change in a resident's ability to perform activities of daily living. Report even the slightest change to the charge nurse.

▶ Monitor the resident's vital signs. Even the smallest changes in temperature, pulse, respiration, and blood pressure may indicate an infection in a resident with COPD.

Some residents may need oxygen occasionally or continuously. To care for residents on oxygen, you should:

▶ Check the resident's nasal passages. Oxygen therapy can be very irritating to tissues in the nose. Report redness, bleeding, or discomfort to the charge nurse (Fig. 24-8).

▶ *Do not* change the oxygen flow rate setting. Only the nurse can do this. Too much oxygen can depress the respiratory centers of the brain and cause a life-threatening situation.

▶ Make sure the head of the bed of this resident is elevated to help him or her breathe more easily.

▶ *Never* allow smoking or flames near oxygen.

▶ Check the tubing and connection to prevent twists.

CIRCULATORY SYSTEM

The circulatory system carries oxygen and vital nourishment to all the cells of the body. It also carries waste products to certain organs, where the body disposes of them.

Common Chronic Illness, Diseases, and Problems
Congestive Heart Failure (CHF)

Congestive heart failure (CHF) occurs when the heart muscle weakens. The heart becomes ineffective in moving blood through the body. CHF is common in people who have had high blood pressure and coronary artery disease for many years.

Signs and Symptoms of Congestive Heart Failure

▶ Shortness of breath

▶ Edema (swelling) of the legs and ankles, fluid weight gain (Fig. 24-9)

▶ Cyanosis Blue

▶ Noisy respirations

▶ Complaints of tiring easily

Nurse Assistant's Role in Intervention and Management

▶ Identify any changes in a resident that suggest a worsening of the condition, such as an inability to perform the activities of daily living.

▶ Monitor vital signs as directed by the charge nurse.

▶ Monitor the resident's weight.

▶ Monitor the resident's dietary restrictions if ordered.

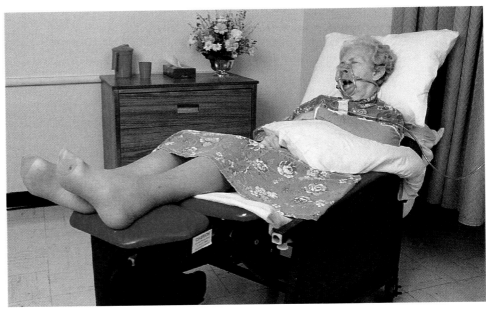

Fig. 24-9. Swelling of the ankles and legs is a symptom of congestive heart failure (CHF).

Goals of Care

▷ Maintain the resident's level of independence.

▷ Maintain the resident's level of respiratory function.

▷ Maintain resident's weight (Fig. 24-10).

Special Intervention or Skills for Care

▷ Provide the resident opportunities to do his or her own personal care.

▷ Have the resident rest frequently.

▷ Encourage the resident to take deep breaths.

▷ Weigh the resident as ordered, and note and report any increase or decrease in weight.

▷ Maintain accurate intake and output records.

To assist a resident with edema in the lower legs:

▷ Have the resident sit with legs elevated on a footstool or lie in bed with legs stretched out for 1-2 hours, three times a day. When legs are elevated, suggest alternating the legs to prevent backache. Legs should be elevated higher than the buttocks.

▷ Encourage the resident to exercise and walk regularly.

▷ Make sure the resident's shoes are not too tight.

▷ If the doctor has ordered support stockings, assist the resident in putting on the stockings before getting up in the morning (before the legs begin to swell) and taking them off at night and more often if ordered. Before assisting him or her with support stockings:

▷ Inspect the skin thoroughly.

▷ Bathe and dry the legs, feet, and between the toes thoroughly.

▷ Make sure the stockings are clean and dry.

▷ You can put the support stockings on most residents while they are lying in bed. The best time is before he or she gets out of bed in the A.M. Assist him or her with putting on support stockings (see Chapter 18).

Stockings should be hand washed in the evening and hung to dry.

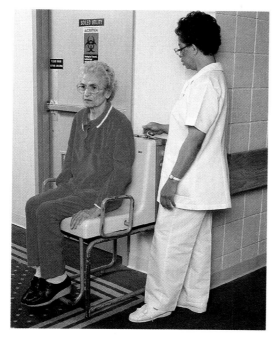

Fig. 24-10.   Maintaining the resident's weight is one goal of care.

Peripheral Vascular Disease

Peripheral vascular disease causes a diminished flow to arms and legs. Tissues in the extremities then receive too little nourishment. This condition is more common in the feet.

Signs and Symptoms of Peripheral Vascular Disease

▷ Change in color of the feet (and sometimes hands)
▷ Complaints of feet (and sometimes hands) being cold
▷ Tingling sensation—"pins and needles"
▷ Loss of sensitivity

Nurse Assistant's Role in Intervention and Management

▷ Identify changes in a resident's skin.
▷ Monitor the environment to prevent injury.

Goals of Care

▷ Promote circulation
▷ Prevent injury

Special Intervention or Skills for Care

▷ Assess the resident's feet.
▷ Feel the temperature of the skin. If circulation is decreased, the skin feels cool.
▷ Observe the color of the skin. Skin looks bluish or pale in a light-skinned person or dusky gray in a dark-skinned person when circulation is decreased.
▷ Observe the color of the nail beds. Poor circulation can cause a bluish tinge to the nail beds.
▷ Feel for pulses in the lower extremities: popliteal behind the knee, posterior tibial at the ankle, and pedal pulse on the upper part of the foot (Fig. 24-11). Report to the charge nurse whether you can feel them or not.
▷ Watch for and report reddened areas, cracked skin between the toes, or skin breakdown.
▷ Encourage the resident to change position every 1-2 hours while awake. If a resident reads or watches television sitting or lying down, encourage him or her to get up and walk around for a few minutes every hour or two.
▷ Encourage the resident to take daily walks and participate in exercise programs at the facility.
▷ Check wounds that do not heal.
▷ Explain to the resident why to avoid the following, which interfere with normal circulation:
  ▷ Crossing legs at the knees
  ▷ Keep legs elevated. Avoid prolonged dangling of feet.
  ▷ Wearing restricting clothing such as tight garter straps or panty girdles
  ▷ Smoking cigarettes or cigars
  ▷ Cold environments, which narrow blood vessels
▷ Encourage the resident to "wiggle" his or her toes and make circles with the feet to promote circulation.
▷ Keep the resident's skin clean, dry, and lotioned.
▷ Provide a safe environment to prevent injury.
▷ Keep a clear path for resident when walking.
▷ Keep the resident's room uncluttered.
▷ Replace any bed attachments that may stick out.
▷ Check bath water temperature for the resident.
▷ Avoid positioning a resident near heaters.

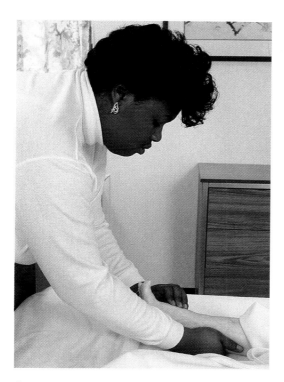

Fig. 24-11. One way of helping to manage peripheral vascular disease is to feel the resident's pedal pulses.

Coronary Artery Disease (CAD)

Coronary artery disease results from decreased blood flow through the coronary arteries, which nourish the heart. The exact cause of coronary artery disease is not known, but several factors can contribute to its development:

- High blood pressure
- Diabetes
- Obesity
- Family history
- Smoking
- Diets high in fat
- Lack of exercise
- Stress

Signs and Symptoms of Coronary Artery Disease

- Complaints of chest pain (angina pectoris pain on effort)
- Change in pulse rate or rhythm
- Change in blood pressure

Nurse Assistant's Role in Intervention and Management

- Educate the resident about risk factors.
- Monitor and watch for changes in the resident's vital signs.
- Follow all treatment programs prescribed.

Goals of Care

- Maintain the person's independence

Special Intervention or Skills for Care

- Encourage the resident to exercise (Fig. 24-12).
- Encourage a diet low in fat.

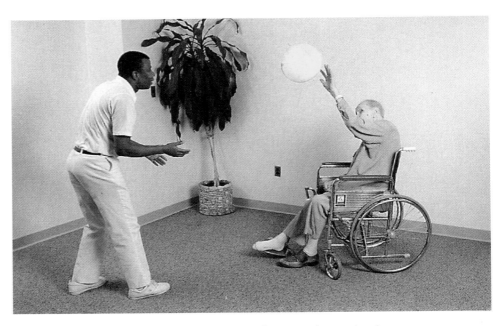

Fig. 24-12. Encourage exercise with a resident who has coronary artery disease (CAD).

▶ Limit stress: talk to the resident about anything upsetting, and work with other staff to help alleviate stress.
▶ If pain occurs:
  ▶ Immediately stop all activity.
  ▶ Have resident sit or lie down. When resident is lying down, elevate the head of bed.
  ▶ Call the charge nurse.
  ▶ Follow the charge nurse's instructions.
  ▶ Monitor the resident's vital signs.
  ▶ Assist with the delivery of oxygen.
  ▶ Reassure resident.
  ▶ Communicate to other staff what factors seem to cause pain (precipitating factors).

Cerebral Vascular Accident (CVA)—Stroke

Stroke occurs when the blood flow to the brain is interrupted. This can be caused by many things, including narrowing of the blood vessel from plaque build-up, blood vessel rupture, or a traveling blood clot that blocks the blood flow.

Signs and Symptoms of Cerebral Vascular Accident (CVA)

Signs and symptoms depend on the extent of the interruption and the resulting tissue damage. The most common results are:
▶ Weakness or paralysis on one side of body
▶ Difficulty swallowing
▶ Difficulty communicating
▶ Change in mental status

Nurse Assistant's Role in Intervention and Management

▶ Support the resident's rehabilitation.

Goals of Care

▶ Prevent complications of paralysis, like muscle wasting and contractures.
▶ Improve the resident's level of functioning and promote independence (Fig. 24-13).

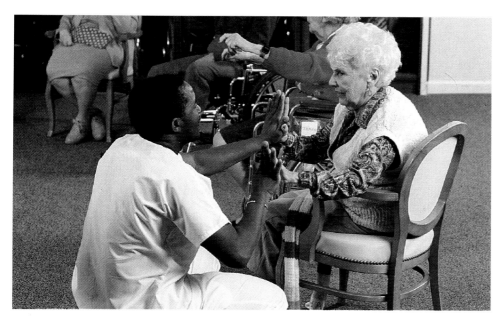

Fig. 24-13. Always promote independence.

Special Intervention or Skills for Care
- To assist a resident with paralysis:
  - Recognize that paralysis changes a person's personality and life drastically, often suddenly. Residents with paralysis may feel very angry and cheated.
  - Assist with ROM exercises 3-4 times a day to prevent contractures and maintain muscle strength. The physical therapist sets the therapeutic plan. Check the care plan or ask the charge nurse for specific guidelines for the ROM exercises.
  - Position and turn the resident at least every 2 hours. Support affected limbs with pillows.
  - Make sure a foot board is in place at the end of the bed and that the resident's affected foot or feet are against it to prevent foot drop.
  - Keep things where the person can see and reach them.
  - Check with the charge nurse about how to reinforce the work of the physical therapist and occupational therapist to retrain the resident in skills such as eating, moving, and dressing.
- For difficulty swallowing:
  - Always put the resident in a high sitting position. *90 degree*
  - Encourage or give small bites of food.
  - Encourage or give small sips of fluid to moisten food.
- Be prepared to perform the Heimlich maneuver if a resident chokes.
  - Offer small sips of fluid often throughout the day to ensure adequate fluid intake.
  - Notify the nurse of:
    - The resident's intake for each meal and snack
    - Worsening of a resident's ability to swallow
    - Signs and symptoms of illness, such as fever or rapid pulse rate
- For difficulty communicating (speaking or understanding) and for residents who do not understand:
  - Check the care plan.

▷ Approach the resident with a calm reassuring manner.

▷ Understand that a resident may understand written messages but not spoken ones.

▷ Point to objects and use gestures as much as possible to show what you want to say.

▷ Remember that even though a resident may not understand the spoken word, thought processes may be normal.

▷ Be patient and gently touch the resident often.

▷ Speak slowly, using simple sentences.

▷ To assist residents who understand speech but cannot put their thoughts in words, you should:

▷ Talk to the person in a normal way. Explain everything you do with the resident.

▷ Remember that the resident can understand you and is not confused.

▷ Allow a resident time to try to speak to you. He may be able to speak some words.

▷ See if the person can write messages. Sometimes residents can still write when they cannot speak.

DIGESTIVE SYSTEM

The function of the digestive system is to provide the body with a continuous supply of nutrients and fluids.

Common Chronic Illnesses, Diseases, and Problems
Constipation

Constipation is a slowing of the bowel that results in difficulty eliminating feces. It is common among residents.

Signs and Symptoms of Constipation

▷ Decrease in the number of bowel movements from a resident's usual pattern

▷ Abdominal distention

▷ Complaints of feeling bloated

▷ Complaints of gas

▷ Loss of appetite

Nurse Assistant's Role in Intervention and Management

▷ Identify change in pattern.

▷ Assist residents in maintaining their regular schedule of bowel movements.

▷ Recognize further complications such as fecal impaction.

Goals of Care

▷ Return to normal pattern of bowel movements

▷ Prevent future problems

Special Intervention or Skills for Care

▷ Encourage resident to drink plenty of fluids.

▷ Encourage resident to eat fruits, vegetables, breads, and cereals, especially those high in fiber like bran.

▷ Encourage exercise, especially walking.

▷ Follow any prescribed orders for enemas or suppositories.

An enema is a procedure for introducing fluid into the rectum to stimulate a bowel movement (Fig. 24-14). Enemas may be commercially prepared (already mixed and ready to administer) or may have to be mixed. There are a number of different mixtures:

▷ Tap water enema

▷ Oil retention enema

▷ Cleansing enema

▷ Medicated enema (the nurse adds the medication and supervises the enema)

▷ Retention enema

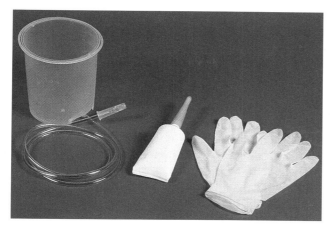

Fig. 24-14. Equipment used during a tap water or fleet enema.

With all types, the procedure and goal are the same. Before beginning, ask the charge nurse what equipment to use, how much water and at what temperature, and how to mix the solution.

Giving an Enema

1. Put on gloves.
2. Place protective pad under resident's buttocks.
3. Position the resident on the left side, helping him or her turn if necessary. Make sure the hips are near the edge of the bed on the side where you're working.
   Note: If the resident cannot hold the enema solution in the rectum, put him or her on the bedpan before giving it. Wear a rubber glove on the hand that inserts the rectal tube.)
4. Hold the rectal tube over the bedpan. Open the clamp on the tubing and let the solution run through into the bedpan until it flows smoothly so that no air is left in the tubing to cause discomfort for the resident. Close the clamp.
5. Turn back the bath blanket so that the resident's hips are exposed and the rest of the body covered.
6. Hold the lubricated rectal tube about 5 inches from the tip. Gently push it into the rectum to the red line on the tube.
7. Raise the container about 15 inches above the resident's hips. Never hold the container any higher.
8. Open the clamp and let the solution run in slowly. If the resident complains of cramps, tell him or her to breathe deeply through the mouth, as you clamp the tubing for a minute or so. You may also lower the irrigating bag.
9. When all the solution has run in, close the clamp.
10. Remove the rectal tube. Wrap the tip with toilet paper. Place the tubing in plastic trash bag.
11. Turn the resident on his or her back and slip the bedpan under him. Ask him or her to try to hold the solution for as long as possible. Raise the head of the bed. See that the call button and toilet paper are within reach.

Left sides [handwritten annotation]

Fecal impaction may occur if a resident's constipation is not treated and continues. It is then necessary to manually remove the feces. This is unpleasant for residents. A resident may have small amounts of loose watery stool that pass by the blockage. You must monitor, record, and report any problems with resident's bowel movements to the charge nurse.

Diarrhea

Diarrhea occurs when the bowel moves the feces through the tract rapidly. Diarrhea is caused by a number of factors: a particular food that did not agree with the person, food allergies, or as a symptom of the flu. These forms of diarrhea are noninfectious. Infectious diarrhea can be a major problem in a facility. This form of diarrhea spreads rapidly to other residents and leads to further complications.

Signs and Symptoms of Diarrhea
- Frequent watery stool
- Complaints of cramping
- Increased gas

Nurse Assistant's Role in Intervention and Management
- Help the person in a regular schedule of bowel movements.
- Identify the change in pattern.

Goals of Care
- Prevent the complications of dehydration and skin breakdown
- Prevent the spread of infectious diarrhea

Special Intervention or Skills for Care
- Offer the person clear liquids to prevent dehydration.
- Ask the charge nurse about keeping a resident well hydrated.
- Keep the resident's skin clean and dry. Apply protective cream to reddened areas to protect the skin.
- Keep the charge nurse informed about the number, color, and consistency of the resident's stools.
- Practice all infection control procedures as instructed by the charge nurse.
- Collect specimens as directed.

Bowel Incontinence

The term "bowel incontinence" is used when a person cannot control or is unaware of bowel movements. Residents with dementia may not recognize the need to have a bowel movement. Some residents with a stroke or spinal cord injury may not be able to feel the urge to have a bowel movement.

Signs and Symptoms of Bowel Incontinence
- Inability to feel the urge to have a bowel movement
- No awareness of the passage of the stool

Nurse Assistant's Role in Intervention and Management
- Help the resident to achieve and maintain a regular pattern of bowel movements.

Goals of Care
- Identify the resident's pattern of bowel movements
- Return to a regular pattern of bowel movement

Special Intervention or Skills
To assist the resident with bowel training and recording the results:
- Record on the bowel training flow sheet (Fig. 24-15):

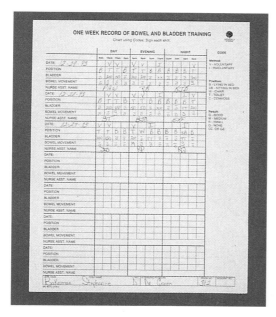

Fig. 24-15.   Example of a bowel training flow chart.

▷ When the resident usually has a bowel movement, such as morning or evening

▷ How often he or she has a bowel movement, such as once a day or every other day

▷ Position the resident on the toilet or bedpan at the time he or she usually has a bowel movement and give plenty of time to finish. Since many residents fall while going to the bathroom, make sure he or she is safe.

▷ Provide plenty of fluids: at least 8 glasses of liquid that hold 8 ounces.

▷ Encourage the person to eat high-fiber foods such as bran cereals and bread, fruit, and vegetables.

▷ Encourage regular exercise, if possible, such as walking, as part of a bowel training program.

▷ Use a laxative or enema as part of the training program as ordered by the physician and directed by the nurse.

▷ Discuss daily with the nurse the results of the bowel training program.

▷ Skin care is important for incontinent residents. Monitor resident's buttocks for reddened areas and apply a protective cream.

URINARY SYSTEM

The urinary system maintains the fluid balance in the body by eliminating waste materials from the blood and reabsorbing the proper amount of water and salt.

Common Chronic Illnesses, Diseases, and Problems
Urinary Tract Infections

An infection in the urinary system is called a urinary tract infection. The bladder is most commonly affected. Urinary tract infections occur more often in women, residents who are incontinent, and residents with poor fluid intake.

Signs and Symptoms of Urinary Tract Infections

▷ Frequent urinating in small amounts (called urinary frequency)

▷ Complaints of burning or stinging urination

▷ Dark yellow or cloudy appearance, or foul odor to the urine

▷ Blood in urine

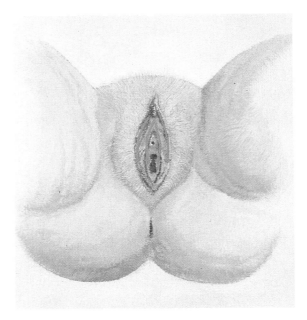

Fig. 24-16.   Encourage proper perineal hygiene.

Nurse Assistant's Role in Intervention and Management
- Identify residents at risk for urinary tract infection.
- Report any changes in a resident's urinary pattern to the charge nurse.

Goals of Care
- Prevent urinary tract infection

Special Intervention or Skills for Care
- Encourage residents to drink enough fluids every day, especially water and fruit juices.
- Encourage residents to urinate at least every 3-4 hours while awake.
- Encourage proper perineal hygiene (such as females wiping from front to back after urination), and daily washing of the perineal area (Fig. 24-16).

Urinary Incontinence

The term "urinary incontinence" is used when a person cannot control when and where he or she urinates. Urinary incontinence can be caused by a number of abnormalities, including:

- Bladder muscle irritability that causes the bladder to contract with little warning
- Damage to the bladder nerves that signal the brain when the bladder is full
- Brain damage preventing the person from feeling the urge to urinate
- Weakness of the sphincter muscles
- Weakness of the pelvic floor muscles (in women sometimes caused by childbirth) causing stress incontinence, which occurs when the person coughs, sneezes, or laughs hard
- Medications
- Urinary tract infection
- Lack of access to a bathroom

Signs and Symptoms of Urinary Incontinence
- Resident found wet from urine and unaware that it occurred.

Nurse Assistant's Role in Intervention and Management
- Identify residents at risk for incontinence.
- Monitor closely the resident's urinary pattern.
- Report any signs of urinary tract infection.

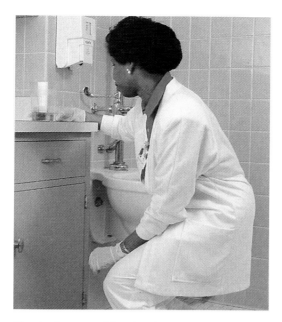

Fig. 24-17. Monitoring a resident's urinary pattern is an important step in managing continence.

Goals of Care
▷ Help residents regain as much control over urinary function as possible through a bladder training program (Fig. 24-17)

Special Intervention or Skills for Care
Begin by keeping a record of the resident's voiding pattern, including:
▷ Time
▷ Amount voided
▷ Fluid voided
▷ Fluid intake
▷ Awareness of need to void

You and the charge nurse set a schedule for expected voiding times based on a resident's voiding pattern. A resident should be toileted about 30 minutes before expected voiding times. Follow these guidelines for a bladder training program:

▷ It takes time, often several weeks, for an incontinent resident to regain control of the bladder. This resident needs continuous encouragement from staff. Staff must be attentive and consistent with the training schedule.

▷ Increasing fluid intake is essential for a bladder training program. A resident should have up to 3 liters (3000 cc) of fluid per day, with the approval of the physician. Often an incontinent resident limits fluid intake so he or she won't urinate so often. However, increasing fluids is essential. Fluids are sometimes increased during the day but limited in the evening to help avoid the need for frequent toileting that is annoying to residents during sleep.

▷ Routine personal care is needed any time a resident is incontinent to prevent skin rashes and breakdown.

Some incontinent residents will not be successful with bladder training. For these, perineal care, use of incontinence pads, and emotional support are important.

Urinary Retention

Urinary retention occurs when a blockage prevents urine from passing. This is more common in older men because the prostate gland often enlarges with aging and can partially block urine from passing down the urethra.

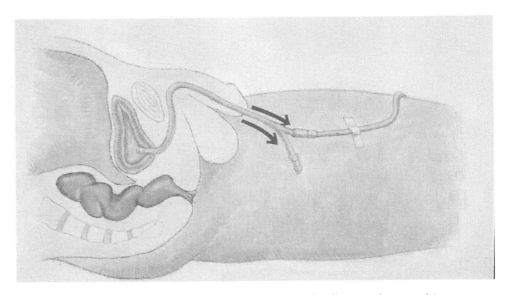

Fig. 24-18. As you clean the resident's indwelling catheter tubing, clean from the urethral opening down.

Signs and Symptoms of Urinary Retention
▶ Difficulty passing urine
▶ Feeling of fullness in the bladder
▶ Urinating in small amounts
▶ Decreased urine output

If a resident complains of difficulty urinating or if you notice a resident's decreased urinary output or swelling in the lower abdomen, report it to the nurse immediately so that the physician can evaluate the problem.

Nurse Assistant's Role in Intervention and Management
▶ Monitor urine output.

Goals of Care
▶ Provide relief from urinary retention

Note: Surgical intervention is most common in men with enlarged prostate gland. You would care for the resident preoperatively and postoperatively when he or she returns from the hospital. A urinary catheter may be used temporarily in both situations.

Special Intervention or Skills for Care

If the physician orders an indwelling urinary catheter, the nurse inserts it, using sterile technique to prevent infection. The catheter is passed through the urethra into the urinary bladder. A small balloon inflated with sterile water keeps the catheter in place. The opening at the tip of the catheter lets urine pass from the bladder through the catheter tube and out into a closed collection bag attached to the bed or chair.

Although the nurse does much of the urinary catheter care, you assist in two ways: perineal care and the positioning of the external catheter tubing and drainage bag. Follow these guidelines when assisting with perineal care:
▶ Put gloves on before beginning perineal care.
▶ Keep the external catheter tube as clean as possible always.
▶ Clean the tubing with antiseptic solution and cotton balls or gauze pads, cleaning the tube first at the urethral opening and then cleansing downward and away from the opening (Fig. 24-18).
▶ Use only one downward stroke at a time. Discard the cotton ball or gauze pad, and clean the next area. *Note:* Avoid pulling on the catheter tube while cleaning, to prevent discomfort for the resident.

▷ Do the rest of perineal care as usual, cleansing with soap and water from front to back.

When you help residents with a urinary catheter change position, follow these guidelines:

▷ The external part of the catheter tube is secured to a resident's inner thigh with tape to prevent pulling of the catheter when he or she moves.

▷ The urinary catheter tube, connecting tube, and drainage bag should not be separated except by a nurse using sterile technique when changing the tubing or collecting a specimen. The drainage system is maintained closed to help prevent infection. Check tubing for kinks and leaks.

▷ The urinary drainage bag is secured to the bed or chair below the resident's bladder, so that the urine flows from the bladder into the bag by gravity. *Note:* Never let the drainage bag touch the floor, which is considered an "unclean" area. Never lift the drainage bag above a resident, as urine could flow back into the bladder, increasing the risk of infection.

▷ The urine from the drainage bag should be emptied at least every 8 hours and the amount of urine recorded. The bag is emptied from the bottom opening only and then resealed.

NERVOUS SYSTEM

The nervous system is like a communication center and helps one make sense of what is happening inside and outside the body.

Common Chronic Illnesses, Diseases, and Problems
Multiple Sclerosis

Multiple sclerosis is a disease that affects the central nervous system's nerve fibers. It is a progressive, disabling disease that often starts in young adulthood.

Signs and Symptoms of Multiple Sclerosis

The symptoms depend on which nerve fibers are affected, but in general they include:

▷ Visual problems
▷ Weakness that progresses to paralysis
▷ Fatigue
▷ Speech pattern changes
▷ Loss of bowel and bladder control

Nurse Assistant's Role in Intervention and Management
▷ Monitor the progression of the disease

Goals of Care
▷ Maintain independence for as long as possible
▷ Prevent complications

Special Intervention or Skills for Care
▷ Give ROM exercises to a resident's arms or legs affected by the disease (Fig. 24-19).
▷ Use proper positioning methods.
▷ Maintain the resident's skin integrity.
▷ Monitor proper nutrition.
▷ Provide adequate fluids.
▷ Identify resident's bowel and bladder patterns and ensure compliance with routines.
▷ Support and listen to resident's concerns about changes occurring in the body.
▷ Attend to any personal requests regarding personal hygiene or social interaction with family and friends.

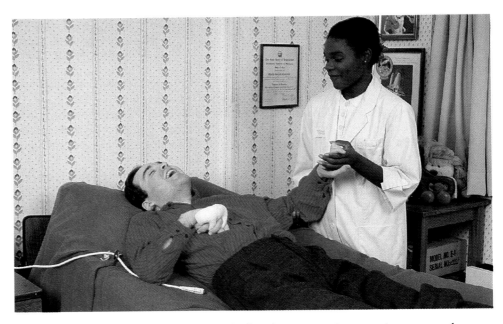

Fig. 24-19. A resident with multiple sclerosis needs to receive range of motion exercises to help sustain affected muscle groups.

Parkinson's Disease

Parkinson's disease is a neurological disease that affects motor skills. The disease usually begins when a person is in his or her 50's or 60's.

Signs and Symptoms of Parkinson's Disease

1. Musculoskeletal changes:
   ▶ Muscle weakness and stiffness
   ▶ Muscle tremors
   ▶ May have slumped, bent-over posture
   ▶ Shuffling walk, poor balance
2. Gastrointestinal changes:
   ▶ Drooling
   ▶ Constipation
   ▶ Difficulty chewing and swallowing
3. Personality changes:
   ▶ Mood changes
   ▶ Confusion

Nurse Assistant's Role in Intervention and Management

▶ Identify changes in a resident's status.

Goals of Care

▶ Maintain mobility
▶ Maintain adequate nutrition and fluid
▶ Maintain a safe environment
▶ Maintain independence

Special Intervention or Skills for Care

▶ Keep the resident's room free of clutter.
▶ Encourage the use of assistive walking devices as ordered.
▶ Encourage frequent rest periods.
▶ Offer small, frequent meals high in fiber.
▶ Encourage fluid intake.
▶ Keep tasks simple.
▶ Support residents by listening to their concerns about their loss of abilities.

Cerebral Palsy

Cerebral palsy results from lack of oxygen to the brain during or immediately after birth.

Signs and Symptoms of Cerebral Palsy

Signs and symptoms depend on the area of the brain affected. Residents with cerebral palsy usually have mobility and coordination problems. Their mental status is usually intact.

Signs include:

▶ Difficulty walking
▶ Paralysis
▶ Incoordination

Nurse Assistant's Role in Intervention and Management

▶ Keep the resident as independent as possible.

Goals of Care

▶ Prevent complications of immobility:
  ▶ Muscle atrophy
  ▶ Skin breakdown
  ▶ Constipation

Special Intervention or Skills for Care

▶ Perform ROM exercises or other exercise programs.
▶ Encourage resident to use assistive devices as ordered.
▶ Encourage adequate food and fluid intake.
▶ Provide good skin care.
▶ If resident is immobile, reposition every 2 hours.

ENDOCRINE SYSTEM

The endocrine system is made up of many glands. Glands are structures that make hormones, chemicals released into the blood and carried throughout the body to regulate and control specific functions. Each hormone has its own job to do.

Following are some of the important glands in our bodies:

▶ Thyroid gland
▶ Pancreas
▶ Ovaries
▶ Testes
▶ Adrenal glands

If a gland cannot secrete the proper amount of hormone to ensure proper body functions, problems can develop.

Common Chronic Illnesses, Diseases, and Problems
Diabetes

The most important endocrine problem is diabetes. In diabetes, either the pancreas is not producing enough insulin or the body is unable to use the insulin that is produced. Insulin's job is to control the use and distribution of sugar in our bodies. When insulin cannot do its job correctly, the sugar level in the blood becomes too high. Diabetes can lead to other complications involving other systems of the body.

Signs and Symptoms of Diabetes

▶ Change in behavior, such as irritability
▶ Excessive thirst
▶ Excessive urination
▶ Blurring vision
▶ Excessive hunger
▶ Itching of the skin
▶ Itching of the vagina and vulva
▶ Tingling and numbness of hands and feet
▶ Slow healing of a sore

Nurse Assistant's Role in Intervention and Management

▶ Identify any changes in resident's behavior.

▶ Closely monitor resident's nutrition. Residents with diabetes are on special diabetic diets.

▶ Monitor and encourage resident's daily exercise program.

▶ Identify and report any physical changes.

▶ Provide a safe environment to limit injury.

Goals of Care

▶ Prevent complications by carefully monitoring resident's status and maintaining proper diet

Special Intervention or Skills for Care

▶ Promptly provide meals and snacks specially prepared for these residents. All diabetics must eat on time and eat the correct amount of foods prepared for them. Report to the charge nurse if a resident is not eating meals and snacks or if he or she is eating foods not on the diet.

▶ When helping a diabetic with personal care, inspect the skin daily and report changes immediately. Wash, rinse, and dry a diabetic's skin thoroughly. Take care especially with a diabetic resident's feet (Fig. 24-20). Clean and dry them thoroughly. Observe skin for any reddened areas or skin breakdown. Report to the charge nurse if a resident's fingernails or toenails need to be cut. A podiatrist is needed to cut a diabetic's toenails.

▶ Observe the resident for any skin discolorations or sores that are not healing, which may indicate decreased circulation to the area. Report immediately to the charge nurse if he or she complains of numbness or tingling in the hands or feet.

▶ Some diabetic residents may have their urine tested each day for sugar and acetone. The test results may show a need for a treatment change. Therefore, test the urine each day at the same time. Record and report the results. (See Chapter 18 on testing a resident's urine for sugar and acetone.)

▶ Pay close attention to the resident's behavior. Note and report any changes. Changes may be significant because they may indicate a problem in blood sugar level.

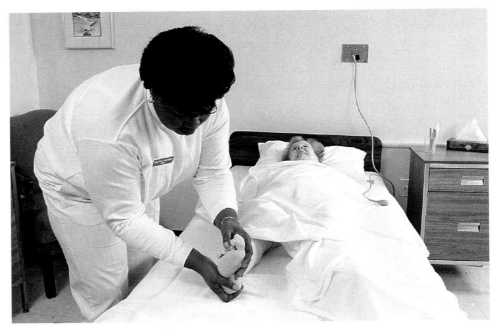

Fig. 24-20. A resident with diabetes needs special care of the feet.

▷ Monitor the resident's physical activity according to his or her physical capabilities. All diabetic residents need physical exercise. However, each resident needs a program designed for his or her individual needs.

SENSORY SYSTEM
Common Chronic Illnesses, Diseases, and Problems
Hearing Loss

Signs and Symptoms of Hearing Loss
▷ Resident may not respond to verbal stimuli
▷ Resident may not interact with other residents
▷ Resident may not participate in activities

Nurse Assistant's Role in Intervention and Management
▷ Report any communication changes you notice when caring for a resident who is hard of hearing.

Goals of Care
▷ Maintain and improve communication with the resident

Special Intervention or Skills for Care
▷ Stand in front of the resident and at eye level when speaking to him or her.
▷ Speak slowly and clearly, as the person may be reading your lips.
▷ Speak in your normal voice, not louder or in changed tone.
▷ Reduce background noise.
▷ Some residents may use a hearing aid. Make sure the resident wears the hearing aid, and check the battery each day before he or she puts it in (Fig. 24-21). Hearing aids should be labeled with the person's name. Always place the hearing aid in a safe place when it is not being worn.
▷ Some residents may not be able to read your lips, so you may have to use writing to communicate.
▷ Point to objects you are talking about.

Cataracts

A cataract is a cloudy area that develops in the lens of the eye and reduces sight. They can occur in one or both eyes.

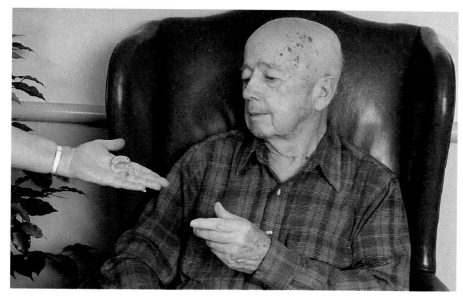

Fig. 24-21. Make sure that a resident who needs a hearing aid remembers to wear it.

Signs and Symptoms of Cataracts
▶ Difficulty in activities of daily living
▶ Difficulty moving from place to place

Nurse Assistant's Role in Intervention and Management
▶ Identify the resident's capabilities.
▶ Ensure a safe environment.

Goals of Care
▶ Improve resident's abilities for activities of daily living
▶ Protect resident from injury

Special Intervention or Skills for Care
▶ Be sure all the resident's items are kept in and returned to the same place.
▶ Help the resident with managing personal belongings. Open lids, apply toothpaste to the brush, assist with color-coordinating clothing, etc.
▶ Describe where foods are on the plate, using clockface directions. For example, "The potatoes are at 3 o'clock, the vegetables are at 12 o'clock, and the meat is at 5 o'clock." (Fig. 24-22).
▶ Make sure a resident wears his or her glasses. Clean and store them properly
▶ Read to resident if necessary.
▶ Keep the room well-lit and uncluttered.
▶ Let the person know when you enter the room and identify yourself.
▶ Stand where the person can see you.
▶ Encourage these residents to touch and feel things.

Blindness

Blindness is the inability to see. Some residents who are called "legally blind" have some sight.

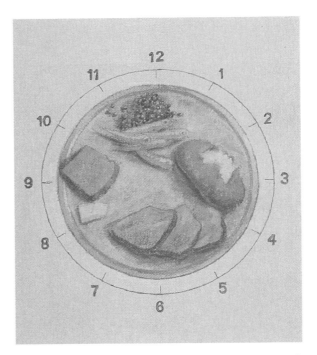

Fig. 24-22.   Use clock-face directions when describing the location of food on a resident's plate.

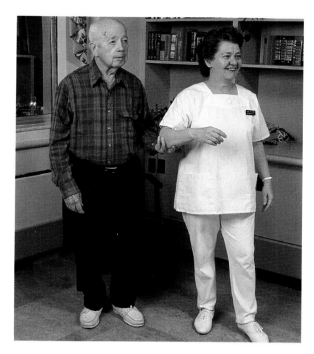

Fig. 24-23. Visually impaired or blind residents will often need a nurse assistant's help to walk.

Signs and Symptoms of Blindness
- Difficulty with activities of daily living
- Difficulty moving from place to place

Nurse Assistant's Role in Intervention and Management
- Identify a resident's capabilities.
- Ensure a safe environment.

Goals of Care
- Improve abilities to perform activities of daily living
- Protect residents from injury
- Help residents to remain active, not isolated

Special Intervention or Skills for Care
- Be sure the resident's things are kept in and returned to the same place.
- Help residents with managing personal belongings. Open lids, apply toothpaste to the brush, assist with color-coordinating clothing, etc.
- Describe the location of foods on the plate, using clockface directions.
- Make sure a resident wears his or her glasses. Clean and store them properly.
- Read to resident if necessary.
- Keep the room well-lit and uncluttered.
- Always let residents know when you enter the room and identify yourself.
- Encourage residents to touch and feel things.
- Assist a resident with walking by having him or her hold your elbow as you guide him or her along or use an assistive device (Fig. 24-23).
- Place furniture in simple arrangements.
- Orient residents to the surroundings.

IN THIS CHAPTER YOU LEARNED TO:
- explain why no one should be labeled
- define the terms acute and chronic
- explain the importance of early detection of cancer
- complete a chart that includes the following: description of any one illness, disease, or problem; signs and symptoms; nurse assistant's role in intervention and management; goals of care; special intervention or skills for care

CHAPTER 25

PULLING IT ALL TOGETHER

IN THIS CHAPTER YOU WILL LEARN TO:

▶ state how nurse assistants contribute to quality care

▶ give examples of things that influence prioritizing

▶ state what to do and what to avoid when working

▶ describe the facility's communication channel

Have you ever put together a jigsaw puzzle? You may have looked at the cover of the box and thought it looked easy, but then you opened the box and found hundreds of little pieces. Perhaps you were overwhelmed and thought "I can't do this, I don't have the time. This is impossible."

Most people who enjoy puzzles devise a plan to avoid being overwhelmed by everything all at once. Maybe you put all the same color pieces together or try to find all the edges and corners first. You always need a plan or some way of organizing the pieces. Otherwise, you wouldn't know where to begin.

This book has given you many pieces of information, including ways to care for a resident mindfully, to assist with meals, to maintain residents' autonomy, and many other ideas and skills. You may feel overwhelmed by all this information, and you may feel it will be difficult to learn it all. But all you need to do is organize all this information as if it were pieces of a puzzle, and then you'll be organized yourself and have a plan to put the pieces together. When you put it all together you will see the whole picture: your job as nurse assistant.

This chapter shows how information can be put together in a typical day in a facility. You will learn to manage yourself and your time, along with tips for how to organize and prioritize your day while you care for residents. Finally, you'll learn about situations to avoid and things to do to stay motivated, to improve the care you give.

THE NURSE ASSISTANT'S CONTRIBUTION TO CARE

You already know that nurse assistants provide about 80% of the care to residents in long term care facilities. Nurse assistants usually make up the largest number of staff. You have more contact with residents than anyone else on the health care team. You are the closest person to a resident, and you gain more knowledge about him or her than anyone else. Does all this sound familiar? You have already learned this in earlier chapters.

You should now have a better understanding of what this all means. Your job description should make more sense now that you're completing this course. Think of the job description as the picture on the cover of the puzzle box: it gives you a look at the puzzle. The information and skills you have learned are the puzzle pieces, each of them important. Leaving out even one piece puts a hole in your picture. Putting the pieces together is a challenge but is well worth the effort.

Once again consider your responsibilities to residents and your employer. As you read the lists in the box titled Nurse Assistant Responsibilities, think of these as the most important aspects of your job.

Think about the introductory chapter to the Application section, Chapter 10, where you learned the concept "It's not what you do, but how you do it." Consider the following:

▶ Who is the first person you see every day?

▶ Who is the last person you see before you go to sleep? Is it the same person?

▶ What kind of influence does this person have on your day? On how you sleep?

If you always saw the same person first thing in the morning and last thing at night, what would you want him or her to be like? Doesn't your day begin more pleasantly when someone says good morning and smiles at you (Fig. 25-1)? Don't you find it easier to sleep if the last person you talk to treats you well? The same

Nurse Assistant Responsibilities

1. Recognize residents as individuals:
   Find out residents' likes and dislikes.
   Ask how they want things done. Get to know their routine.
   Learn about residents' cultural background.
   Find out if residents have cultural preferences about their care.
2. Promote residents' autonomy (independence):
   Know and respect residents' rights.
   Be sure your nursing care practices are in keeping with residents' rights.
   Encourage and work with residents to maintain their optimal level of functioning.
   For personal care:
   Be sure you give residents choices.
   Let residents participate in all care decisions.
   Maintain residents' privacy and dignity.
3. Provide mindful caregiving:
   Balance the skill and the art of caregiving.
   Observe residents closely.
   Watch for any changes in attitude or behavior.
   Let residents determine their own routines.
   Report any changes carefully to the charge nurse.
4. Be a good employee:
   Be reliable.
   Be healthful.
   Be considerate of others.
   Cooperate with other team members.
   Be efficient with your time and supplies.
   Follow all personnel policies.
   Dress appropriately, neat and clean.
   Pay attention to personal hygiene.
   Do not use drugs or drink alcohol.

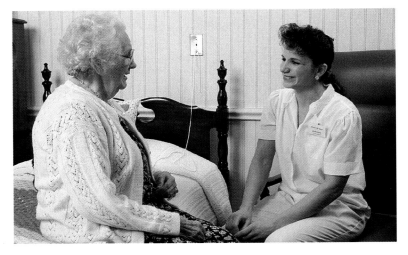

Fig. 25-1. Always try to greet the resident with a cheerful smile.

thing is true for residents. You can influence the quality of their care like no other person in the facility because you are the one who spends the most time with them. You and other nurse assistants are the first person a resident sees and the last. Read the following example and think about how that nurse assistant has influenced a resident's day.

It is 6 A.M. and most of the residents in the facility are just waking up. The night shift nurse assistants are making their rounds, recording measurements on intake and output sheets and starting A.M. care for residents who want an early start. One of the nurse assistants, Mary, decides it would be a good idea to weigh residents before the next shift arrives. She checks the weight chart and makes a list of residents to be weighed.

When Mary arrives at the first room on her list, she knocks on the door and introduces herself, and as she walks in she tells Mr. Sinclair she wants to weigh him. Mr. Sinclair wakes to find Mary in his room with the scale. Without apologizing for waking him or even saying "Good morning," Mary says again she wants to measure his weight. He hesitantly agrees and climbs out of bed onto the scale.

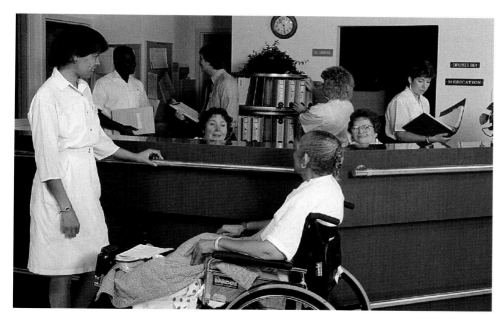

Fig. 25-2. The day shift is often very busy.

How would you feel if someone woke you this way? Would you think that the person who woke you this way cared about you? Is this a pleasant way to start the day?

Mary had good intentions to help the day staff with some of their work, but she did not consider this resident's needs. Mary forgot that Mr. Sinclair is a person, not just something on a list to check off.

A DAY IN A FACILITY

Nursing care is continuous, going on 24 hours a day, seven days a week, 365 days a year. This care in a long term care facility is typically organized in a day of three shifts, with nursing staff assigned to one of the three. Shifts usually include the day shift (7 A.M. to 3:30 P.M.), the evening shift (3 P.M. to 11:30 P.M.), and the night shift (11 P.M. to 7:30 A.M.). The shifts overlap to allow the shift leaving to communicate with the one beginning and ensures that residents are never without someone to care for them.

Day: 7 A.M. to 3:30 P.M.

The day shift is often very busy because most of the other team members work during the day shift (Fig. 25-2). On this shift you are responsible for the personal care needs of residents. You assist with two meals, scheduled appointments, and recreational activities. Most staff meetings, care plan meetings, and doctor visits occur during the day. New equipment and care procedures are first tried and evaluated on the day shift. Visitors typically start arriving before lunchtime.

Evening: 3 P.M. to 11:30 P.M.

The evening shift is a time when many family members and friends often visit. Fewer staff are on duty, and scheduled appointments are fewer. Residents relax after their appointments. The evening meal is served, and P.M. care, which prepares residents for bed, is usually the focus of the shift. This includes undressing, partial bathing, oral hygiene, toileting, and specific comfort measures for residents. Comfort measures may include straightening out or changing linens, providing back rubs, reading to residents, turning on soft music, and dimming the lights.

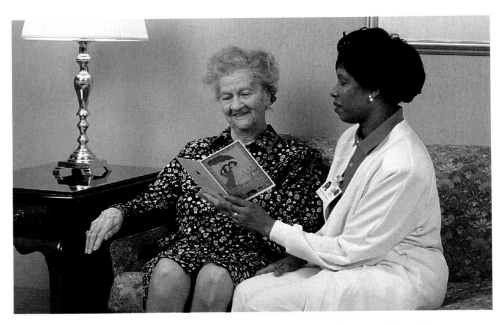

Fig. 25-3. You will have an opportunity to spend time with residents and their families if you work the evening shift.

This shift gives you the opportunity to spend time with residents and their families (Fig. 25-3).

Night: 11 P.M. to 7:30 A.M.

This shift is often considered the quiet shift, but that's not always the case. During the night most residents do sleep, but there are always some who nap during the day and stay awake at night. The night shift has specific duties, such as completing tasks the evening shift could not complete, checking supplies, comforting residents who cannot sleep, and dealing with unexpected emergencies. You may have responsibility of preparing paperwork needed for the next 24-hour shift's work (Fig. 25-4). You would total input and output sheets, collect vital signs and BM charts, and replace them with new ones. You would make a list of residents that may need showers or tub or whirlpool baths. You have important tasks to prepare for the next day's activities. For example, you may have pre-operative orders for a resident who will have a surgical procedure the next day. The most common pre-operative order is keeping a resident "NPO p̄ MN," which means a resident cannot drink anything after midnight. Another night shift responsibility is A.M. care. For residents who rise early, A.M. care includes helping them wash their face and hands, brush their teeth, and go to the bathroom.

All Shifts

Throughout the 24 hours of care, consider each residents' needs. The shifts themselves are only a framework. Although each shift has its specific duties, never insist on a task if a resident does not want it done at that time. Similarly, if a resident wants you to do something normally scheduled for the next shift, make every effort to help.

MANAGING YOUR TIME: THE BALANCE OF ART AND SCIENCE

To begin to learn how to manage yourself and your time, consider the following pieces of the "nurse assistant puzzle." These are three sets of responsibilities you learn to balance.

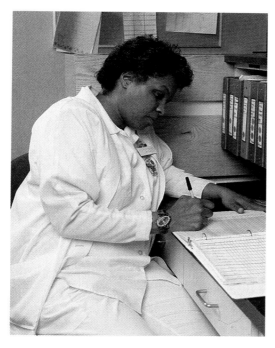

Fig. 25-4. The night shift has specific duties, which often include preparing the paperwork needed for the next 24-hour shift.

1. Resident's Preferences and Routines

As this book discusses throughout, residents should always have a say in their own care. Let residents perform as much as their own care as they can. Also let residents choose how they want things done.

2. Shift Responsibilities

On your shift you have set duties. For example, on the day shift you get residents ready for an X-ray or appointments, on the evening shift you serve dinner, and on the night shift you total the 24-hour intake and output records. You will learn your tasks and responsibilities during your orientation to the job.

3. Assignment

You receive your daily assignment from the charge nurse. You should then ask the following questions:

▶ Do residents have any special needs I should know about?
▶ Do I need to call the charge nurse for any treatments?
▶ Does the charge nurse want certain activities done first?
▶ Do residents have any specific appointments to keep?

These three sets of tasks help you make a plan you can follow to give care. You are giving quality care when you balance all three responsibilities together. The example in the following case study shows how a resident's preferences, shift responsibilities, and daily assignments make up your job.

Case Study

You are working the 3 P.M. to 11:30 P.M. shift and are assigned by the charge nurse to care for the six residents listed below. Your assignment also includes other shift responsibilities. The charge nurse gives you the following information at report time (Fig. 25-5).

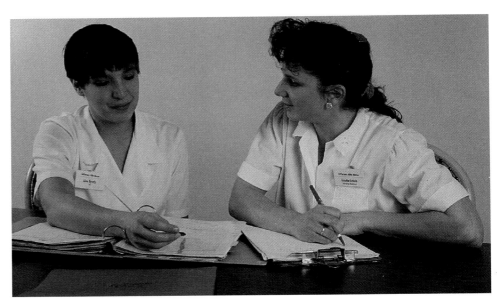

Fig. 25-5. The charge nurse gives you specific information at report time.

Residents

▶ Room 1, Mrs. Green—Had an uneventful day. Her daughter visited her at lunch. Appetite has been poor, but is better today.

▶ Room 2A, Mrs. Rose—Had chest X-ray today at local hospital for cough and shortness of breath, which she has had for one week. Seems anxious about results.

▶ Room 2B, Mrs. Brennan—Slept all day because she "did not sleep a wink the night before." Has no other complaints.

▶ Room 3A, Mr. Gilbert—Uneventful day. Day 6 Post-op; dressing dry and intact.

▶ Room 3B, Mr. Goldberg—Scheduled for removal of his prostate in A.M. Seemed withdrawn on day shift.

▶ Room 4, Mrs. Beck—New admission to facility. Lived with her daughter. Has a scheduled meeting with family members and social worker this P.M.

Additional Assignments

▶ Add up all intake and output sheets at the end of shift.
▶ Supervise unit residents in the dining room.

Miscellaneous

▶ Dinner break 7:00-7:30 P.M.

With this information and a clear understanding of your shift responsibilities, you can plan an order for your tasks that gives a sense of direction for your caregiving. You are thus prioritizing your responsibilities. You decide what to do first and what is the most important thing you must do. Prioritizing involves first making a list and then ordering the list by what to do first, second, third, etc. resident's preferences and routines primarily determine what to do first, second, or third, but you must also consider the shift responsibilities and the timing of some of these. For example, you can prioritize things to be done before dinner, things in preparation for dinner, and things after dinner and before bedtime.

Below is detailed information on the six residents, including information from the charge nurse's report, questions to ask the charge nurse, and residents' preferences and routines.

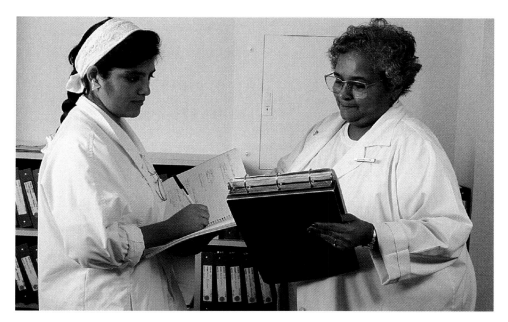

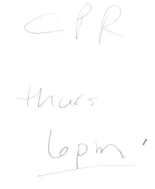

Fig. 25-6. Ask the charge nurse any necessary questions.

Room 1, Mrs. Green

Information from report:
▷ Her daughter visited today instead of this evening, when she usually does.
▷ Her appetite is better.
Questions for charge nurse (Fig. 25-6):
▷ Was Mrs. Green's appetite poor because she was ill, or was it something else?
▷ Should I check with Mrs. Green about what foods she wants to eat?
▷ Does she have an intake and output sheet?
Resident's preference and routine:
▷ You know that Mrs. Green usually likes to get ready for bed after her daughter visits.
▷ She needs assistance with P.M. care.

Room 2A, Mrs. Rose

Information from report:
▷ Mrs. Rose has been short of breath and has had a cough for one week.
▷ Today she had a chest X-ray and is very concerned about the results.
Questions for charge nurse:
▷ When will the results of the chest X-ray be told to Mrs. Rose?
▷ Is there anything I can do to relieve Mrs. Rose's shortness of breath, like encouraging deep breathing, providing frequent rest periods, offering fluids, and elevating the head of the bed?
Resident's preference and routine:
▷ Mrs. Rose enjoys hot tea before bedtime.
▷ She has a favorite TV show that she watches with other residents every night at 7:30.
▷ She likes her bed turned down by 9 P.M. so she can go to bed without assistance.
▷ She likes some assistance with P.M. care.

Room 2B, Mrs. Brennan

Information from report:
▷ Mrs. Brennan slept all day.

▶ She had trouble sleeping the night before.

Questions for the charge nurse:

▶ Did something happen to cause Mrs. Brennan to have trouble sleeping?

▶ Is she not feeling well?

▶ Should I spend time with Mrs. Brennan to find out what is bothering her?

Resident's preferences and routine:

▶ Mrs. Brennan is usually independent and does not ask for assistance.

▶ She likes toast with jelly before bedtime.

▶ She likes to read in the lounge after dinner.

Room 3A, Mr. Gilbert

Information from report:

▶ Mr. Gilbert is doing well after surgery.

▶ He has a dressing, which is dry and intact.

Questions for the charge nurse:

▶ Is Mr. Gilbert in any pain?

▶ Can he get up in a chair?

▶ What can he eat?

▶ When should I call you for the dressing change?

Resident's preference and routine:

▶ He needs complete assistance with P.M. care.

▶ He can get from bed to chair with assistance.

▶ He needs encouragement with eating.

Room 3B, Mr. Goldberg

Information from report:

▶ Mr. Goldberg is being transferred to the hospital for surgery in the morning.

▶ He seemed withdrawn during the day shift.

Questions for the charge nurse:

▶ Is there anything I should do for this resident this evening?

▶ What is the surgery?

▶ How can I comfort this resident?

Resident's preferences and routine:

▶ He needs complete assistance with P.M. care.

▶ He can get from bed to chair with assistance.

▶ He loves to listen to the radio after dinner.

Room 4, Mrs. Beck

Information from report:

▶ New admission.

▶ Lived with her daughter.

Questions for charge nurse:

▶ What is Mrs. Beck like?

▶ What is her level of independence?

▶ Does she need any supplies?

▶ Has she been oriented to the facility?

Resident's preference and routine:

▶ Not known. You begin to gather information tonight.

You use each of these pieces of information to put together your plan for the evening. Below is an example of how you can organize the care you need to provide.

1. Make rounds and say hello to all residents you are caring for this evening, introducing yourself to the newly admitted Mrs. Beck. You now find out how residents are feeling this evening, what needs they may have, and whether any resident has a particular need that becomes your top priority.

2. If no resident has a pressing need, you can go back to the first resident and begin care to prepare for dinner. At this time you can ask residents about their day, focusing on information of concern to a resident. Fox example, you say to Mrs. Rose, "I understand you had a chest X-ray today. How was it?" This gives her an opportunity to talk about her feelings. You tell Mrs. Rose that the charge nurse said the result would be back tomorrow. Maybe you offer her a cup of tea before dinner, knowing how much she enjoys it. This gesture also shows Mrs. Rose you care about her.

   You also continue to gather other information about residents' preferences and routines. For example, you could ask Mrs. Rose when she would like to get ready for bed after the 7:30 show tonight. If you follow this procedure with each resident, you will find what care you need to do and when to do it. Encouraging Mrs. Rose to take deep breaths, checking Mr. Gilbert's dressing, and talking to all residents are all part of your before-dinner care.

3. Staff dinner breaks are usually scheduled around the residents' meal. Knowing you are responsible for the unit supervision in the dining room, you scheduled your break for after this time. You meed to take your breaks and eat so you will stay healthy and able to keep giving the best care.

4. The planning you did before dinner will help you organize the care you give after dinner and in preparation for bedtime. Because Mrs. Green's daughter visited during the day, she might want to go to bed earlier tonight. Checking on what she ate at dinner and talking about her likes and dislikes would be very important for Mrs. Green's care, because her appetite has been poor lately.

   Knowing when and what residents like to do and how much assistance they need will help you in your planning. For example, both Mr. Gilbert and Mr. Goldberg, who are in the same room, need complete assistance with P.M. care. You need to plan much time for their care and still make sure that while you're caring for them, your other residents are taken care of. You need to tell the charge nurse when to come in for Mr. Gilbert's dressing change. You want to talk to Mr. Goldberg about his surgery because letting him talk about his fears will help him greatly.

5. When you have completed P.M. care for all these residents, you can now do your other assignments. You can assist other staff members and discuss any questions you may have with the charge nurse.

6. Before ending your shift, make rounds again, complete all the I & O sheets, and be sure each resident's needs are met, your assignments are completed, and you have reported and recorded all information necessary.

This example shows you one way to organize your time by prioritizing your three responsibilities:
1. A resident's preference.
2. Your shift responsibilities.
3. Your assignment to complete the job while caring for residents.

MANAGING YOURSELF AND STAYING MOTIVATED

Managing yourself is as important as managing your time. When you are managing yourself you are taking care of yourself. Part of managing yourself is staying motivated.

If you look at every day as a new opportunity to learn and grow, you will be less likely to get bored or feel you're in a rut. It's easy to become bored if you don't have a positive attitude toward your job or if you get involved in nonproductive activities like gossiping and cutting corners. A large part of staying motivated and happy about your job involves doing things that make you feel good and avoiding certain pitfalls. Think about the lists in the box titled Staying Motivated and Happy on the Job. If you keep in mind all the things to do, you will stay motivated and enjoy your job more.

Staying Motivated and Happy on the Job

THINGS TO DO:

1. Take advantage of all opportunities to learn.
2. Ask questions, get involved, be concerned.
3. Be open to change and be willing to offer change.
4. Participate in evaluation exercises.
5. Try new products and techniques.
6. Stay healthy.
7. Find balance between work and home.
8. Work with others to help them grow.

THINGS TO AVOID:

1. Cutting corners—like feeding two residents at the same time, skipping assignments, guessing about information.
2. Gossiping about residents or staff, especially the charge nurse.
3. Alienating individuals or not cooperating with co-workers.
4. Bringing personal problems into the facility.
5. Discussing your frustrations with residents.
6. Not being open to try things differently or to change.
7. Having a negative attitude about your work or residents.

If you feel you're falling into a rut or find yourself saying, "I don't want to do this any more," take some time and review the lists above to see if you have slipped into things to avoid and have forgotten things to do. This self-evaluation can help you identify what is wrong. Discuss your concerns with a close friend or, if necessary, with the charge nurse.

Sometimes just talking out loud about your problems can help you find what the real issue is. Making changes and solving problems are easy if you don't let things go on too long. If you do find it necessary to take action about a concern, be sure to communicate through the proper channels.

PROPER COMMUNICATION AND PROBLEM RESOLUTION

Communicating through proper channels is important for all employees in a facility. Because you work in the facility's nursing department, you should understand its chain of command. The chain of command begins with the Director of Nursing.

If you have any grievances, complaints, concerns, or questions about your caregiving or that of a co-worker or team member, first discuss the issue with the charge nurse. Be clear about what you feel is the issue, be accurate in your description, and give as many examples as possible. Be willing to discuss solutions and if needed put your issue in writing.

If the charge nurse is unavailable and immediate action is necessary, go directly to the nursing office and request a meeting with the Assistant Director or Director of Nursing. Examples requiring immediate attention are incidents of resident abuse or injury. The charge nurse can handle most complaints. Give the charge nurse every opportunity to deal with your concerns before going to the Director of Nursing. If you find it necessary to go to the Director or facility administrator, be sure you have all your information straight and can state the facts, give examples, and suggest solutions.

Sometimes it is necessary to file a formal grievance or complaint about something related to your job or care practices you are concerned about. If so, be sure to follow your facility's policy for grievances. The procedure is in your facility's personnel policy manual. Follow each step accurately. Grievance policies give all staff members a way to state complaints and find solutions for improvements in quality care.

IMPROVING QUALITY CARE

This text often mentions the concept of quality care. Quality care is individualized care provided in a mindful manner. If you consider a resident's needs, incor-

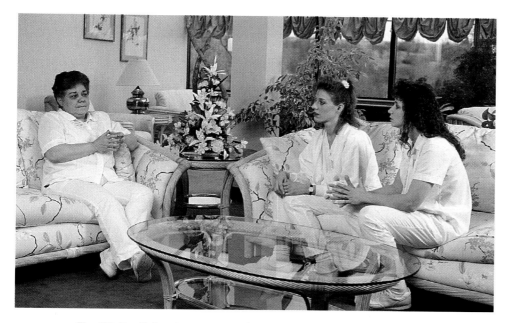

Fig. 25-7. Take time to openly communicate with other staff.

porate the themes of care, and every day treat residents mindfully, you are providing quality care. You can keep improving the quality of care by seeking feedback from your customers—residents, their families, your co-workers, and your supervisors. Feedback lets you know how well you are doing. It helps you improve your work, and it can also let you know when you're doing a good job.

The following is an example of what supervisors look for when evaluating a nurse assistant:

▶ Does the nurse assistant complete all the work assigned?
▶ Does the nurse assistant ask questions?
▶ Are all residents comfortable?
▶ Does the nurse assistant check on all residents frequently?
▶ Does the nurse assistant report changes in residents immediately?
▶ How do the nurse assistant's co-workers feel about the nurse assistant's work?
▶ Is the nurse assistant a team player?

In addition to considering these questions about yourself, you can take the initiative yourself to ask your supervisor questions such as the following:

▶ "Did you check my work today? How did I do?"
▶ "Could I show you how I do this to see if it's the most effective way?"
▶ "I seem to have a problem in this area. Can you help me?"

Your open communication with other staff will help you grow as a nurse assistant (Fig. 25-7). You will also feel better about your work if you seek feedback. Also ask residents questions like, "Have I met all your needs? Is there anything else I can do for you?" Ask family members how they think their loved one is responding to your care. Do they like the schedule for activities and other aspects of your care?

Most important, accept the feedback you receive in a positive way. Make changes you can, or get help in areas you find difficult.

Improving Care Through Education

Inservice education is an important part of quality care. Inservice education can be formal or an informal dissemination of information. Residents' needs change, technology improves, and nursing care practices are updated. Facilities are required to offer at least 12 hours per year of inservice education. But you need to take re-

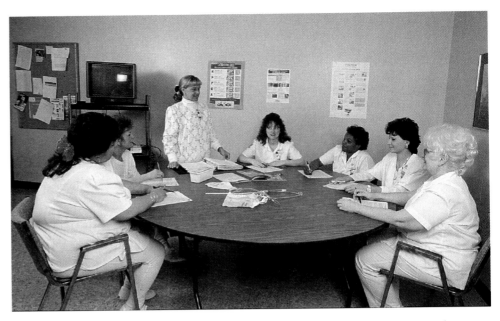

Fig. 25-8. Continuing your education will help you improve your quality of care.

sponsibility for your own learning. Inservice education gives you an opportunity to grow, to change, and to improve. It is the best way to stay challenged and motivated. Take advantage of one of your best employee benefits.

We all learn in many different ways. Attending inservice education classes in the facility is the best way to gain new hands-on knowledge. Going back to school and subscribing to professional magazines are other ways to continue your education and improve the quality of the care you give (Fig. 25-8).

MEDICAL TERMINOLOGY

abuse   to hurt, injure, or damage

abduction   moving away from the body

activities of daily living   tasks needed for daily living, like dressing, hygiene, eating, toileting, and bathing

acute   illness that occurs suddenly

adduction   moving toward the body

alignment   to put in a straight line

ambulation   moving about; walking

aphasia   defective or absent language ability

apical pulse   pulse measured at the heart through auscultation

aspiration   inhaling fluid or food into the lungs

assault   to touch the body of another person without consent

assessment   an evaluation of a condition or resident

auscultate   to listen to body system sounds with a stethescope

axillary   armpit area

blood pressure   the measure of the force of the blood against the walls of a blood vessel

body mechanics   using the body properly to prevent injury when lifting, moving, and bending

cardiac arrest   the stoppage of the heart

catheter   a small tube used to drain fluid

chronic   illness that is of a long duration or frequent recurrence

chart   collection of medical records

clean   free of germs that cause infection or disease

colostomy   surgical opening of the colon or bowel on the surface of the abdomen where fecal contents collect in an external appliance

communicable disease   disease that is spread from one person to another

confidentiality   a resident's right to limit others' awareness of personal information, to keep information free from public knowledge

constipation   difficulty in passing stool

contaminated   no longer clean or sterile

contracture   a muscle that is drawn or shortened

continence   control of bladder or bowel function

cyanosis   blue color of any part of the body due to lack of oxygen

decubitus ulcer   breakdown of layers of skin to form a wound; also known as bed sore, pressure sore

defecate   to have a bowel movement, to pass stool

dehydration   a condition in which the body has less than normal fluid

dementia   a severe state of cognitive impairment characterized by memory loss, difficulty with abstract thinking, and disorientation

diarrhea   liquid or semi-liquid stool

diastolic pressure   the bottom number in the blood pressure reading; reflects the pressure of blood in vessels when the heart is at rest

dirty   contaminated with germs

disinfection   process of killing most germs

dysphagia   difficulty swallowing

dyspnea   difficulty breathing

edema   swelling of parts of the body from fluid accumulation

emesis   vomit

enema   insertion of fluid into the bowel to stimulate a bowel movement

extremities   parts farthest from the center of the body, usually the arms and legs, hands and feet

extension   straightening of an extremity

fecal impaction   inability to dispel feces from the bowel

feces   stool, bowel movement

flexion   bending of an extremity

force fluids   encourage fluid intake

Fowler's position   sitting upright

fracture   a broken bone

guard belt   belt used for safety to transfer and ambulate residents (also referred to as a gait belt, transfer belt)

hemorrhoids   enlarged blood vessels at the anus that look like flat or swollen tags of skin

hospice   care given to someone who is terminally ill

hypertension   high blood pressure; leading cause of stroke

ileostomy   surgical opening of the ileum (small intestine) on the surface of the abdomen where fecal contents are collected in an external appliance

incontinence   loss of control of bladder or bowel function

indwelling catheter   a plastic tube inserted into the body to drain fluids (usually urine)

infection   invasion of the body by disease-causing germs

interdisciplinary team   professionals from different fields and departments who work together with the resident to develop and implement an individualized plan of care

invasion of privacy   an interruption of a resident's right to privacy or intimacy

legal   according to law

long term care facility   part of the health care system that provides rehabilitation, continuous supportive, high level nursing, respite, or hospice care

lubricant   a slippery substance such as petroleum jelly, which facilitates passage of instruments into body orifices

microorganism   a tiny cell or organism only seen with a microscope

mindfulness   interacting with others by paying attention to details, looking at situations openly, and being observant and flexible

multidisciplinary team   another name for the interdisciplinary team

negligence   a form of resident abuse by failing to act as a reasonable person would in a similar situation

nonpathologic   not disease-causing

nonverbal communication   communication through body language

nurse assistant   a trained member of the health care team who provides the majority of hands-on resident care

objective observations   undisputable facts

observation   use of the senses to gather information

ombudsman   resident representative who investigates reported complaints and helps to achieve agreement between parties (i.e. resident/family and staff)

oral   in the mouth

orientation   (1) to be shown something new (as a new job); (2) ability to accurately identify person, place, and time

palpate   use of touch to assess

paralysis   loss of voluntary movement

pathologic   disease-causing pathology

penis   the external male sex organ

perineal care   cleansing of the perineum

perineum   area between the thighs, the external genitals and anus

post-mortem   after death

prosthesis   artificial body part

prone   lying flat, face down

pulse   heart beat

radial pulse   pulse felt at the inner wrist

range of motion   extent to which a joint can be moved safely

rehabilitation   process by which residents improve their functional abilities

residents' rights   legal protections ensuring residents' physical and mental well-being

respiration   the process of breathing in and breathing out

restraint   device used to restrict movement

role   the part that one plays in relationship to others

sexuality   the quality of being male or female

significant others   all people important to a resident

sphygmomanometer   instrument of measure blood pressure; (cuff and gauge)

sputum   mucus from the lungs

sterile   free of all germs

stool   feces, bowel movement

subjective observations   individual guesses or hunches based on objective information

supine   lying flat, face up

systolic pressure   the top number of the blood pressure reflects pressure in vessels when the heart is beating

transfer   to move from one place to another

urine   fluid waste formed by the kidney and excreted from the bladder

vital signs   temperature, pulse, respirations, and blood pressure

void   to urinate

B

COMMON MEDICAL ABBREVIATIONS

$\overline{a}$ before
abd   abdomen
a.c. or $\overline{ac}$ before meals
ADL   activity of daily living
ad lib   as desired
Adm   administrator
AM   morning
amb   ambulate
amt   amount
AP   apical
ASAP   as soon as possible
bid   two times a day
BM   bowel movement
B/P BP   blood pressure
BR   bedrest
BRP   bathroom privileges
BSC   bedside commode
$\overline{c}$ with
cath   catheter
cc   cubic centimeter
c/o   complains of
CPR   cardiopulmonary resuscitation
CVA   cerebrovascular accident; stroke
DC or D/C   discontinue, stop
DNS   Director of Nursing Service
DON   Director of Nursing
drsg or dsg   dressing
dx   diagnosis
F   Fahrenheit
FF   force fluids
ft.   foot, feet
h or hr   hour
H₂O   water
HA or H/A   headache
HOH   hard of hearing
hs   hour of sleep; bedtime
ht   height
I&O   intake and output
ICP   interdisciplinary care plan
IV   intravenous
kg   kilogram (2.2 kg = 1 lb.)
L or lt   left
lb   pound

MD   medical doctor
midnoc   midnight
ml   milliliter (1 ml = 1 cc)
NA   sodium (salt)
NAS   no added salt
neg.   negative
noc   night
NPO   nothing by mouth
OD   right eye
OOB   out of bed
OS   left eye
OT   occupational therapy
$\overline{\textbf{p}}$ after
p.c., $\overline{\textbf{pc}}$ after meals
PM   afternoon or evening
PO   by mouth
PR   per (or by) rectum
PRN   as needed
PT   physical therapy
q   every
qd   every day
qhs   every hour of sleep
qid   four times a day
qod   every other day
q2h, q3h, etc   every 2 hours, 3 hours, etc.
R or **rt**   right (R can also mean rectal)
RCP   resident care plan
res   resident
ROM   range of motion
$\overline{\textbf{s}}$ without
SOB   shortness of breath
spec   specimen
Stat   immediately
tid   three times a day
TPR   temperature, pulse, respiration
u/a, U/A   urinalysis
VS   vital signs
W/C   wheelchair
wt   weight
x   times

C

COMMON MEDICAL PREFIXES AND SUFFIXES

Prefix/ Suffix	Translation	Example
a-, an-	without, lack of	anemia (lack of blood)
ab-	away from	abduct (move extremity away from body)
ad-	toward, near	adduct (move extremity toward the body)
-al	pertaining to	dermal (pertaining to the skin)
-algia, -algesia	pertaining to pain	myalgia (muscle pain)
ante-	before, forward	antecubital (before or in front of the elbow)
anti-	against	antidepressant (drug to counter depression)
arter-	artery	arteriosclerosis (hardening of arteries)
auto-	self	autoinfection (infection by organism already in the body)
bi-	twice, double or	bifocal (two points of focus)
bio-	life	biology (study of living things)
brady-	slow	bradycardia (slow heart rate)
-cele	herniation, pouching	mucocele (cavity containing mucus)
cent-	hundred	centimeter (hundredth of a meter)
-centesis	puncture and aspiration	thoracentesis (puncture through thoracic cavity to remove fluid)
-cid(e)	cut, kill	germicide (kills germs)
-cise	cut	incise (cut into)
circum-	around	circumcision (incision removing foreskin around penis)
con-	with	concurrence (agree with)
contra-	against, opposite	contraception (against conception)
-cyte	cell	erythrocyte (red blood cell)
de-	down, away from	dehydrate (remove water)
dia-	across, through	diameter (distance across a circle)
dis-	apart from, separate	disinfection (apart from infection)
dys-	difficult, abnormal	dysfunctional (not functioning normally)

Prefix/ Suffix	Translation	Example
ecto-	outer, outside	ectoderm (outer layer of tissue)
ectasis	dilation	telangiectasis (dilation of capillaries)
-ectomy	removal of	tonsillectomy (removal of tonsils)
-emia	blood condition	anemia (lacking iron in blood)
en-	in, into, within	enclave (tissue enclosed inside other tissue)
endo-	inside	endoscope (instrument for looking inside the body)
epi-	over, on	epidermis (outer layer of skin)
eryth-	red	erythrocyte (red blood cell)
-esthesia	sensation	paresthesia (abnormal sensation)
ex-	out, out from	extract (to remove)
extra-	outside of	extracellular (outside the cell)
-genesis	development	pathogenesis (development of disease)
-genic	producing	pathogenic (disease-causing)
-gram	printed recording	arteriogram (diagnostic picture of an artery for visualization)
-graph	instrument for recording	audiogram (device to evaluate hearing)
hemi-	half	hemiplegia (half of body paralyzed)
hyper-	over, excessive	hypertension (high blood pressure)
hypo-	below, deficient	hypoglycemic (low blood sugar)
iasis	condition of	nephrolithiasis (condition of kidney stone)
il-	not	illegible (not readable)
in-	into, within or not	injection (forcing liquid into)
inter-	between	intercostal (between the ribs)
intra-, intro-	within	intravenous (within the veins)
-ism	a condition	rheumatism (condition of rheumatoid arthritis)
-itis	inflammation	appendicitis (inflamed appendix)
-logy	the study of	psychology (study of the mind)
-lysis	destruction of	hemolysis (destruction of blood cells)
leuk-	white	leukocyte (white blood cell)
macro-	large	macromastia (abnormally large breasts)
mal-	illness, disease	malabsorption (inadequate absorption of nutrients)
-megaly	enlargement	acromegaly (enlargement of head, hands and feet)
-meter	measuring instrument	spirometer (instrument that measures breathing)
-metry	measurement	telemetry (measurement using remote transmitter)

Prefix/ Suffix	Translation	Example
micro-	very small	microorganisms (very small organisms)
mono-	one, single	monoplegia (paralysis of one extremity)
neo-	new	neoplasm (tumor growing new cells)
non-	not	noninflammatory (not causing inflammation)
olig-	small, scanty	oliguria (low excretion of urine)
-oma	tumor	granuloma (tumor consisting of granulation tissue)
-oscopy	look into	gastroscopy (look into the stomach)
-osis	condition	fibrosis (condition of fibrous tissue formation)
-ostomy	opening into	colostomy (opening into the colon)
para-	abnormal	paralgesia (abnormal painful sensation)
-pathy	disease	myopathy (disease of muscle)
-penia	lack	leukopenia (lack of enough white blood cells)
per-	by, through	perfusion (passage of fluid through an organ)
peri-	around, covering	pericardium (the sac around the heart)
-phasia	speaking	aphasia (speaking or language disorder)
-phobia	exaggerated fear	hydrophobia (fear of water)
-plasty	surgical repair	myoplasty (repair of a muscle)
-plegia	paralysis	quadriplegia (paralysis of arms and legs)
poly-	much, many	polyuria (much urine)
post-	after, behind	post-operative (after surgery)
pre-,pro-	before, in front of	pre-operative (before surgery)
-ptosis	falling, sagging	ptosis (drooping eyelid)
re-	again, back	reinjure (injure again)
retro-	backward	retrograde (moving backward)
-rrhage	excessive flow	hemorrhage (heavy bleeding)
-rrhaphy	suturing	colporrhaphy (surgical suturing of vagina)
-rrhea	profuse discharge	diarrhea (heavy discharge of water stool)
-scope	examination instrument	microscope
-scopy	examination using a scope	endoscopy (looking inside body with endoscope)
semi-	half, part	semi-reclined (partly lying down)
-stasis	control, stop	hemostasis (stopping bleeding)
-stomy	creation of opening	colostomy (opening of bowel to abdomen)
sub-	under	subcutaneous (under the skin)
super-	above, excessive	superinfection (excessive infection occurring during the treatment of another infection)

Prefix/ Suffix	Translation	Example
tachy-	fast, rapid	tachycardia (fast heartbeat)
-tomy	incision	sinusotomy (incision of a sinus)
trans-	across	transdermal (across the skin)
uni-	one	unilateral (one side)
-uria	condition of the urine	polyuria (passing abnormally large amount of urine)

D

EMERGENCY TRANSFER TECHNIQUES

Blankets are the most useful of all the evacuation equipment available, for several reasons:

▶ They can serve as a stretcher for moving residents quickly.
▶ They can be used to smother fires.
▶ They can be used in different evacuation techniques.

EVACUATION TECHNIQUES

There are six different evacuation techniques you should know. Which you use in an evacuation depends on the particular situation and the availability of help from others.

One Nurse-Blanket Carry

This carry should be used for a resident who is smaller than you when you are doing the carry alone.

1. Fold blanket diagonally with point downward and long ends on either side of resident.
2. Help the resident into a sitting position on bed.
3. Wrap the blanket around the resident's back and under the arms (like a shawl), and then tie the ends of the blanket in a knot. Cross resident's arms.
4. Insert your right arm between the knotted blanket (below knot) and resident's chest.
5. Turn your back to the resident, bend your knees, and adjust the blanket comfortably over your right shoulder.
6. Straighten your knees to lift resident from the bed with minimum amount of strain or effort. Carry the resident on your back. Support resident's legs with your left arm.
7. Carry the resident to safety.

Blanket Drag

1. Unfold the blanket on the floor.
2. Help the resident onto the blanket diagonally.
   Note: If the resident is wearing shoes, remove them. This eliminates the possibility of heels catching on stairs and floor obstructions.
3. Lift the corner of the blanket nearest the resident's head. This keeps the resident's head off the floor.
4. Using one or both hands, pull the resident, head first, to a place of safety.

Pack Strap Method

1. Help the resident to a sitting position.
2. Grasp the resident's right wrist with your left hand and left wrist with your right hand.
3. Place your head under the resident's arms without releasing wrists and turn, placing your back against the resident's chest so that your shoulders are lower than his or her armpits.

4. Then pull the resident's arms over your shoulders and across your chest for leverage. Keep the resident's wrists firmly grasped.
5. Lean forward slightly, straighten your knees, and transport the resident to safety.

Hip Method

1. Turn the resident on his or her side facing you, sit on the bed, and place your back against the resident's abdomen.
2. Grasp the resident's knees with one arm and slide your other arm down and across his or her back.
3. Begin to stand while drawing the resident up onto your hips.
4. Carry the resident to safety.

Cradle Drop (To Blanket)

1. Unfold the blanket on the floor; face the side of the bed. Resident should be in supine position.
2. Lift under resident's knees with one arm and under his or her shoulders with the other. Guide resident toward you.
3. Bend one knee at a right angle, and press it against the bed, keep foot firmly on floor.
4. Lower the resident to the floor by bending back leg to the floor. Keep the other knee against the bed.
5. Pull resident toward you and ease him or her to the blanket.
   Note: Your raised knee will support the resident's knees and legs, and your arm will support the shoulders and head. The cradle formed by your arm and knee will protect his or her shoulders and head.

Kneel Drop

1. Unfold the blanket on the floor. Resident should be in supine position.
2. Face the side of the bed and lower your body to both knees in a kneeling position.
3. Grasp the resident's knees with one arm, his or her head and shoulders with the other.
4. Pull the resident straight out from bed until his or her body contacts your chest, and allow the resident to slide down your body to the cushion formed by your knees.
5. Ease the resident to the blanket and move to safety.

BIBLIOGRAPHY

Abraham I and Neudorker M: Alzheimer's disease: a decade of progress, a future of nursing challenges, *Geriatr Nurs (New York)* pp 116-119, May/June 1990.

American Health Care Association: *Quest for quality* ed 2, 1991, The Association.

American National Red Cross: *Nurse assistant training*, Washington, 1989, American Red Cross.

American Red Cross Instructor Candidate Training Participants' Training Manual, 1990, the American Red Cross.

Arking R: *Biology of aging*, Englewood Cliffs, NJ, 1991, Prentice-Hall Inc.

Back tips for health care providers, Daly City, Calif, 1986, Krames Communications.

Back to backs: a guide to preventing back injury, San Bruno, 1988, Krames Communications.

Benenson AS, editor: *Control of communicable diseases in man*, ed 15, Washington, DC, 1990, American Public Health Association.

Bennett JV and Brachman PS, editors: *Hospital infections*, ed 3, Boston, 1992, Little Brown and Co.

Brown M: Nursing assistants' behavior toward the institutionalized elderly, *QRB*, pp 15-17, Jan 1988.

Brubaker TH: *Aging, health, and family long-term care*, Newbury Park, NJ 1987, Sage Publications.

Burgener S and Barton D: Nursing care of cognitively impaired, institutionalized elderly, *J Geriatr Nurs* 17:37-43, 1991.

Burger S: (1993) *Avoiding physical restraint use: new standards in care*, 1993, The National Citizens' Coalition for Nursing Home Reform.

Caudill M and Patrick M: Nursing assistant turnover in nursing homes and need satisfaction, *J Gerontol Nurs* 15:24-30, 1989.

Centers for Disease Control: CDC Guideline for isolation precautions in hospitals, *Infection Control* 4(4):245-325, July/August 1983.

Centers for Disease Control: Update: universal precautions for prevention of transmission of HIV, HBV, and other bloodborne pathogens in health-care settings, *MMWR* 37(24):377-388, 1988.

Centers for Disease Control: Guideline for prevention of transmission of HIV and HBV to health-care and public-safety workers. *MMWR* 38(Suppl S6):1-37, 1989.

Centers for Disease Control: Recommendations for prevention of HIV transmission in health-care settings, *MMWR* 36(Suppl 2S):1-18, 1987.

Charnes LS and Moore PS: Meeting patients' spiritual needs: the Jewish perspective, *Holistic Nurs Pract* 6(3):64-71, 1992.

Consultant Dieticians in Health Care Facilities: *Dining skills*, 1992, funded by The Retirement Research Foundation.

Coons D, editor: *Specialized dementia care units*, Baltimore, 1991, Johns Hopkins University Press.

Dawson P et al: Preventing excess disability in patients with Alzheimer's disease, *Geriatr Nurs*, pp 298-301, Nov/Dec 1986.

Drugay M: Influencing holistic nursing practice in long-term care, *Holistic Nurs Pract* 7(1):46-52, 1992.

Elias M: Sexuality: late love life, *Harvard Health Letter* 18(1):1-3, 1992.

Evans L and Strumpf N: Tying down the elderly, *J Am Geriatr Soc* 37:65-74, 1989.

Fraser D: Patient assessment: infection in the elderly. In Jackson MM, guest editor: Special issue: infection in the elderly, *J Gerontol Nurs* 19(7), July 1993.

Gagnon M, Sicard C, and Sironis JP: Evaluation of forces on the lumbosacral joint and assessment of work and energy transfers in nursing aides lifting patients, *Ergonomics* 29(3):407-421, 1986.

Gallagher-Allred CR: *OBRA: a challenge and an opportunity for nutrition care*, Columbus, OH, 1992, Ross Laboratories.

Garg A, Owen BD, and Carlson B: An ergonomic evaluation of nursing assistants' jobs in a nursing home, *Ergonomics* 35(9):979-995, 1992.

Gould J and Davies GS: *Orthopaedic and sports physical therapy*, St. Louis, 1985, Mosby.

Gwyther LP: *Care of Alzheimer's patients: a manual for nursing home staff*, Washington, DC, American Health Care Association and Alzheimer's Disease and Related Disorders Association, 1985.

Health Care Financing Administration: *Interpretative Guidelines*, Washington, DC, 1989.

Hegland A: Resident assessment: means justifies ends, *Contemporary Long Term Care*, pp 54-56, Jan 1991.

Hegner B: *Nursing assistant: a nursing process approach*, ed 6, Albany, NY, 1992, Delmar Publishers.

Herbert R: The normal aging process reviewed, *Int Nurs Rev* 39(3):93-96, 1992

Heriot C: Spirituality and aging, *Holistic Nurs Prac* 7(1):22-31, 1992.

Hiatt-Snyder L, et al: Wandering, *Gerontologist* 18:272-80, 1978.

Hirst S and Metcalf B: Why's and what's of wandering, *Geriatr Nurs* pp 237-238, Sept/Oct 1989.

Hoffman SB and Platt CA: *Comforting the confused*, Owings Mills, Maryland, 1990, National Health Publishing.

Hussian R: Severe behavioral problems. In Terri L and Lewinsohn P, editors: *Geropsychological assessment and treatment*, New York, 1985, Springer.

Jackson MM and Lynch P: Infection control: too much or too little? *Am J Nurs* 84:208-210, 1984.

Jackson MM and Lynch P: An alternative to isolating patients. *Geriatr Nurs* 8:308-311, 1987.

Jackson MM and Lynch P: In search of a rational approach. *Am J Nurs* 90(10):65-73, 1990.

Jackson MM and Lynch P: An attempt to make an issue less murky: a comparison of four systems for infection precautions. *Infect Control Hosp Epidemiol* 12:448-450, 1991.

Jackson MM and Schafer K: Identifying clues to infections in nursing home residents: the role of the nurses' aide. *J Gerontol Nurs* 19(7):33-42, July 1993.

Jackson MM et al: Clinical savvy: why not treat all body substances as infectious? *Am J Nurs* 87:1137-1139, 1987.

Jernigan AK: *Nutrition in long term care facilities*, Chicago, IL, 1987, The American Dietetic Association.

Jewish Home and Hospital: *Retrain don't Restrain*, prepared for the National Restraint Minimization Project at The Jewish Home and Hospital for Aged under a grant from the Commonwealth Fund, 1991.

Johnson-Pawlson J: *How to be a nurse assistant*, ed 2, Washington, DC, 1990, American Health Care Association.

Kass M: Sexual expression of the elderly in nursing homes, *Gerontol* 78(18):372-378, 1992.

Kisner C and Colby LA: *Therapeutic exercise: foundation and techniques*, Philadelphia, 1985, FA Davis.

Lancaster E: Tuberculosis comeback: Programs for long-term care. *J Gerontol Nurs*, 19(7):16-21, July 1993.

Langer: *Mindfulness*, Reading, MA, 1989, Addison-Wesley.

Larson E: APIC guideline for use of topical antimicrobial agents. *Am J Infect Control* 16(6):253-266, December 1988.

Levy L: Psychosocial intervention and dementia: part I: state of the art, future directions, *Occupational Therapy in Mental Health* 7:69-107, 1987.

Lewis CB: What's so different about rehabilitating the older person, *Clinical Management* 4(3)10-13, 15, 1984.

Lewis CB and Knortz KA: *Orthopedic assessment and treatment of the geriatric patient*, St. Louis, 1993, Mosby.

Lift With Care (videodisc), Redwood City, CA,1987, VISUCOM Productions, Inc., for Beverly Enterprises.

Lucero M: *Products for Alzheimer's self-stimulatory wanderers, Phase 1 Final Report,* Bethesda, MD, National Institute on Aging Research Project (1R43AGO7759-O1A1), 1990.

Lyman K: Bringing the social back in: a critique of the biomedicalization of dementia, *Gerontologist* 29:597-605, 1989.

Lynch P et al: Rethinking the role of isolation practices in the prevention of nosocomial infections. *Ann Intern Med* 107:243-246, 1987.

Lynch P et al: Implementing and evaluating a system of generic infection precautions: body substance isolation. *Am J Infect Control* 18:1-12, 1990.

Lynch P et al: Letter: handwashing versus gloving. *Infect Control Hosp Epidemiol* 12:139, 1991.

Marton WJ and Garner JS, guest editors: Proceedings of the third decennial international conference on nosocomial infections. *Am J Med* 91 (special issue 3B), pp. 15-3335, September 16, 1991.

Maslow A: *Toward a psychology of being,* New York, 1962, D. Van Nostrand.

McCracken A and Fitzwater J: The right environment for AD, *Geriatr Nurs (New York),* pp 243-244, Nov/Dec 1989.

Mery B: Healthy aging: why we get old, *Harvard Health Letter* 10(9):9-12, 1992.

Mourad LA and Droste MM: *The nursing process in the care of adults with orthopedic conditions,* ed 2, New York, 1988, Wiley Medical.

Newsburn VB: Failure to thrive: a growing concern in the elderly, *J Gerontol Nurs* 18(8):21-25, 1992.

Niemoller J: Change of pace for AD patients, *Geriatr Nurs (New York),* pp 86-87, March/April, 1990.

Nutrition interventions manual for professionals caring for older Americans, Washington, DC, 1991, Greer, Margolis, Mitchell, Grunwald & Associates, Inc.

Parke F: Sexuality in later life, *Nurs Times* 87(50):40-42, 1991.

Perspectives on dysphagia, Evansville, Ind, 1990, Bristol-Myers Squibb Company.

Pritchard V: Infection control programs for long-term care. *J Gerontol Nurs,* 19(7), July 1993.

ProCare: *How to be a nurse assistant* (videodisc), Atlanta, 1990, Interactive Health Network.

ProCare: *Body mechanics* (videodisc), Atlanta, 1991, Interactive Health Network.

Pugliese G, Lynch P, and Jackson MM, editors: *Universal precautions: policies, procedures, and resources,* Chicago, 1990, American Hospital Publishing.

Rader J: *Magic, mystery, modification and mirth: the joyful road to restraint free care,* Mt. Angel, OR, 1991, The Benedictine Institute for Long Term Care, under a grant from the Robert Wood Johnson Foundation.

Rader J: *Magic, mystery, modification, & mirth.* Mt. Angel, OR, 1992, Benedictine Institute for Long Term Care.

Rader J, Doan J, and Schwab M: How to decrease wandering behavior: a form of agenda behavior, *Geriatr Nurs,* pp 196-99, July/Aug 1985.

Reed PG: Spirituality and mental health in older adults: extant knowledge for nursing, *Fam Comm Health* 14(2):14-25, 1991.

Reisberg B and Ferris S: The global deterioration scale for assessment of primary degenerative dementia, *Am J Psychiatry* 139:1136-1139, 1982.

Reisberg B et al: Stage specific incidence of potentially remediable behavioral symptoms in aging and Alzheimer's disease, *Bull Clin Neurosci* 54:95-112, 1989.

Rutala WA: APIC guideline for selection and use of disinfectants. *Am J Infect Control* 18(2):99-117, April 1990.

Saunders DH and Melnick MS: *Self help manual: save your back,* Minneapolis, 1987, Educational Opportunities Publishers.

The 7 habits of highly effective people, New York, 1989, Simon & Schuster.

Sine R et al: *Basic rehabilitation techniques: a self instructional guide,* Rockville, Md, 1988, Aspen Publishers.

Smith PW, editor: *Infection control in long-term care facilities,* ed 1, New York: 1984, John Wiley and Sons; 2nd edition to be published in 1993.

Smith PW and Rusnak PG: APIC guideline for infection prevention and control in the long-term care facility. *Am J Infect Control* 19(4):198-215, August 1991.

Sorrentino S: *Textbook for long term care assistants,* St. Louis, 1988, Mosby.

Spechko PL: Bloodborne pathogens: can you become infected from your older patient? In Jackson MM, guest editor: Special issue: infection in the elderly. *J Gerontol Nurs* 19(7), 12-15, July 1993.

Stolley J, Buckwalter K, and Shannon M: Caring for patients with Alzheimer's disease, *J Gerontol Nurs* 17:34-38, 1991.

Sunshine Terrace Foundation Policy Manual: *Policy & procedures for safeguarding residents' belongings*, Logan, UTAH, June 1992.

Tellis-Nayak V and Tellis-Nayak M: Quality of care and the burden of two cultures, *Gerontologist*, 29:307-313, 1989.

Thornbury J: Cognitive performance on Piagetian tasks by Alzheimer's disease patients, *Res Nurs Health* 15:11-18, 1992.

Tideiksaar R: *Fall prevention in the home, Topics in Geriatric Rehabilitation* 3(1):57-64, 1987.

Troya SH et al: A survey of nurses' knowledge, opinions, and reported uses of the body substance isolation system. *Am J Infect Control* 19:268-276, 1991.

U.S. Department of Labor, Occupational Safety and Health Administration: Occupational exposure to bloodborne pathogens: final rule (29 CFR Part 1910.1030). Federal Register 56(235), December 6, 1991.

U.S. Department of Labor, Office of Health Compliance Assistance. OSHA Instruction CPL 2-2.44C: Enforcement procedures for the occupational exposure to bloodborne pathogens standard, 29 CFR 1910.1030, March 6, 1992.

United States Federal Register: *Rules and Regulations*, Vol. 56, No. 187, Sept 26, 1991.

Waxman H et al: How nurse aides perceive quality care, *Nursing Homes*, pp 12-16, Sept/Oct 1990.

Wenzel RP (editor): *Prevention and control of nosocomial infections*, ed 2. Baltimore, 1993, Williams & Wilkins.

Williams CO'B and Feldt K: A nursing challenge: methicillin-resistant *Staphylococcus aureus* in long term care, *J Gerontol Nurs* 19(7), 22-27, July 1993.

Yurick A et al: *The aged person and the nursing process*, ed 3. Norwalk, CT, 1989, Appleton & Lange.

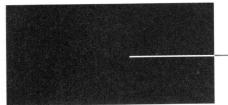

INDEX

NOTES

NOTES

NOTES

NOTES

NOTES

NOTES

NOTES

NOTES

NOTES

NOTES

NOTES